Spinal Cord Injury

A Guide for Living

A JOHNS HOPKINS PRESS HEALTH BOOK

SPINAL CORD INJURY

SECOND EDITION

Sara Palmer, Ph.D.

Kay Harris Kriegsman, Ph.D.

Jeffrey B. Palmer, M.D.

with contributions by
John W. McDonald, M.D., Ph.D.
and Cristina L. Sadowsky, M.D.

THE JOHNS HOPKINS UNIVERSITY PRESS
Baltimore

Note to the Reader. This book is not meant to substitute for medical care of people with spinal cord injury, and treatment should not be based solely on its contents. Instead, treatment must be developed in a dialogue between the individual and his or her physician. Our book has been written to help with that dialogue.

© 2008 Sara Palmer, Kay Harris Kriegsman, and Jeffrey B. Palmer
All rights reserved. Published 2008
Printed in the United States of America on acid-free paper
9 8 7 6 5 4 3 2 1

The Johns Hopkins University Press
2715 North Charles Street
Baltimore, Maryland 21218-4363
www.press.jhu.edu

Library of Congress Cataloging-in-Publication Data
Palmer, Sara.
    Spinal cord injury : a guide for living / Sara Palmer, Kay Harris Kriegsman, Jeffrey B.
Palmer ; with contributions by John W. McDonald and Cristina L. Sadowsky. — 2nd ed.
        p. ; cm. — (Johns Hopkins Press health book)
    Includes bibliographical references and index.
    ISBN-13: 978-0-8018-8777-2 (hardover : alk. paper)
    ISBN-10: 0-8018-8777-1 (hardcover : alk. paper)
    ISBN-13: 978-0-8018-8778-9 (pbk. : alk. paper)
    ISBN-10: 0-8018-8778-X (pbk. : alk. paper)
    1. Spinal cord—Wounds and injuries—Popular works. 2. Spinal cord—Wounds and
injuries—Psychological aspects. 3. Paraplegia—Psychological aspects. 4. Quadriplegia—
Psychological aspects. I. Kriegsman, Kay Harris. II. Palmer, Jeffrey B. III. Title.
IV. Series.
    [DNLM: 1. Spinal Cord Injuries—rehabilitation. 2. Adaptation, Physiological.
3. Adaptation, Psychological. WL 400 P176s 2008]
    RC400.P35 2008
    617.4'82044—dc22   2007035741

A catalog record for this book is available from the British Library.

Illustrations on pages 12 and 13 are by Jacqueline Schaffer. Illustrations on pages 4, 38, 68, 98, 124, 168, 200, 236, 282, and 308 are by Else Lennox. Illustration on page 244 by Edmond Alexander.

Special discounts are available for bulk purchases of this book. For more information, please contact Special Sales at 410-516-6936 or specialsales@press.jhu.edu.

The Johns Hopkins University Press uses environmentally friendly book materials, including recycled text paper that is composed of at least 30 percent post-consumer waste, whenever possible. All of our book papers are acid-free, and our jackets and covers are printed on paper with recycled content.

This book is dedicated to those who,
living life with spinal cord injury or loving someone who does,
shared their stories with us in the hopes of offering creative
solutions, dispelling myths, and opening horizons
for fellow travelers. We thank . . .

Art . . . Bailey . . . Bella . . . Billy . . . Bob
Cecily . . . Chelsea . . . David . . . Don
Elliott . . . Flip . . . Franklin . . . Gwen . . . Hannah
Jack . . . Jane . . . Jeff . . . Jim . . . Joan
Lamar . . . Lark . . . Laura . . . Lee
Melinda . . . Michaela . . . Mike
Noah . . . Nora . . . Patty . . . Pauline . . . Peter
Randy . . . Richard . . . Robert . . . Sally
Scott . . . Sonia . . . Steve . . . Susanna . . . Sylvia
Ted . . . Tom . . . Tricia . . . Vanessa*

---

* All names have been changed to protect the privacy of individuals.

I believe our son made a very deliberate choice.
That choice is the choice to be free.
He's chosen not to hide out in self-pity.
He's chosen not to hide out behind the label "disabled."
He's chosen not to hide out in the guise of "poor little victim."
He's chosen to be a member of his community.
He is taking scary risks and those risks will help him grow
From the inside out.
The point is not: not being scared.
The point is being scared and going through the fear.
Doing what you have to do anyway.
To me, that's freedom.

—Jane's tribute to her son (see Chapter 7)

Contents

Preface

Working in the field of rehabilitation medicine and psychology, we have seen many people grapple with physical, social, and emotional changes after spinal cord injury. We have seen some people overwhelmed by emotional despair or bogged down by a lack of resources to meet their physical, economic, and social needs. But we have also seen many people finish their rehabilitation and go on to live successful, fulfilling lives.

For some people, adjustment to spinal cord injury is relatively smooth and easy. Others can resume a stable and productive life only after a period of emotional upheaval and economic or social struggle. The difficulties presented by a spinal cord injury often stimulate a period of soul-searching and spark a person's capacity for creative problem-solving. These processes can lead to a renewed sense of personal strength, transcendence of loss, and development of a more meaningful "way of being in the world."

Our experience in working with people with spinal cord injury tells us that physical and emotional recovery and successful living after injury go more smoothly when people know what to expect. Being able to recognize and cope with medical and emotional difficulties, and having an idea of how to deal with changes in social relationships, really does help. In our current health care climate, priority is given to providing basic medical care and physical rehabilitation. Sometimes, not enough time and attention are given to helping people learn psychological, sexual, social, and vocational coping skills. A person may leave the hospital with the physical equipment for a changed way of life but be unprepared for the emotional and social upheavals that lie ahead.

We wrote this book as a guide for understanding and navigating the journey from the initial trauma of spinal cord injury through rehabilitation, return to the family and community, and development of the personal strengths and talents that help ensure a successful future. We describe the trauma of spinal cord injury, what to expect in the rehabilitation process, and how to meet the psychological, medical, social, and spiritual challenges of life with the injury. The primary purpose of the book is to help people with spinal cord injury and their families. Students in rehabilitation nursing, counseling, medicine, or physical and occupational therapy can also benefit from the information and personal perspectives, which can help promote a better understanding of spinal cord injury and the recovery process.

Learning to live successfully with a spinal cord injury and its associated disability is a long and challenging process. Unlike most acute medical crises, such as a broken leg or appendicitis, spinal cord injury cannot be completely "fixed," and its consequences do not go away once the immediate medical crisis is over. In almost all cases, even with the best medical or surgical intervention, a spinal cord injury results in some enduring physical disability that affects one's life in many ways. The process of adapting to a spinal cord injury continues throughout life.

If you are newly injured, this book can help you and your family prepare yourselves for what is to come or find answers to questions or problems that you are experiencing at this moment. If you've lived with a spinal cord injury for some time, this book can help you cope more effectively with emotional and social problems that surface at various stages of life. It can inform you about new technologies and medical advances and help you anticipate the challenges that come with aging. We provide essential information, but we also want to raise new questions and new possibilities that you can discuss with your health care providers.

The information in this book is based on clinical reports, research studies, popular articles and autobiographical accounts, individual case studies, and our own experiences working with individuals with spinal cord injury (sources used in the text are listed, by page number, in the Notes section at the end of the book). We have also included the invaluable insights of people who volunteered to be interviewed for the book. They have graciously shared their fears and frustrations, challenges and triumphs, obstacles and solutions. Their practical tips for day-to-day living, their emotional insights, and their social experiences should prove both instructive and inspiring.*

The book is divided into three parts. Within each part, the chapters roughly follow the chronological sequence of events and issues that arise in the course of recovery: initial injury, acute hospitalization, rehabilitation, self-image, return home, sexuality, independent living, education and employment, lifestyle choices, and ongoing adjustment issues. Chapter 5 is addressed to the families of people with spinal cord injury and is devoted to their special needs and concerns. Chapter 8 describes the latest clinical and research innovations in rehabilitation technology, prevention and treatment of medical complications, activity-based therapies, and spinal cord regeneration.

You can read the chapters in any order you like. If you have a particular interest in one area, such as early rehabilitation, depression, or sexuality, you can go directly to the relevant chapter. Each chapter has references to other places in the book where you can find more information on particular subjects. Or, you may want to read the book "straight through." Whether you are a seasoned veteran of spinal cord injury or a newly injured person, we hope the book will provide a fresh perspective, some new insights and practical tips, and some help in anticipating future problems and possible solutions.

It is important to note that the consequences of spinal cord diseases, such as spinal tumors, disruption of blood supply to the spinal cord, or transverse myelitis (an inflammatory disease), can have functional consequences that are very similar to those experienced after a traumatic injury. The prognosis for recovery may be different than with traumatic spinal cord injury, especially in transverse myelitis, in which symptoms sometimes resolve completely and sometimes recur. However, many nontraumatic spinal cord injuries result in permanent functional deficits (in mobility, bowel and bladder function, and so forth) that are identical to

---

* In all cases, the identities of the interviewees have been disguised to protect their privacy, and all names used are pseudonyms. Case examples have been similarly altered to protect confidentiality, and many are composites.

those associated with trauma. This book is relevant for people with all types of spinal cord damage. Sections on psychological and social adjustment are applicable to people with related neurological disorders or disabilities that result in a sudden change in function or inability to walk (such as multiple sclerosis or lower limb amputation).

Spinal cord injury has a tremendous impact on physical, psychological, social, and economic aspects of life. After the injury, most people spend a significant period of time in the hospital, undergoing emergency treatment, acute medical care, and rehabilitation. In Part I we explore the physical and emotional effects of spinal cord injury from the time of injury through emergency treatment, acute care, and hospital rehabilitation. Chapter 1 explains different types of spinal cord injury in detail. It also describes early medical and surgical procedures that may be used to stabilize the injury, medical complications and their prevention, and how to understand and negotiate life in the hospital.

To a great extent, self-image and identity are intertwined with the experiences of the body. Spinal cord injury interferes with these experiences by disrupting normal movement, sensation, and sexual function, and sometimes by causing pain. Spinal cord injury can make your favorite activities impossible, limit your choices, and increase your physical dependence on others. Chapter 2 deals with the hospital-based rehabilitation process, which is designed to help you begin to cope with these changes. We describe therapies, explore the emphasis on mobility, and examine the psychological changes that might occur at this time, including depression, anger, and altered body image.

The disruptions and limitations caused by spinal cord injury can affect the sense of self, personal relationships, and social roles. Chapter 3 explores more fully these changes in self-image and identity, offers several paths for making sense of the changes, and deals with the transition from hospital patient to member of the family and community.

The road to recovery has many pitfalls. Losses and changes brought about by the injury can produce lowered self-esteem, depression, family conflicts, and social isolation. Passivity, self-pity, self-neglect, and substance abuse are some of the problems that may derail your progress. Social stigma and prejudice, environmental and social barriers, and problems with the delivery of health care and economic benefits compound the emotional and physical struggles and create further obstacles to living successfully. In Part II we look closely at these obstacles and how to overcome them. The adjustment process continues with the return to family and social relationships, resumption of sexual activity, and return to the workplace.

In Chapter 4 we discuss the initial challenges of life outside the hospital. These include changing roles and expectations within the family, testing physical limitations and abilities, working with personal care attendants, and improving family communication and goal-setting. Families are frequently called on to provide physical care, emotional support, and economic assistance for people with spinal cord injury. Chapter 5 focuses on the emotional and social impact of the injury on family members and the needs of family caregivers. Chapter 6 deals with the impact of spinal cord injury on sexuality and sexual function. It explores ways to enhance sexual pleasure and communication, ways to deal with dating and establishing a new sexual relationship, and treatments for sexual dysfunction and infertility. In Chapter 7 we explore some paths to greater physical and economic independence, such as access to housing, transportation, and vocational rehabilitation; adaptations for work; and awareness of one's legal rights under the Americans with Disabilities Act.

Spinal cord injury, like any major life crisis, can be a catalyst for positive change. You'll find that it can shake up old ways of thinking and doing and inspire a reassessment of your values, goals, and relationships. It can sharpen the appreciation of your mind, spirituality, and emotional connections to others. It can bring a family closer together. A spinal cord injury challenges you to find new and creative channels for self-expression and to discover new pathways to a full and satisfying life. Part III provides some guidance on how to integrate the impact of spinal cord injury with other aspects of living so you can move into the future with creativity and personal strength. It also covers the latest innovations in medical research and rehabilitation technologies.

In Chapter 8 we discuss advances in research on spinal cord regeneration and rehabilitation technologies, how to interpret research, and how to maintain your physical health as you age. Chapter 9 examines the process of "finding yourself" after spinal cord injury through greater self-acceptance and by nurturing your individuality, staying connected to other people, and developing a lifestyle that suits your abilities and interests. Finally, Chapter 10 examines strategies for adaptation over the life span, building on your unique strengths, adjusting to new stresses, and sharing your wisdom with others.

Resources listed at the end of the book can help you locate organizations, publications, and Internet sites devoted to people with spinal cord injury. These resources will allow you to keep up with the newest developments in spinal cord injury treatment and research; share information, opinions, and support with other people with spinal cord injuries; and find additional resources for adaptive equipment, economic benefits, legal advice, and other practical assistance.

Finally, a note on terminology. The suffix *plegia* means paralysis. The medical term for paralysis affecting two limbs (the lower body only) is *paraplegia,* and in the past, the term for paralysis affecting all four limbs (upper and lower body) was *quadriplegia.* Recently, the medical community has adopted the term *tetraplegia* for the latter condition. The switch in terminology was an attempt to be more consistent in labeling spinal cord injuries. The prefixes *para* (two) and *tetra* (four) both come from Greek, whereas the prefix *quadri* (also meaning four) comes from Latin. The term *quadriplegia* is still used by many people who have spinal cord injuries, and will be found in older medical articles on spinal cord injury. You should be aware that *quadriplegia* and *tetraplegia* are interchangeable terms with identical meanings. For the second edition of this book, we have chosen to use the newer term, *tetraplegia,* because it is the accepted medical term and will be found in current and forthcoming medical and rehabilitation literature on spinal cord injury. In the future, *tetraplegia* is likely to become a "household" term, as *quadriplegia* is now.

BEFORE THE MIDDLE OF THE TWENTIETH CENTURY, the complexities and complications of spinal cord injury were not well understood. Effective medical treatments and rehabilitation methods had not yet been developed. Most people with spinal cord injury died within a few years of the injury, usually because of medical complications such as kidney failure or pneumonia.

The picture is *very* different today. With advances in emergency medicine, the initial survival rate for people with traumatic spinal cord injuries is much higher. And developments in medical treatment and rehabilitation have greatly reduced the incidence of fatal complications.

About 250,000 people in the United States are living with spinal cord injury, and about 11,000 new injuries occur each year. Rehabilitation therapies and advanced technologies allow many people not just to survive, but to lead active, fulfilling lives and to participate in a broad range of activities.

This book can help you find or create solutions to medical and psychological problems and overcome physical and social barriers that stand in the way of a productive and satisfying life. Share the book with your family and friends as a way of inspiring better communication and understanding about your spinal cord injury. Use the information you read here to form a working partnership with your health care providers, to ask pertinent questions, and to seek out additional knowledge and resources. Wherever you are along your journey, we hope this book makes the next steps a little easier as you discover your own path to living successfully with spinal cord injury.

Acknowledgments

We are grateful to our friends, patients, and colleagues with spinal cord injury who have taught us so much about life. Special thanks go to those who volunteered to be interviewed for this book. Their unique insights, practical solutions, and philosophies of living contribute immeasurably to the substance of the book.

Many individuals have guided us in the development of our ideas and approaches, including Beverly Celotta, Barbara de Lateur, Nell Kirby, David Hershenson, Paul Powers, Bobbie Stewart-Larson, Steven Stiens, and the late Arthur Siebens. We appreciate the help of Sue Harris, Kevin Fang, Thea Spiers, and Stephen Wegener, who opened doors to information and resources. Charleene Frazier and Margaret Roffee provided valuable assistance for updating the Resources section and identifying potential interviewees. The late William Kriegsman gave us thoughtful feedback and support during the preparation of the first edition.

We thank our colleagues and co-workers at the Johns Hopkins University Department of Physical Medicine and Rehabilitation, the Good Samaritan Hospital of Maryland, and the International Center for Spinal Cord Injury for their support and encouragement.

We are indebted to the Christopher and Dana Reeve Foundation for their support of the second edition through a Quality of Life Grant. Jacqueline Wehmueller, executive editor at the Johns Hopkins University Press, encouraged us to write a book on living with spinal cord injury, gave thoughtful comments on the first edition, and supported our efforts throughout the preparation of the second edition. The final manuscript was improved by Maria denBoer's copy editing.

Last, but by no means least, we thank our parents, Suzanne and Irving Sarnoff, Elizabeth B. Harris, and Barbara and Walter Palmer; our children, Joshua and Noah Palmer, Bill and Christy Kriegsman, and Katie and Jerry Peters; our grandchildren, Kyle Kriegsman and Darby, Raymond, and Addy Peters; and our many dear friends for their love, support, and patience during the years of writing and revising this book.

PART I

TRAUMA, HOSPITALIZATION, AND REHABILITATION

Spinal cord injury strikes like a lightning bolt. In a flash, the ground seems to be pulled from beneath you, your body no longer works the way it should, your life is turned upside down. The far-reaching consequences of your injury will take a long time to assimilate. Initially, you may have awareness only on an emotional, feeling level. Or you may have a rational understanding with or without any feeling attached. How can you understand this new reality? How can you adapt to your new physical limitations? How will you adjust emotionally to changes in your body's appearance and function?

In Part I we focus on these questions and their answers. The reality of a spinal cord injury is often intensified by other life-threatening injuries. Initially, your mission is to survive physically; then later, emotionally. You will enter a world of hospital and medical systems, rehabilitation routines, and complex, surprising emotional reactions in yourself and your family members.

In Chapter 1 we discuss trauma, emergency care, and acute hospitalization. We explore many of the questions you may have about the initial aftermath of spinal cord injury: What is my injury? What treatments and procedures will be used? What medical complications and physical challenges can I expect? What new concepts and schedules will I need to master? What kinds of equipment will become part of my life? How will I react to this change in my life circumstances?

Chapter 2 begins the discovery process, as you find out what you can do and how you feel. We discuss various types of physical, occupational, and other therapies that are part of rehabilitation, explore the range of emotional reactions and changes in self-image that follow a spinal cord injury, and suggest some coping skills for this part of your recovery.

This discovery process continues in Chapter 3 as you begin to integrate your new self-image into your personality and your "old" life. We look at various pathways for making sense of what has happened to you, finding the motivation to go on with your new life, and making the transition from patient to person.

In essence, Part I describes some of the experiences you may have as you begin to feel the impact of disability on your life and some of the tools you can use to start finding your way out of the wilderness.

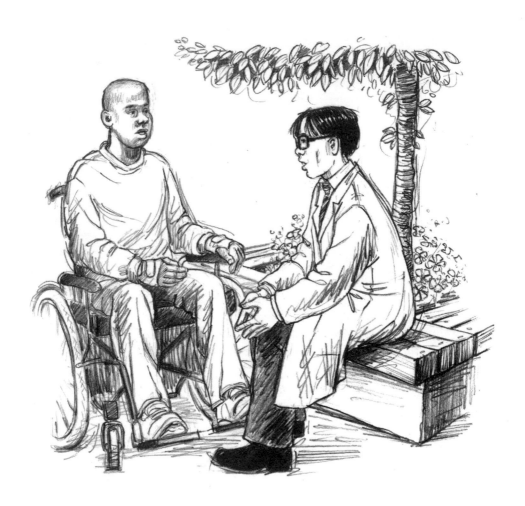

1

Into the Wilderness
Trauma, Hospitalization, and Acute Care

with contributions by Cristina L. Sadowsky, M.D.

Scott was a Marine sergeant in charge of a military unit blowing up Iraqi ord-nance in the U.S. conflict in Iraq. The unit had detonated some explosives and were driving away when their Humvee rolled over. Scott fell out of the Humvee, breaking his neck and his right wrist. His right index finger was cut off, and his right rotator cuff was torn. The corpsman, knowing that Scott should be trans-ported carefully, took a seat out of the Humvee to make a flat board for him and put two Meals-Ready-to-Eat on each side of his head to keep it secure. Scott was transported to another city in Iraq, and then was taken by a series of two heli-copters to an army hospital outside of Iraq. He remembers bits of the process as he drifted in and out of consciousness. Scott had injured his spinal cord at C6 (the sixth cervical level of the spinal cord) and had paralysis of his legs and most of his arms (tetraplegia). He spent one day in the MASH hospital, where he was put in a halo brace and traction. He recalls being awake and in pain during the halo placement (see page 16 for an explanation of the halo). He believes that his paralysis would not have been quite so severe if doctors in the hospital had adhered to spinal cord treatment protocols more strictly.

Scott was then flown to a large armed forces medical center in Europe, where he remained for three weeks. He recalls little of that stay because of medical complications. Back in the United States, he had a five-day stay in the ICU. He required a tracheostomy (a surgical opening made in the trachea) because of breathing difficulties.

Finally, he was moved to a major naval hospital for rehabilitation. He found the hospital very supportive; staff challenged him to get up and be active. Scott notes that the nurses there were "my age or younger and treated you like you're human, with dignity and respect." Although still wearing the halo, he was up in a wheelchair after only two days in the rehabilitation hospital.

Along with his wife, his parents and siblings were at the hospital every day. Staff talked with him and his family in a team conference, with all his therapists and care providers included. After the first month, when his parents and siblings returned to their home in the Midwest, medical conference calls kept them up to date; this was a big relief to Scott.

One of the things that Scott disliked most was insertion and removal of the tracheostomy tube (which maintains the opening). Eventually, he was able to have the tube removed, but because his respiratory muscles were weak, coughing to clear his lungs was difficult. The rehab hospital staff taught his wife how to take a hand to push hard on his diaphragm, while he pushed at the same time, forcing phlegm out of his lungs. "That was the biggest thing I learned. It was a lifesaver."

Although he spoke with a psychologist at the hospital, Scott didn't feel comfortable with her or find the discussions useful. At first he felt, "I'd rather deal with it myself." Eventually, he found it helpful to talk with someone else with a disability. His roommates, ages twenty and twenty-nine when injured, were and still are important to him. "We visit and talk all the time; they are my release valve."

Injuring your spinal cord transports you into a whole new territory. What can you expect during the "wilderness" phase? This depends on the individual. Each person's experience, and each person's base of knowledge, is different. And spinal cord injury affects people differently, depending on the location and type of the damage. The level of injury (where on the spinal cord the injury occurs) defines the point below which paralysis and changes in sensation can occur. Whether the spinal cord is completely or partially damaged determines the extent of the weakness or paralysis. How quickly emergency intervention begins and the quality of medical care received also affect outcome. Age, prior medical problems, and psychological outlook can have an impact on physical recovery and personal experience after injury.

Nearly everyone with spinal cord injury requires emergency room care, acute hospitalization, and inpatient rehabilitation. In many cases, surgery is required to stabilize the spine; other people do not require surgery. Some have long hospital stays; others, short. In this chapter we explore the early encounters with the world of the hospital.

INITIAL TRAUMA AND TREATMENT AT THE SCENE OF AN ACCIDENT

If you are reading this book, you or your loved one are already over the initial trauma, the moment when sensation, movement, strength, bodily function, and, generally speaking, control over your physical existence changed. Events surrounding initial spinal cord injury are often hard to recall, and your understanding of the physical effects may be limited, even later in your recovery. So, it might be helpful to recap the sequence of events and understand what happened in that fateful moment when, in an instant, trauma left your body unable to properly move or feel.

When spinal cord trauma is suspected at the scene of an accident, it is imperative that proper handling of the spine, with careful immobilization of the structures that house and protect the spinal cord, occurs. Removal from the accident site should always be done by professionals properly trained in spine immobilization. They will use a backboard, a cervical (neck) collar/brace, and sand bags, and they will try to maintain the spine in proper alignment, as further and unnecessary movement might continue to damage the spinal cord. If a young child is injured, use of a mattress to raise the torso in relationship to the head is recommended because young children have larger heads in comparison to the rest of the body. In these first hours, saving your life and protecting the spine from more damage are priorities. The ABCs of emergency treatment require Airway management and ensuring proper Breathing and Circulation. A breathing tube might be inserted into the mouth (intubation) if the breathing muscles are paralyzed. "In the field," that is, before you get to a hospital that has a mechanical ventilator, the outside end of the tube will be connected to a bag that is manually inflated and deflated by EMS personnel and provides oxygen to the lungs. In some states, EMS personnel are trained to administer steroids (methylprednisolone or Solumedrol), to help decrease the swelling of the spinal cord inside the spinal canal.

After making sure that the ABCs are taken care of and the spine is properly stabilized, transport to the nearest hospital occurs. Transport can be done by ambulance or helicopter or both. The first hospital is not always the hospital where all the treatment will be rendered. If steroids were not administered "in the field" by the EMS personnel, then it will most likely occur at the acute hospital. Solumedrol is administered to most people with spinal cord injury. Studies have shown that it has a small but positive effect on the neurological recovery of individuals with spinal cord injury compared with no intervention. However, side effects, like increased risk of infections and stomach ulcers, can occur with steroid use, and newer guidelines for spinal cord injury management may eliminate steroid use from their protocols.

EMERGENCY ROOM TREATMENT AND SURGERY

Because spinal cord injuries are complex in nature and require specialized medical and surgical treatment, patients will frequently be transferred to a bigger hospital, designated as a "trauma center," that is not only capable of handling the stabilization phase (keeping breathing and blood pressure under control, treating all associated complications, keeping the patient alive), but also has highly trained surgeons (neurosurgeons or orthopedic surgeons) capable of making decisions about surgical interventions to stabilize the spine.

In the emergency room, physicians will determine the level and extent of the injury utilizing a standardized neurological assessment recommended by the American Spinal Injury Association (ASIA). At the end of the careful examination, a neurologic level and severity of injury will be assigned (for example, T4 ASIA A). The level—say, C (cervical)5—signifies the lowest level of the spinal cord that is functioning normally on both sides of the body, and a letter (A through E) is assigned to signify the severity of damage to the spinal cord (A is most severe, E is normal).

ASIA A, also called complete, does not mean that the spinal cord has been completely severed. It only means that there is no motor or sensory function (light touch and pinprick are the only ones assessed by the ASIA examination) at and around the anal area, which receives nerve messages from the lowest segment of the spinal cord. The individual might still retain ability to move the legs (and frequently does so when the cauda equina, a bundle of nerve roots in the lower back, is injured) or feel deep sensation.

ASIA B means there is some preserved sensory function below the level of the injury, including the anal area. The sensation might be normal, but most frequently it is somewhat impaired.

ASIA C means there is some residual motor function below the injury level, including the anal muscles. Typically, the movements are weak and individuals have a tough time raising their limbs against gravity. Sometimes, these movements are only flickers, barely seen and impossible to use for function. But the fact that they exist means there are some nerve fibers passing through the level of injury that continue to function and there is hope for more and better strength. We don't know exactly what percentage of connections need to be maintained in the human spine in order to walk, but animal studies done in the 1990s showed that cats and rats with about 10 percent of their connections through the spinal cord can walk. Humans probably need a higher percentage of connections in order to walk.

ASIA D means that there is good strength in the muscles below the level of injury, although there is some weakness, and sensation might not be normal. In children younger than seven years of age, performing an ASIA neurologic examination might prove to be challenging and less reliable.

Doctors use the ASIA system to help establish prognosis for recovery of function. By analyzing hundreds of individuals with well-defined (by ASIA) neurologic level and following them throughout their recovery period, patterns of functional recovery were established so medical professionals could predict what type of neurologic outcome could be achieved using the ASIA examination at twenty-four and seventy-two hours. These studies were initially conducted ten to thirty years ago, and advances in medical and rehabilitative care are increasing the likelihood of recovery (see Chapter 8). These days, the ASIA examination at seventy-two hours is used to predict the potential for recovery in individuals with traumatic spinal cord injury, because of the difficulty of obtaining an accurate exam at twenty-four hours.

To help with defining the injury, x-rays, MRI (magnetic resonance imaging), or CT (computerized tomography) scans are done as soon as possible after arrival in the ER. The x-ray or CT scan reveals any signs of injury to the vertebral column (the spinal bones). The MRI scan shows the structural damage to the spinal cord (nerves) and surrounding tissues, which is important for planning treatment. In MRI, powerful magnets apply a magnetic field to the body while you lie perfectly still in a large machine. Specialized detectors pick up changes in the field, and this information is fed into a sophisticated computer. The computer then reconstructs detailed three-dimensional images of the spinal cord and related structures. In children under ten years of age, spinal cord injury can occur without signs of damage on x-rays or CT scanning. Today, when MRI is used often in the assessment of the traumatized spine, MRI abnormalities (such as ligament rupture, fractures, spinal cord bleeding, or swelling) are commonly seen in patients with normal x-rays and CT scans. Unlike the adult population with spinal cord injury, MRI abnormalities in children correlate with the severity of the neurological deficit and the prognosis for recovery.

The majority of people with trauma-induced spinal cord injury will undergo surgical stabilization to remove bone fragments from the spinal canal, to restore the alignment of the bones, and to reduce pressure on the swollen spinal cord. Surgery can occur in the first seventy-two hours (early stabilization) or later, after the body has been medically stabilized and prepared to undergo the surgical intervention (delayed stabilization). There is no consensus on which timing is better, and neurological outcome is similar in both situations. Advocates of early stabilization argue that, once surgery is performed, the patient can move quicker to the next phase, rehabilitation, and the cost of initial care is reduced by minimizing the stay in the intensive care unit. Early stabilization also decreases the likelihood of prolonged immobilization in cumbersome braces, like a halo (see page 16). Surgery helps in the recovery of the nervous system but does not cure the spinal cord injury.

Surgery is usually performed to relieve compression (squeezing) of the spinal cord or to stabilize the vertebral column. The spinal cord can be decompressed by removing pieces of bone or other materials that are pressing against it. When the vertebral column is unstable, a bone graft (also called a spinal fusion) may be performed. In this procedure, small pieces of bone (taken from the patient's pelvis or leg or from a cadaver) are implanted in the spine to provide extra support. These pieces eventually fuse with the bones of the spine, but the vertebrae must be held absolutely still while the bones and ligaments are healing, a process that can take months. Metal plates, screws, or rods are attached during surgery to hold the vertebral bones in place. Braces may be necessary to provide external support. Although these procedures improve the chances for recovery, decompressing the spinal cord and stabilizing the bones of the spine do not ensure any improvement in strength or sensation below the level of injury.

In children, early surgical stabilization may be necessary when there is a severe fracture or dislocation of the vertebrae, progressive weakness, or complex wounds. Early fusion of a child's developing spine can cause problems later on, such as stunted growth of the trunk or curvature of the spine.

ANATOMY OF THE SPINAL CORD

A review of the anatomy of the spinal cord will help you understand what happens when the cord is injured. The spinal cord and the brain form the central nervous system, or CNS. The spinal cord is composed of a delicate bundle of nerve fibers connecting the brain to the rest of the body. It is surrounded by a long, tubular structure of bones, cartilage, and ligaments called the vertebral column. (The vertebral column is also known as the spine. It is important to understand that the spine is a bony structure surrounding the spinal cord.) The vertebral column consists of a series of small bones called vertebrae, which form a column extending from the base of the skull to the lower back. The vertebrae are cushioned and separated by small gelatinous blocks of cartilage called intervertebral disks.

The vertebrae are named by region of the body, with seven cervical (C) vertebrae in the neck, twelve thoracic (T) vertebrae in the upper back, five lumbar (L) vertebrae in the lower back, and a fused block of vertebrae, called the sacrum (S), at the base of the spine. The vertebrae are also numbered from top to bottom within each of these regions: the lowest cervical (neck) vertebra, C7, sits atop the highest thoracic (upper back) vertebra, T1 (Figure 1.1).

Most people with a spinal cord injury also have an injury of the vertebral column, such as a fracture or dislocation of a vertebra. A spinal fracture is a broken vertebra; a dislocation of the spine is movement of a vertebra out of its normal alignment. When any vertebra is fractured or dislocated, there is a high risk of spinal cord injury. Ligaments hold the bones together. If ligaments are destroyed, bones can move out of

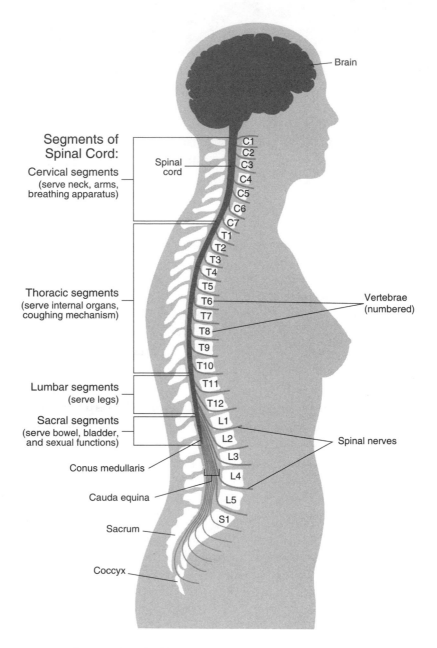

Segments of Spinal Cord:

Cervical segments
(serve neck, arms,
breathing apparatus)

Thoracic segments
(serve internal organs,
coughing mechanism)

Lumbar segments
(serve legs)

Sacral segments
(serve bowel, bladder,
and sexual functions)

Conus medullaris

Cauda equina

Sacrum

Coccyx

Brain

Spinal cord

C1
C2
C3
C4
C5
C6
C7
T1
T2
T3
T4
T5
T6
T7
T8
T9
T10
T11
T12
L1
L2
L3
L4
L5
S1

Vertebrae
(numbered)

Spinal nerves

Figure 1.1. The spinal cord. This sketch shows the adult spinal cord and vertebral column (backbone). The vertebrae are numbered and segments of the spinal cord are labeled, along with the functions associated with each level or segment of the spinal cord. The adult spinal cord is much shorter than the vertebral column, ending at vertebral level L1 or L2. The cauda equina carries the nerve roots from the lumbar, sacral, and coccygeal segments of the spinal cord. These nerve roots emerge from the vertebral column in the lower back.

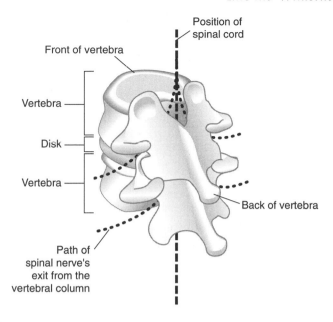

Figure 1.2. Two stacked vertebrae. Shown here are two adjacent vertebrae, viewed from the back and slightly to the left. Between the vertebrae is an intervertebral disk (made of cartilage). The position of the spinal cord in the vertebrae is indicated by a dashed vertical line. The spinal nerves emerge from the vertebral column on each side, between the adjacent vertebrae. At the very back of each vertebra is a prominence that can be felt through the skin.

proper alignment and compress the spinal cord. The forces involved in serious accidents—car accidents, for example—can tear or stretch vital ligaments. Some people need bracing until ligaments heal; others require surgery. Ensuring the stability of the vertebral column is essential to the care of individuals with spinal cord injury.

The spinal cord, like the vertebral column, has segments from cervical to sacral. Two pairs of nerve roots (bundles of nerve fibers) connect with the spinal cord at each level. Each pair of nerve roots consists of a sensory (or dorsal) root and a motor (or ventral) root, which join to form a mixed spinal nerve. These spinal nerves pass through the vertebral column between the vertebrae, carrying sensory information from and motor information to the arms, legs, and trunk (Figure 1.2).

In newborns, the spinal cord is the same length as the vertebral column, so the L4 level of the spinal cord lies next to the L4 vertebra, for example. During childhood, the skeleton grows tremendously, but the spinal cord grows only a little longer. By the time we reach adulthood, the spinal cord is much shorter than the vertebral column. Because the top of the spinal cord is still attached to the brain, the C1 level of the spinal cord lies next to the C1 vertebra. But the S3 level of the spinal cord is near the L1 vertebra, only about two-thirds of the way down the back. This means that the level of a vertebral injury may be quite different from the level of the spinal cord injury it causes. For example, when the T10 (middle back) vertebra is fractured, it may result in L3 spinal cord injury. Injuries of the lower lumbar and sacral parts of the vertebral column are below the bottom of the spinal cord, because the cord extends only to about L1. Thus lower injuries may cause damage to the nerve roots in the lower back (called the cauda equina) but do not affect the spinal cord itself. Upper cervical injuries are more common in infants and young children because of their proportionately larger heads, less developed neck muscles, and immature vertebral columns.

Because the spinal cord is the main connection between the brain and the nerves supplying the arms, legs, and trunk, spinal cord injury usually results in both motor and sensory loss. Motor loss refers to weakness or paralysis. Sensory loss refers to the absence of bodily sensation (such as the senses of pain, touch, and temperature), a condition called anesthesia, or to a reduction in this sensation. Both kinds of loss usually affect all or part of the body below the level of the injury. Other types of sensory changes include paresthesia (tingling, or "pins and needles"), and dysesthesia (pain) caused by damage to the nervous system (discussed later in Chapter 8 under Chronic Pain). Bowel and bladder control may also be affected.

The location of the spinal cord injury determines the parts of the body that are paralyzed or that lose sensation or function. To help you understand your injury, consider the effects of injury in the four main regions of the spinal cord.

Cervical spinal cord (C1 through C8) injury causes paralysis or weakness in both arms and legs (tetraplegia). All regions of the body below the neck or the top of the back can be affected. Frequently, though not always, tetraplegia is accompanied by loss of physical sensation, loss of bowel and bladder control (incontinence or retention), and sexual dysfunction.

Thoracic spinal cord (T1 through T12) injury is less common because the rib cage protects and stabilizes this middle area of the body. When these injuries do occur, they again affect the area below the level of injury. Thoracic spinal cord injuries can cause paralysis or weakness of the legs (paraplegia), loss of sensation, sexual dysfunction, and problems with bowel and bladder control. Arm and hand functions are usually unaffected.

Lumbar spinal cord (L1 through L5) injury usually results in paralysis or weakness of the legs (paraplegia), loss of sensation, sexual dysfunction, and problems with bowel and bladder control. Shoulder, arm, and hand functions are unaffected by lumbar spinal cord injury.

Sacral spinal cord (S1 through S4) injury primarily causes loss of bowel and bladder control and sexual dysfunction. Some sacral injuries may also cause weakness or paralysis of the hips and legs.

Incomplete spinal cord injuries result in a large variety of neurological impairments. Most spinal cord injuries are incomplete, causing greater weakness and sensory loss in some areas of the body than others. Some individuals have only minor weakness and numbness but no bowel or bladder problems. In others, the spinal cord is damaged on one side only, producing weakness of muscles on the same side and a complex pattern of sensory loss. Injuries of the central region of the spinal cord typically result in greater weakness of the arms than the legs. Injuries of the cauda equina may cause weakness, paralysis, and sensory loss in the legs, as well as loss of bowel and bladder control.

The specifics of early treatment for spinal cord injury depend on the level and type of damage to the vertebral column and spinal cord, as described below.

SPINAL CORD INJURY LEVELS AND THEIR TREATMENTS

Cervical Spinal Cord Injury

The immediate course of action for injury at this level often includes placement of "tongs" on the head for treatment of a dislocated vertebra. The two arms of the tongs are attached directly to the skull (under local anesthesia) with a pin on each side of the head. Weights are connected to the tongs by a pulley system, and the device is used to apply traction to (stretch) the cervical spine. With increasing weight, the traction al-

lows the dislocated bones to slip back into their proper positions gradually, thus preventing damage that could result if the bones were forced
into position. Tongs are useful for realigning the spine, but surgery and/
or bracing are necessary for long-term stability.

Because the neck is highly flexible, it is difficult to stabilize it with a
brace. The most effective kind of neck brace is called a halo brace. A ring
of metal (the halo) is attached around the circumference of the head
with small pins drilled directly into the skull (under local anesthesia).
The pins are tightened to hold the halo firmly in place. The patient wears
a hard plastic vest that fits close to the upper body, and the vest is attached
to the halo by metal bars and joints. This type of bracing virtually eliminates any movement of the spinal column, allowing the bones and ligaments to heal in their proper positions. The halo can cause some pain,
but this usually decreases with time and can be controlled with mild pain
relievers. In children, external stabilization devices include hard collars
and halos for cervical injuries; however, halo use is more difficult in children, because the skull is thin.

Thoracic Spinal Cord Injury

The thoracic spinal cord is protected by vertebrae that are stabilized by
a natural anatomical bracing system—the rib cage. Because of this protection, thoracic spinal cord injuries are uncommon, but this region can
be injured in shootings, stabbings, and severe accidents. Some patients
require surgery to decompress the thoracic spinal cord, and surgery can
be difficult because this part of the spinal cord is so close to the lungs
and kidneys. Most patients need to wear a brace on the trunk after surgery, to provide extra stability to the healing vertebral column. Traction
is typically not needed, given the stability provided by the rib cage.

Lumbar or Sacral Spinal Cord Injury

With trauma to the lower back (lumbar or sacral vertebrae), injury often
occurs in the cauda equina, not the spinal cord itself. Injury involving
the uppermost part of the lumbar vertebrae can damage the lowermost
portion of the spinal cord, the conus medullaris (see Figure 1.1). Inju-

ries of the conus medullaris and the cauda equina can cause weakness of the lower limbs and loss of bowel and bladder control.

These injuries often require surgery and external spinal stabilization, because the lower back has no bony protection to hold the vertebrae in alignment. Several kinds of external stabilization are used. The first is the thoraco-lumbar-sacral orthosis (TLSO), or "clam shell," brace. The TLSO is a custom-molded, form-fitting device that surrounds the body, front and back, extending from the upper back and chest down to the lower back and groin. It usually has Velcro straps so that it can be removed for bathing. For lesser degrees of external stabilization, various other back braces and corsets with metal stays are used. These are more comfortable than the TLSO but provide less support to the spine. TLSO braces are sometimes used for thoracic injuries, too, to provide additional stabilization after surgery.

ACUTE HOSPITALIZATION AND MEDICAL MANAGEMENT

An injury to the spinal cord affects not only movement of the limbs and sensation, but also the function of internal organs and regulatory systems of the body. In fact, most systems of the body are affected in some way by spinal cord injury.

Cardiovascular System

Hypotension

Immediately following the traumatic injury, hypotension (low blood pressure) is likely to occur. This is usually managed by giving intravenous fluids and sometimes medications that raise the blood pressure temporarily to keep an adequate blood flow to the brain and vital organs. More persistent changes to the cardiovascular system affect mainly individuals with an injury at or above T6, as the heart is controlled from the T1–T5 spine level. After the initial trauma, low blood pressure, sometimes accompanied by dizziness or nausea, will occur with changes in body position (orthostatic hypotension). The use of tight support stockings or an abdominal binder, a higher intake of salt, or even medication may be necessary to alleviate low blood pressure.

Autonomic Dysreflexia

Sometimes, unusually high blood pressure occurs. Autonomic dysreflexia (AD), or hyperreflexia, is an abnormal reaction of the part of the nervous system that controls vital functions (breathing, heart beat, blood pressure, etc.) and can cause very high blood pressure. AD often results from unpleasant body stimuli. Normally, when there is an unpleasant stimulus to the body we feel it and we act to remove it (for example, feeling a small stone in your shoe). After a spinal cord injury, there is loss of sensation, so you may not always be aware that something needs to be done. It is important to learn how your body reacts to noxious stimuli, so you can protect yourself from them. Typically, head, back, or neck tingling, blurred vision, facial flushing, sweating above the paralysis level, nasal congestion, goose bumps, or a pounding headache can occur, signaling that something is bothering the body. In 85 percent of cases, the person's bladder is full and needs to be emptied. Sometimes, the person needs to have a bowel movement. And sometimes, there is another unpleasant stimulus to the body below the injury level, like tight clothing or shoes, an ingrown toenail, or too much pressure on the skin. Other causes include trauma (for example, a broken bone), infection, severe menstrual cramps or contractions during labor, or temperature changes. Learning to "read" your body and know when something needs to be done becomes very important. You can use the tingling sensation in your neck to know that it is time to empty the bladder or look for another cause for your symptoms. You also need to know if your blood pressure rises to dangerous levels, because, if the stimulus is not removed, the body can react more violently, elevating the blood pressure to a point where a stroke can occur.

Treatment is usually simple. Once it starts, an attack of autonomic dysreflexia is best treated by finding and removing the cause. When the cause is eliminated, the attack usually resolves almost immediately. Not everybody is familiar with AD so you should carry a card in your wallet explaining about AD and its treatment. While adults and school-aged children are able to report headache or discomfort, younger children are not, so the possibility of an AD episode should be considered whenever a child with spinal cord injury displays symptoms such as flushing, sweating, or high blood pressure. Blood pressure varies with body size and age; parents should know their child's normal blood pressure range and how to monitor it with home equipment. Children with cervical injuries will normally exhibit lower blood pressure than those without spinal cord injury.

Deep Vein Thrombosis

The deep veins are the large blood vessels chiefly responsible for returning blood to the heart. A deep vein thrombosis—or blood clot—in the legs is common in the first few months after spinal cord injury. Normally, walking and otherwise moving the legs promotes circulation and prevents clots, but when the legs are immobilized, the risk of blood pooling and clotting in the legs increases.

Typically, deep vein thromboses occur only in the veins of the lower leg and are not a serious problem. If they spread to the thigh, however, there is a risk of pulmonary embolism, a potentially serious complication in which a piece of a blood clot breaks off and travels through the bloodstream to the lungs. Lodged in the lung, the embolism (clot) damages lung tissue by disrupting its blood supply.

The risk of blood clotting is smaller in children before the age of puberty. The risk of deep vein thrombosis is reduced by wearing TED (thrombo-embolic deterrent) stockings, a special type of support hose that helps prevent swelling and discourages formation of blood clots in the legs. TED hose are tight fitting and maintain a constant pressure on the legs, which helps to prevent blood from pooling. A sequential compression device is sometimes used to supplement TED hose, but can be used only when lying in bed. This machine uses air bags to put intermittent pressure on the legs, another way to reduce swelling and prevent thrombosis. For some patients, elastic wrappings around the legs work better than TED hose. A low dose of a blood thinner such as heparin or enoxaparin (Lovenox) also helps prevent blood clots.

Temperature Regulation

Internal body temperature regulation is another major concern for people with tetraplegia. Spinal cord injury affects two mechanisms for maintaining body temperature: shivering, which generates heat, and sweating, which cools the body. (You can still sweat above the level of the injury, because the spinal cord can communicate with the skin above this level.) Having lost these mechanisms of temperature control, people with tetraplegia cannot regulate their internal body temperature. They are dependent on external temperature control, a condition called poikilothermia.

If you have tetraplegia you will need to be vigilant in monitoring your body temperature and will need to rely more on clothing, covers, and heaters to stay warm. When the environment is hot, you'll develop a high temperature. Fever does not necessarily indicate infection for a person with tetraplegia. It may mean that a blanket needs to be removed or the body cooled down. When you are out in the sun, you must carefully monitor your body temperature. Similarly, exposure to cold may cause a drop in body temperature. Without the ability to shiver, the body can't warm itself. You will need to anticipate clothing needs carefully when going outside in cold weather. If you lack sensation in your feet, they must be adequately protected by warm boots to prevent frostbite.

Pulmonary System

Respiratory complications are the most common medical problems in people with spinal cord injury. The diaphragm is the main muscle for inhaling air: contraction of the diaphragm sucks air in but does not push it out. The chest is elastic and springs back into place when we stop breathing in, and as the chest springs back, air is naturally pushed out of the nose and mouth. The muscles of the chest and abdomen allow us to exhale air forcefully, as in coughing, shouting, or clearing the throat.

Ventilators

The diaphragm receives its nerve supply primarily from the C4 level of the spinal cord via the phrenic nerves. Spinal cord injury affecting the C4 level or above can cause permanent weakness or paralysis of the diaphragm, so that the injured person cannot breathe. A mechanical ventilator (breathing machine) is then needed to pump air into the lungs, substituting for the diaphragm.

An endotracheal (breathing) tube carries the air from the ventilator into the lungs, and a tracheal suction tube is used to clear phlegm from the windpipe. The endotracheal tube temporarily makes speaking impossible, and if left in place too long it can damage the larynx (voice box). Damage to the larynx can be prevented by a minor operation called a tracheostomy, the formation of a small opening in the front of the neck that allows air to enter the windpipe directly. The tracheostomy is usually held open with a small plastic tube.

Several different types of tracheostomy tubes are available. Some include a small plastic cuff that inflates, thereby directing air into the lungs and preventing it from leaking out of the nose and mouth. This is important to provide adequate airflow to the lungs, especially during surgery when the patient may be unconscious. The problem with this cuffed tracheostomy tube is that it generally makes speech impossible. When the individual exhales, all the air flows out through the tracheostomy tube and none through the larynx. If a cuffless tracheostomy tube is inserted, airflow through the larynx is possible. Individuals who require long-term use of a tracheostomy tube or a mechanical ventilator can usually learn to speak with a cuffless tracheostomy tube and special techniques for breathing and speaking. This often requires the use of a tracheostomy speaking valve, which helps to direct airflow through the larynx. If the strength of breathing muscles improves, the tracheostomy is easily reversed by simply removing the tube and allowing the opening to heal.

After use of a mechanical ventilator for more than a day or two, the resumption of independent breathing may be difficult. This problem is handled by a process called ventilator weaning. During the weaning process, the amount of respiratory support provided by the ventilator is gradually reduced, and the individual is permitted to have short periods of time off the ventilator. The length of these periods is gradually increased until the ventilator is no longer necessary.

People with permanently paralyzed breathing muscles must use a ventilator for the rest of their lives. This is especially common in cervical spinal cord injuries above the C4 level. (Some people with lower spinal cord injuries also need a ventilator, if only temporarily.) Long-term dependence on a ventilator has a significant effect on mobility, can require attendant care, and may affect psychological adjustment.

Coughing and Clearing the Lungs

In people with spinal cord injury, difficulty coughing (and thus clearing the lungs), prolonged bed rest, and decreased mobility all contribute to an increased risk of developing pneumonia. Several treatments are used for patients who contract pneumonia. A combination of antibiotics and vigorous respiratory therapy is the first choice. The respiratory therapist pounds with both hands on your chest or back while you are tilted at an angle to help drain the affected lobe of the lung. This is called postural drainage. Inhalants are also used to help dilate and clear airway passages.

People with tetraplegia usually need assistance with coughing to prevent or treat pneumonia. In a technique known as quad coughing, the caregiver pushes on your upper abdomen while you cough, and this helps to expel air forcefully from the lungs. Pneumonia vaccine should be given to all adults and children over two years old who have respiratory dysfunction, and influenza (flu) vaccination should be administered yearly starting at six months of age. Children and adults who require lifelong ventilatory support and have a neurologic lesion at C3 or above may be candidates for a diaphragm pacemaker. This can provide periods off the mechanical ventilator for some individuals (see Chapter 8).

Gastrointestinal System

Dysphagia

Abnormal swallowing, known as dysphagia (pronounced *dis-fay-juh*), affects about one-third of individuals with tetraplegia. It can cause pneumonia, dehydration, or malnutrition. The higher the spinal cord injury is located, the greater the likelihood of dysphagia. The causes for dysphagia in spinal cord injury are not well understood, but can include direct injury to the structures of swallowing or damage to the nerves that control swallowing. Either type of injury can occur as a direct result of the trauma or as a consequence of cervical stabilization surgery.

Dysphagia can be identified by a variety of symptoms. People with dysphagia can experience difficulty swallowing with coughing, choking, drooling, or the feeling of food sticking in the throat or chest. In severe cases, food or liquids may go into the lungs, an event called aspiration.

Aspiration can cause pneumonia or other complications. The normal response to aspiration is a strong cough. So-called silent aspiration, in which the person is not aware of aspiration and does not cough, is particularly worrisome, because it commonly causes complications.

When a problem with swallowing is identified, a speech language pathologist (SLP) is usually consulted. An SLP is specially trained in evaluation and treatment of problems with speech, language, swallowing, and cognition. The SLP takes a history and does a thorough examination of the mouth and throat. When dysphagia is significant, additional testing is necessary, because it is difficult to know what is happening inside the throat without looking at it with x-rays or a special scope. The usual test for swallowing is called a videofluoroscopic swallowing study (VFSS), also known as a modified barium swallow (MBS). In this test, the patient eats and drinks solid and liquid foods containing barium, a substance that allows the food to be seen on x-rays. The doctor and SLP can observe and record the swallowing mechanism with videofluoroscopy, which is a video x-ray. The VFSS shows the mechanism of swallowing in detail. It also allows testing of therapeutic and compensatory maneuvers that may improve swallowing. These include modifying the consistency of the food as well as special positions of the head and neck, special ways of breathing, and exercises to stretch and strengthen the muscles of swallowing.

Most people with dysphagia after spinal cord injury recover their ability to swallow, but it can take several months. In the most severe cases, when a patient is not able to safely eat and drink, it may be necessary to use tube feedings to put food directly into the stomach. For short-term feeding (usually just a few days) a nasogastric tube can be used. This tube passes through the nose and down to the stomach. But a different type of tube is needed for longer-term use. Most common is a PEG (percutaneous endoscopic gastrostomy) tube. This tube is put into the stomach through a hole in the abdomen in a simple operation. A liquid diet can be easily put through the tube into the stomach. These tubes do not prevent swallowing. For example, if a person has dysphagia and can only eat a little bit of food each day, the PEG tube can be used to supplement oral feeding. Then, when the person is able to eat enough food by mouth, the tube can easily be removed.

Bowel Function

Immediately following the spinal cord injury the bowel might slow its activity to the point of paralysis. This is called ileus and requires keeping the bowel "at rest"—specifically, not taking any food by mouth and maintaining nutrition through intravenous feeding. Reintroduction of food is done slowly, starting with clear liquids and gradually advancing to solid foods. Spinal cord injury often results in permanent dysfunction of the bowel's ability to empty spontaneously. Stimulation of the bowel on a regular schedule is called a bowel program; this can "train" your bowel to empty on a schedule and help avoid accidents. Restoration of scheduled bowel movements depends on the level of injury to the spine. For injuries above the lumbar level, stimulation of the anal sphincter with a suppository or a gloved finger is usually required. In some cases, a person may initially need to have stool removed manually by a nurse or aide. Suppositories, stool softeners, and laxatives may also be required. If the injury occurred at or below the lumbar level, manual removal of the stool and use of stool softeners are usually needed.

Stomach Ulcers and Bleeding

Because trauma is such an overwhelming event, stress ulcers of the stomach can occur. The lining of the stomach thins out in certain places, followed by bleeding into the stomach cavity. In people with normal sensation, this process causes significant warning pain, but loss of sensation after spinal cord injury makes it more difficult to detect the danger. By the time there are outward signs (decrease in already low blood pressure, increase in heart rate), the blood loss could be significant. Treatment requires intravenous fluids, drugs called H2 blockers (ranitidine, cimetidine, etc.) or proton pump inhibitors (omeprazole, lansoprazole), blood transfusions, and sometimes surgery. These drugs are also given prophylactically in order to prevent stress ulcers in all individuals that have suffered significant trauma.

Genitourinary System

Some people find the loss of control of basic bodily functions—urination and bowel movements—one of the most difficult and frustrating aspects of their injury. Use of a urinary catheter becomes part of the daily routine for many people with spinal cord injury. The catheter is a rubber tube that is inserted into the bladder through the urethra, the opening through which urine leaves the body. Going to the bathroom is part of daily human life, and a private one at that. It is not usually a planned part of the day. Now you may have to empty your bladder on a timed schedule to prevent incontinence (a bladder accident).

Your level of injury dictates whether you'll be able to manage the insertion, emptying, and cleaning of the catheter yourself. Most people with paraplegia can care for themselves, but some people with damage higher in the spinal cord cannot, and they require the help of a family member or attendant. Some patients use a Foley or indwelling catheter, which empties into a drainage bag that can be taped to the leg or be hung over the bed rail at night. An external catheter (sometimes called a condom catheter) can be used by some men whose bladder empties spontaneously but unpredictably.

Some individuals with spinal cord injury are prone to developing urinary tract infections (UTIs), for two reasons. First, the nerves that signal when the bladder is full and those that control the sphincter muscles between the bladder and the urethra can be damaged by the injury. When the bladder does not empty completely, there is a greater risk of infection. Second, the use of a urinary catheter can introduce bacteria into the bladder. Infections can be minimized by proper bladder care and the use of sterile catheters but may occur despite your best efforts. A UTI requires treatment with antibiotics, usually for about a week. A mild UTI involves only the bladder and typically responds to oral antibiotics. A severe UTI with fever may involve the kidneys and can cause serious kidney damage if not treated aggressively. It usually requires intravenous antibiotics and a short stay in the hospital.

Skin

Pressure sores, or decubitus ulcers (also known as bed sores), develop on the skin in areas subjected to prolonged pressure that temporarily decreases the blood flow to that area. The skin can easily recover if the pressure is relieved, but when pressure persists, pain and eventually irreversible damage can result.

Decubitus ulcers are a potential problem in the absence of normal sensation in the skin, because the individual does not feel discomfort after putting pressure on one area for too long. The first approach to preventing decubitus ulcers when you are confined to bed is to change position every two hours, turning onto your side or your back. Once you begin sitting up in a chair, regular pressure releases will get pressure off the sensitive areas. These exercises will become part of your daily routine for the rest of your life. Several kinds of pressure releases relieve the pressure of body weight from particular areas of skin. A common type of pressure release for those who can use their arms is a wheelchair pushup, using both arms to lift your body above the seat for about a minute to relieve pressure on the buttocks. If you cannot use your arms, pressure can be relieved by using an electric wheelchair that automatically tilts back your upper body and thus shifts your weight. To prevent decubitus ulcers from forming while you sleep, you may need to change position every few hours. This may require assistance from another person.

Pain

Most individuals with spinal cord injury have to deal with pain at some point during the recovery process. For some, the pain is transient and is associated with the initial trauma (for example, the pain caused by a vertebral fracture or an associated injury). This pain may persist for weeks, but it generally is responsive to traditional analgesic medications (painkillers) and resolves over time. However, many individuals have chronic pain after spinal cord injury that is disabling and difficult to treat (see Chapter 8 for more information on pain in spinal cord injury).

Nutritional and Metabolic Abnormalities

Spinal cord injury produces changes in the body's metabolism and nutritional needs. The energy requirement decreases, as does lean body mass, so the need for calories in the diet is reduced. Fluid balance changes as more fluid tends to pool in the legs during the day and urine output increases at night. Immobilization can lead to hypercalcemia (high levels of calcium in the blood), especially in children with spinal cord injuries, usually occurring one to two months after injury. The excess calcium causes impaired kidney function, which leads to even higher calcium levels. Symptoms include nausea, vomiting, and decreased alertness. Prompt treatment is essential to prevent complications such as bladder and kidney stones and kidney failure.

Muscle Tone

Spasticity, or abnormally increased muscle tone, affects most individuals with spinal cord injury at the T12 level or higher. It often increases over time and can cause a variety of problems, including muscle stiffness, sudden involuntary contraction of muscles (spasms), or rhythmic, repetitive muscle jerks. These uncontrolled movements may be jarring, annoying, and painful, and may interfere with positioning and transfers or cause falls from the wheelchair.

Several drugs are used to treat spasticity that is interfering with comfort or activities. Lioresal (Baclofen), diazepam (Valium), tizanidine (Zanaflex), clonidine, and dantrolene sodium (Dantrium) are the most common. Other treatments for spasticity include stretching, splinting, and injections of phenol or Botox. Because some medications for spasms have unpleasant side effects and because spasms are not necessarily dangerous, some people with spinal cord injury choose not to use medicine for spasms. Some learn to control spasms by changing position, applying pressure to a limb, or using other physical means. A few people can learn to harness spasms for useful purposes, intentionally eliciting particular spastic movements that help with pressure releases, transfers, or other functional activities.

Damage to the spinal cord itself usually causes spasticity, an increase in muscle tone, as noted above. Damage to the cauda equina (the bundles of nerve roots located below the spinal cord but inside the lower vertebral column), however, usually causes decreased muscle tone. (Muscle tone can also decrease in some cases of true spinal cord injury.) When tone is reduced, the muscles become flaccid and may atrophy (lose bulk). Flaccid legs can become very thin and bony. Loss of the cushioning normally provided by muscle increases the risk of developing pressure sores on the skin.

Traumatic Brain Injury

Traumatic injuries to the spinal cord are sometimes accompanied by other injuries, such as broken bones, damage to internal organs, or brain injury. The same jerking or compressing force that damages the spine may also cause trauma to the head. For severe brain injury resulting in a coma or significant impairment of mental function, the course of treatment and subsequent rehabilitation is quite different from that for spinal cord injury alone. Rehabilitation of moderate to severe brain injury is a complex topic, beyond the scope of this book.

Sometimes, because the primary focus of treatment is on the spinal cord injury, a mild injury to the head may be undiagnosed. It is useful to be aware of symptoms that can result from a mild head injury so that you can report them to your doctor and get appropriate treatment. Symptoms of mild head injury include dizziness, headache, difficulty remembering recent events, and poor concentration. Mood swings and increased irritability or emotionality (for example, crying, laughing, or becoming angry more readily than usual) can also occur. Most symptoms get better spontaneously over time, but if your injury is diagnosed early, your rehabilitation program can be better tailored to help you learn and to avoid unnecessary frustration. Medications may be helpful to lessen emotional swings and irritability and to improve concentration.

REHABILITATION

Rehabilitation usually begins in the acute hospital and continues with more intensity in a rehabilitation facility. Early rehabilitation efforts focus on maintaining the health of the body systems affected by spinal cord injury by helping patients learn how to move, breathe, and talk and how to manage the myriad of medical challenges they face in the early period after spinal cord injury. (Later rehabilitation efforts will focus more on recovery of activities of daily living [ADLs], such as bathing, dressing, and transferring from bed to chair, and more advanced instrumental activities of daily living [IADLs], such as driving, cooking, banking, and other skills necessary to living independently with a disability.) There are several important therapies that may be part of your treatment in the acute hospital, depending on your particular injury and needs.

Physical, Respiratory, Occupational, and Speech Therapies

Physical therapists, respiratory therapists, speech therapists, and occupational therapists all help the patient intensively during the early days of hospitalization. Every patient with a spinal cord injury will work with a physical therapist. Physical therapy involves the use of physical exercises and techniques such as massage or the application of heat or ice. The physical therapist has the major responsibility for maintaining your strength and flexibility and for teaching you mobility skills. The therapist will test each body part to determine muscle function and strength before initiating an individualized exercise program.

As you begin physical therapy, you'll encounter different terms for the various exercises. Range of motion exercises are the bedrock of the therapy, and these begin immediately. Range of motion refers to the degree of flexibility of a joint and is quantified by measuring (in degrees) the joint's limits of motion in each direction. Various exercises are used to maintain or improve range of motion. If you cannot move your own limb and the therapist does it for you, it is called passive range of motion exercise. In active range of motion exercises, you control your own movement. There are also active resistance exercises in which you move against a force with your own energy. In active assisted exercise, the therapist helps you move weakened muscles. Range of motion exercises will become part of your daily routine for the rest of your life. They prevent contracture, a condition in which soft tissues around joints shorten, stiffen, and lose flexibility, leading to a loss of joint motion that may be permanent.

Physical therapists also teach you and your family the proper positioning of your body and proper movement so that pressure sores, or decubitus ulcers, do not develop. After a few days in the hospital, you'll probably begin to sit up, and your physical therapist will be there to help with positioning and to ensure that you do not experience complications (such as low blood pressure) from sitting up too quickly.

If necessary, respiratory therapy is initiated early in your hospitalization. This therapy involves the use of machinery and the therapist's hands to help you breathe and cough. If you are using a ventilator, respiratory therapy is essential to monitor proper use of the ventilator equipment and management of the tracheostomy, and to begin weaning you off the ventilator when appropriate. If you do not need a ventilator but your injury is above T12, you may need respiratory therapy to help keep your lungs clear of fluid, because the muscles for coughing are weakened. This therapy includes inhaling medications to help expand the small airway passages in the lungs, along with breathing exercises and techniques to help keep your lungs clear.

Speech therapy may be part of your early rehabilitation if you have any problems that affect your ability to talk, such as damaged vocal cords or a tracheostomy. Speech therapists work closely with respiratory therapists to ensure that proper ventilation is maintained during speaking valve trials and other procedures. Speech therapists may also be involved in evaluation of cognitive, or thinking, abilities, for example, if you have had a mild head injury in association with your spinal cord injury or have had changes in your thinking due to other medical problems. Finally, speech therapists will work with you if you have difficulty swallowing, which may occur after spinal surgery. Speech therapists can evaluate your swallowing abilities, determine which types of foods and liquids are safe to swallow, and provide mouth and tongue exercises to improve your swallowing.

Occupational therapy focuses on use of the upper body, arms, and hands for self-care activities such as feeding, bathing, and dressing, and for functional activities such as writing, balancing a checkbook, and cooking. The occupational therapist may begin work on basic self-care activities in the acute phase of your treatment, but you will work more intensively with occupational therapists in the rehabilitation hospital.

WHAT YOU CAN EXPECT AS A HOSPITAL PATIENT

Now that you have some grounding in the medical and physical realities of spinal cord injury, what can you expect as a patient in a hospital? How do you deal with medical personnel? What are their roles?

As a patient in a hospital, you have entered a new world. It consists of predetermined schedules for visitors, therapies, meals, and waking and sleeping. It has a defined hierarchy of authority. It gives you more (or less) personal care than you probably expect and minimal privacy.

Schedules and Time Management

First, let's consider the hospital timetable. Hospitals have their own schedules. You're awakened early and have your meals early. You usually order your meals from a limited number of offerings. Technicians may come into your room at any time to give you a variety of tests, or you may be removed from your room for tests or therapies. Visiting hours may be set, and at some hospitals, phone service is cut off early in the evening. Just when you get the schedule under your belt, a weekend arrives and the whole itinerary changes!

You may find the disruption of some routines and the rigidity of others disorienting during your first weeks in the hospital. You may also experience time as compressed or slowed down, because many tasks will take much longer to accomplish soon after your injury. Yet your situation may seem to change every day as early recovery unfolds.

Doctors and Nurses

Doctors usually make their rounds at fairly specific times. Because doctors are not mind readers, make sure you have your questions or concerns at hand when they visit. It helps to write your questions down so you can remember them when the doctor visits. Some patients are reluctant to ask questions or present problems. Remember that your concerns help the doctors to focus on your specific issues and to have a more informed view so that they can make more educated decisions. As Scott discovered, "the squeaky wheel gets the grease . . . If I don't [tell them], they don't know what's bothering me."

You'll interact with and receive care from a number of doctors, including orthopedists (specialists in the muscular and skeletal systems), neurosurgeons (surgeons who operate on the nervous system), and physiatrists (pronounced *fizz-ee-aah-trists*—specialists in physical medicine and rehabilitation, who usually lead the rehabilitation team). You'll encounter doctors at various levels of training and experience, especially if you are in a teaching hospital. After graduating from medical school, doctors do a residency for several years. During this time they learn to practice a specialty and are called residents. First-year residents are sometimes called interns. Residents are on call in the hospital at all times, especially at night!

Nursing care is an especially important consideration for people with spinal cord injury, because the care required is usually more intense and frequent than for other patients. The nursing staff includes individuals with differing levels of training and experience. Registered nurses (RNs) usually have the equivalent of a bachelor's degree and carry management responsibility for the floor or ward. A certified rehabilitation registered nurse (CRRN) has extra training and experience in rehabilitation of individuals with spinal cord injury and other disabling conditions. Licensed practical nurses (LPNs) have graduated from shorter courses and do much of the hands-on work. Other members of the nursing staff (such as aides, assistants, and technicians) have less training and carry out most of the bathing, toileting, and feeding duties.

Nursing care has changed over time, partly as the result of cost-cutting in this era of managed care. You can no longer expect the comforting extras, such as a back rub at night. However, your relationship with your nurse is still likely to be one of your closest connections with hospital staff, because he or she will provide so much of your personal care. Your nurse can be a good source of information about various aspects of spinal cord injury.

Because children and adolescents require significant supportive help with understanding and adapting to their new condition, a psychologist knowledgeable in changes that are common following a spinal cord injury often becomes part of the day-to-day treatment team (see Chapter 2 for information on the role of psychologists in adult spinal cord rehabilitation).

PARTICIPATING IN YOUR OWN CARE

In many ways you may feel like a passive bystander during your acute hospitalization, and in some ways you are. There you are, immobilized, cared for, having things done to you and for you. Now it is time to begin investigating what medical choices you and your family can make.

Although you may seem to have few choices, in reality you are always the arbiter of your treatment. Remember that you, the patient, are also the consumer of services and have the obligation to understand the treatment and to determine whether the service is satisfactory. Don't hesitate to ask questions about your care, and ask again and again if you don't understand the answers. You are dependent on your doctors and nurses at the beginning of your recovery, but you'll gradually become a partner in the management of your own care. Again, remember that the hospital staff is working for you and it is their job to take care of you both emotionally and physically. You have the final say about what tests you undergo and what procedures are performed. If you do not understand why a test is necessary, ask for an explanation.

How Can My Family Help during the Acute Hospital Phase?

In the initial stages of your hospitalization, how can you and your family take some control of the situation? Here are some suggestions for how family members can assume responsibility for supporting you (and each other) and for seeing that you get the best care.

1. Form your own family team, with each member responsible for information and input about a certain aspect of your care. For instance, one member could be with you each morning to talk with the doctors on their rounds. Another member could talk with rehabilitation centers about the second stage of your recovery to get the information necessary for making the best decision.
2. Ask questions until you really understand procedures, medications, and any side effects of treatments and medications. This is how you'll become an informed consumer and a partner in the decision-making for your care.
3. Ask family members to accompany you to therapies to observe,

assist, and give you feedback. They can reinforce your progress and will also be better prepared to help you with exercises when you return home.

4. Advocate for your own care. If your voice is not heard, ask family members to speak up for you.

5. Ask family members to listen to you and understand your observations and needs. And listen to your family. Listening to each other will keep you attuned to one another's emotional states so that you can support each other when needed.

6. If you have questions or concerns that are not being answered or addressed to your satisfaction, request a meeting with the physician. In a rehabilitation hospital or in an acute care setting that uses a team approach to patient care, you can request a family conference with the care team. This is a meeting that pulls together all the medical personnel involved in your care. You and your family will be included in the conference so that you can hear the different strategies being integrated to form the core of your care. Carefully consider every aspect of your care or prognosis so that you can ask just the right questions.

What Emotional Reactions Should I Expect from Myself and My Family?

When the extent and consequences of your spinal cord injury are explained to you and your family, individual reactions will vary greatly. Some will react with tears, others with profanity, frozen shock, a feeling of emptiness, saintly acceptance, humor, stoic resolve, complete denial, anger, confusion, or a feeling that life is unfair. Many other feelings and consequent behaviors, some seemingly bizarre, can also be experienced.

Don't be concerned if you and your family are "all over the map" in your reactions to your spinal cord injury. Whatever feeling erupts or seeps through is a normal reaction to one of life's abnormal events. You and each family member are entitled to feel however you do. This happens because each of you has different expectations, coping skills, and relationships. Expressing your feelings may help to unload that big bag you feel is weighing you down. Paradoxically, you sometimes need to give yourself permission to lose control in order to maintain control.

At this early stage, family members need to accept and support each other wherever they are emotionally. Support from friends, neighbors, and extended family may also be vital to the immediate family members. Scott's wife, Michaela, recalls feeling alone and scared when he was injured. Although confident that Scott was getting good care, she felt "lost, in waiting . . . ditched," in part because of the distance between her home and the hospital. By contrast, one mother recalls the value of having a number of friends with her when her son was first injured. "Without them, I'd have melted on the floor. They kept me grounded."

You—and your family—are experiencing one of life's unplanned wilderness experiences; you are a frontiersman. You have no map for this new phase of life. You and those around you need to express all your feelings, including feelings of uncertainty, and seek support from friends and hospital staff when needed. Doing so will bring much relief. You can then concentrate your energy on the next difficult steps toward your recovery.

WHAT HAPPENS NEXT?

After the initial shock and trauma of entry into the ER, and the twilight zone of acute hospitalization, the reality of your life begins to sink in. It is a reality that includes all the elements of living with a disability. For most people with spinal cord injury, the next step toward recovery is further treatment in a rehabilitation program, where the primary focus is learning how to live with the consequences of your injury.

Your level of injury and its medical complications, your age at injury, and other factors all play a role in what type of rehabilitation facility will be recommended, how quickly you complete your rehabilitation, and whether you can resume your pre-injury activities. Many other psychological, family, and social factors also influence your mood, self-image, and overall emotional adjustment to your injury.

Changes in the delivery of health care and insurance constraints mean shorter stays in many inpatient hospital rehabilitation units (technically called acute rehabilitation). People with severe spinal cord injuries, who need a very gradual period of recovery before they are ready for intensive rehabilitation efforts, may go from the acute medical hospital to a sub-acute rehabilitation program. These are usually housed within a nursing home but provide rehabilitation therapies. Some people will start rehabilitation at an acute setting and finish up at a subacute facility, where they may continue working toward their goals. After they return home, most people with spinal cord injury will have a period of in-home and/or outpatient rehabilitation in order to maximize their potential.

In the following chapter we explore the practical and emotional aspects of early rehabilitation, guiding you through your exploration of this new territory. You may feel lost at first, but the search for solutions will soon begin as you enter the next phase of your unique journey into the world of living with spinal cord injury.

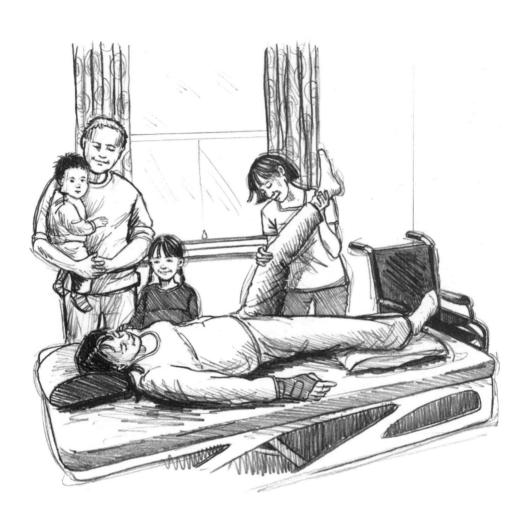

2

Lost and Searching
Rehabilitation

Jim was feeling on top of the world as he drove down the highway to a new job site. He was twenty-eight, had been married a few years, and was enjoying success in his job as foreman in a large construction company. He loved working outside, using his physical strength and mental abilities at the same time and being around people. He had dreams of owning his own company, starting a family, vacationing in the Rocky Mountains.

Jim was almost at his exit when he noticed a truck coming up behind him a little too fast. He figured it was just a case of tailgating intimidation, but before he could change lanes, the truck smashed into his car. Jim lost consciousness. When he came to, he heard ambulance sirens and felt pain in his neck. His legs wouldn't work. He was trapped in a crushed car and had to be extracted by the Jaws of Life machine.

At the hospital Jim was found to have an incomplete cervical spinal cord injury causing significant weakness in both legs. After his neck was stabilized surgically, he was transferred to an inpatient rehabilitation facility. He couldn't walk and had to use a wheelchair to get around. He couldn't urinate normally and had to be catheterized several times a day. His neck hurt, and he couldn't lift anything heavy. He noticed that he didn't have "morning erections" anymore, and he wondered if his sex life was over. He was pretty sure he could never return to his construction job.

Jim's friends were working and didn't have much time to visit. His wife came every day, but she couldn't sleep at the rehabilitation facility. They had no privacy, and Jim couldn't share his fears and frustrations with her. He was humili-

ated by his dependence on others, but at the same time he was lonely and felt isolated from people. He wanted more than anything to get well, to walk again, but at times he was so overwhelmed by anger, grief, embarrassment, and fear that he had to force himself to do his physical therapy. Jim felt his dreams were dashed. It would be easy just to give up. Who would care anyway? He was useless to everyone.

After emergency treatment and acute hospitalization, most people with severe spinal cord injury spend some time in an inpatient rehabilitation program. During this period, further assessment is done to determine the effects of the injury on physical function. Doctors, nurses, physical and occupational therapists, and other staff members work with the injured person to prevent complications, maximize remaining physical abilities, develop techniques to compensate for lost abilities, and increase proficiency in the use of assistive devices (such as wheelchairs, braces, and splints). At the same time, family and other caregivers are taught how to assist the injured person in areas where he or she cannot become completely self-sufficient.

The inpatient stay generally ends when the injured person and his or her family have learned the skills and obtained the equipment needed for living at home. However, in some cases, due to insurance coverage or state and federal restraints on payment for acute rehabilitation care, further inpatient rehabilitation at a subacute facility (usually located within a nursing home) will be needed to meet this goal. After discharge, home-based or outpatient physical therapy and other types of treatment may continue for a brief time or an extended period, depending on individual needs.

For many newly injured persons, entry into the rehabilitation hospital inspires an odd mixture of hope and uncertainty. After surviving the initial trauma and hospitalization, they may see the rehabilitation process as the next step to recovery and getting back to normal, a sign of no longer being in imminent danger. Most of the time, however, the real challenge has just begun. No longer is the injured person a passive recipient of care, a broken body waiting to be healed by doctors. Full recovery depends on the ability to shift from a passive to an active role, to do more for oneself, to make decisions and choices about care and management, and to take a hard look at how to *live with* the disability.

As a person with spinal cord injury, you are expected to start doing things for yourself from the first day in the rehabilitation program. You won't be treated as a sick person. But in trying to be self-sufficient after so recently being so dependent on others, and having undergone a dramatic change in function since last being independent, you are immediately confronted with the impact and extent of your physical limitations.

The game plan is different in rehabilitation—instead of submitting passively to treatments that are done to him or her, the injured person is expected to participate actively in tasks that teach how to manage daily activities with, or in spite of, the disability. This is when you come face to face with the altered reality of your life. In the acute hospital you may have wondered, "Will I survive?" Now the question becomes, "How will I live, and what can I do?"

PHYSICAL CHANGES AND LIMITATIONS

At this stage in your recovery, awareness of physical changes and limitations is a primary concern. You may not be able to walk to the bathroom, tie your shoes, or eat your food without assistance from another person. Like Jim, you may not be able to walk at all. If your cervical spine is damaged, your arms and hands may be weak or paralyzed. You may not be able to turn over in bed, feed yourself, or hug your child.

For many people with spinal cord injury, being unable to walk is the most frustrating part of their disability. Persons with incomplete injuries can sometimes learn to walk with (or sometimes without) crutches and metal braces, but this is not for everyone. Brace-walking may require weeks and weeks of intensive physical therapy, because it is quite different from normal walking. It requires a whole gamut of new physical skills, and it can be slow and extremely strenuous. Even with sophisticated braces, lightweight crutches, and extensive physical therapy, some individuals with paraplegia find that walking with crutches and braces is simply too difficult, too strenuous, and too slow for use in the real world.

Some other possible consequences of spinal cord injury were outlined in Chapter 1. Individuals with injury at a very high level of the spinal cord may need to use a mechanical ventilator (respirator), because the muscles that control breathing are partially paralyzed. Some need special help to cough or clear fluids from the throat and chest. Some people have difficulty communicating because the ventilator and tracheostomy tube interfere with speech, and paralysis of the arms prevents them from writing. Weeks of speech therapy and specialized speaking valves or other equipment may be needed to learn to talk again.

Depending on the type of spinal cord damage, you may have mild or profound changes in sensation. If you are tetraplegic, you may be unable to regulate your body temperature, perhaps experiencing fluctuations from hot to cold (even developing a fever in hot weather) and having to rely more on air conditioners, heaters, blankets, and so forth. You may experience bowel or bladder incontinence, inability to empty your bowel or bladder spontaneously, or a combination of these, requiring bladder catheterization or a bowel program to maintain healthy elimination. And your sexual function and sensation may be affected. Men may have changes in their ability to have an erection, experience sexual pleasure, or ejaculate. Women's menstrual cycles may be temporarily interrupted, although periods and fertility generally return after some months, and they may have changes in genital sensation and the ability to lubricate or have an orgasm.

Rehabilitation is the period in which you confront and come to understand the full range of your limitations, disabilities, and complications. This is one of the most physically difficult tasks a person can undertake. It is also emotionally disruptive, intellectually demanding, and a challenge to your personality, social skills, and spiritual beliefs. One of the keys to success is being able to cope with a variety of emotional responses while simultaneously focusing your energy on physical recovery.

BALANCING PHYSICAL AND EMOTIONAL NEEDS

As rehabilitation begins (and especially in the current climate of shortened hospital stays and pressure to get patients home as quickly as possible), tension often exists between the goals of the rehabilitation program and the psychological needs of the injured person. Both you and the hospital staff share the same ultimate goal of maximizing your health and physical abilities, but you may be on a different psychological timetable.

Enthusiastic staff will present you with an array of therapeutic methods and technological supports to help you learn new ways of caring for yourself, performing daily living activities, and getting around (mobility). They won't hesitate to point out the areas in which you are permanently impaired (or at least for the foreseeable future) and to show you different ways of compensating for your lost abilities. You'll be expected to take part in a rigorous program of exercise and self-care training (such as dressing or bathing), as well as planning for economic assistance, vocational retraining, and perhaps home modifications or personal assistance after you return home. You may be told to learn to rely on a wheelchair for mobility and not to count on walking again.

At the same time, you are experiencing an emotionally traumatic event. You may be so overwhelmed by your feelings about the injury that you have difficulty participating in any activity. While the rehabilitation professionals urge you on to success in using your wheelchair, you may still be reeling from the loss of your ability to walk. While they are promoting compensatory measures, you may be hoping for a return to fully normal functions. And while they are demanding action and learning, you may feel too depressed to get out of bed or too anxious and scared to face another day of therapy.

Your ability to make the best use of the inpatient rehabilitation period depends on at least a partial resolution of these tensions. Although everyone with a spinal cord injury experiences some emotional upheaval and loss, the effects of emotions on ability to function are not necessarily disastrous. Many people can focus on progress and the excitement of meeting new goals. Some view their disability as an opportunity for changing their direction in life or strengthening their character. Some people initially feel depressed and defeated in rehabilitation, whereas others see it as a battle they have just begun to fight. With some understanding of the range of feelings you can expect, how to talk them through, and how to get emotional support, you'll be better equipped to begin your emotional adjustment and healing while you are going through physical adjustments and therapies.

HOW DO I FEEL?

In this section, we explore in more detail the range of emotional responses to disability associated with a spinal cord injury. Feelings and reactions vary from person to person. While all the reactions described below are common and in many cases expected, you may experience only some of them. Despite the common notion about a set sequence of emotional reactions to loss, individuals vary widely in when, whether, and how intensely they experience these emotions. We provide a sample of some typical feelings and give some examples to show how individuals have experienced and ultimately coped with strong emotions following spinal cord injury.

Denial and Hope

Many people go through a period of emotional shock following a paralyzing spinal cord injury. This may include a period of disbelief ("This can't be real, this can't be happening to me") and distrust in the doctors' diagnosis or prognosis ("They must be mistaken—this is only temporary. I just need time to heal"). Professionals often speak of this reaction as denial, and indeed some patients literally deny that they are impaired. In our experience, however, this type of total denial is quite rare. More typically, patients simply question the permanence of their injuries and may not be able to accurately anticipate the impact the injuries will undoubtedly have on every aspect of their lives. The positive, flip side of this phenomenon is hope. Hope for recovery is normal and emotionally adaptive, even while recognizing the likelihood that some of your limitations will be permanent. In fact, hope has been shown to be important in motivating individuals to work toward achieving their full potential and in improving quality of life after spinal cord injury. Many people with incomplete spinal cord injuries recover significant functional abilities weeks or months after their initial injury. And in fact (as we discuss in Chapter 8), medical advances may one day lead to partial or total cures for the paralysis of spinal cord injury.

> Lark (whose story you'll read in Chapter 8) developed incomplete C5–C6 tetraplegia after a diving accident. Soon after her hospitalization, some of the staff asked her if she'd like to meet with a former patient who could act as a role model for living with paralysis. She declined. "You don't know that I won't recover," she said. "Why should I make myself miserable now when I don't know what recovery there will be? I can wait two years and be miserable then!"

She rejected a "disabled role model," feeling that her denial at that point, com-bined with hope, helped her cope emotionally and motivated her efforts at rehabilitation.

Elliott (see Chapter 6) had an injury almost identical to Lark's. For the first three months after his injury, he recalls, he was told that he was going to walk. "When I first got hurt, I was fed a lot of lies. Maybe they thought I wouldn't be able to handle it or they were doing me a favor by bringing it on slowly." But Elliott felt that confronting the reality of his disability was just what he needed so that he could set goals and put his all into rehabilitation. "You need to know the truth, the facts. You've got to start dealing with it right away."

Communicating with your doctor about these issues—what to expect *now*, what you need to function in the *immediate* future, and what may be available in the *distant* future—is probably the best way to develop an attitude of hopefulness combined with realism. This will help you focus on what you need to do to live with your current abilities without taking away your motivating vision of a better future. Expressing your feelings and communicating your confusions and questions about your injury is the surest way to avoid a more entrenched denial that could prevent your getting full benefit from the rehabilitation program.

Jim hated using his wheelchair. Throughout his early rehabilitation he struggled with feelings of shame and depression about needing to use it. How-ever, he quickly progressed to the use of forearm crutches, and because he had strong arms and had been in excellent physical condition before his injury, he soon developed a relatively speedy and efficient gait. Jim's doctors praised his accomplishment, while telling him that he would probably always need crutches. But Jim would not give up on his dream of walking "normally." He became obsessed with this goal, spending many hours beyond his allotted therapy time on practicing his walking and exercising his arms, often to the point of exhaustion.

When he was discharged from the rehabilitation hospital, Jim requested a referral for daily outpatient physical therapy, much more time than most peo-ple would want. His doctor worried about Jim's denial of his limitations. He seemed to be spending all his effort on the elusive goal of "normal" walking, leaving little energy for dealing with important vocational and family concerns. Jim's psychologist was also concerned with his social withdrawal and seeming inability to "lighten up" and enjoy himself during this period.

Working together, his physician and psychologist discovered that, in Jim's mind, easing up on his physical therapy regimen would mean "accepting that I'm okay like this." To Jim, that was the same as giving up hope, and he still needed the hope of full recovery, or normalcy, in order to carry on both physically and emotionally. And being disciplined and perfectionist by nature, he needed to be absolutely sure that he'd left no stone unturned, that he'd put as much effort into his rehabilitation as was humanly possible.

The doctor agreed to prescribe extra therapy time, as long as Jim was showing progress in strength and efficiency. Jim's psychologist helped him examine his negative self-image and fears of being rejected socially, and helped him accept the need to change to a less physically demanding career.

Ultimately, Jim gained a great deal of physical strength and confidence. He was able to use a single crutch or cane on occasion. He felt better about himself because of his persistence. As he became involved in other aspects of living and put himself in situations where people responded positively to him as a person, he became less focused on either denying or conquering his limitations. Jim continued to hope for full recovery. But now he also had hope for living a full and satisfying life with his disability. He began to accept himself, pursue alternative job plans, and go out with friends again.

Grief and Depression

How do you feel when reality begins to sink in and you are confronted with so many losses, changes, and disruptions? Many people experience a sense of grief in the wake of becoming disabled. Sadness, unhappiness, and feeling "down" or "blue" are normal responses to any loss. With the onset of a physical disability, many people also feel inadequate, useless, and unattractive and suffer a loss of self-esteem or self-worth. Added to the impact of the physical and functional losses, these feelings can lead to a downward spiral of self-pity, self-recrimination, and despair.

Many people with spinal cord injury become depressed at some point after their injury. Estimates vary across studies, but the rate of depression is thought to be higher in people with spinal cord injuries than in the general population. Clinical depression, or depressive disorder, is distinguished from sadness or "the blues" by the way in which it impairs function, above and beyond the effects of the physical disability itself. Symptoms of a clinical depression include changes in sleep and appetite, loss of interest or pleasure in most activities, feelings of worthlessness or guilt, frequent crying spells, social withdrawal, suicidal thoughts, and a decreased ability to care for oneself. Depressive disorders are very common and highly responsive to treatment with psychotherapy and antidepressant medications. If you or your family think you may be depressed, discuss your symptoms and feelings openly with your physician, psychologist, or social worker. You can then get effective treatment and avoid any disruption in your rehabilitation.

Depression can be a fatal illness. The risk of suicide is also higher for people with spinal cord injury than for the general population. The first three years appear to be the time of greatest suicide risk: about 80 percent of all suicides in people with spinal cord injury occur during this period. Early recognition and treatment of depression and prompt evaluation of suicidal thoughts can help prevent suicide.

If you are having any thoughts about hurting or killing yourself, talk about them immediately with your doctor, psychologist, nurse, or other health care provider. Your doctor may want to consult a psychiatrist or psychologist to determine whether you are clinically depressed and whether your suicidal thoughts pose a serious risk. Being open about your thoughts is the best way to get proper treatment. Talking about your feelings will also help you sort them out.

While one should err on the side of caution by considering treatment or safety precautions when suicidal ideas occur, it may be reassuring to know that not all suicidal thoughts are necessarily dangerous or pathological. For someone confronted with complete tetraplegia, dependence on a ventilator, and the need for assistance twenty-four hours a day, thoughts such as "I don't know how I can live like this" or "How can life be worth living in this state?" may be quite reasonable. And thoughts such as "It would be easier or better if I were dead" might arise in individuals who don't have the slightest intention of actually hurting themselves.

Robert, at age twenty-four, sustained a T4 spinal cord injury when he fell asleep at the wheel of his truck. He remembers his first thoughts after transfer to a rehabilitation hospital. "I laid in bed thinking, Do I want to go on? I could read people's faces and see how bad things were. I knew I had messed up, done some stupid things." But soon after, Robert became highly motivated, in part by his realization of his mother's sadness about his accident. "I knew I had to turn things around, make her proud. I said to myself, I'll figure it out."

Speaking your concerns aloud has another advantage: it will prompt the rehabilitation staff to teach you how people *do* live with tetraplegia. They can discuss and find answers to your particular questions about how to get through the day, how to improve your experience of life, and how to make it meaningful to yourself and others. And sharing concerns with loved ones gives them the opportunity to validate your worth as a person and allows you to search for solutions together.

Most people with spinal cord injuries don't become severely depressed, but grief and sadness are common. Grief and mourning are normal responses to any significant loss. Normal grieving usually involves feelings of sadness related specifically to the lost person, object, or function. Crying spells, some transient sleep disturbance, and feelings of guilt or regret are usual. Normal grieving does *not* involve persistent and pervasive feelings of worthlessness, suicidal thoughts, or loss of pleasure in all activities. During a period of sadness or grief, the grieving person can respond positively to comfort and support from others, can benefit from talking about the loss, and can continue to perform everyday functions such as dressing, eating, and doing chores.

Recognizing that sadness and grief are normal responses to loss, allowing yourself a period of mourning, and above all talking to your loved ones about your feelings will help you work through your loss more quickly. In the rehabilitation hospital, social workers and often psychologists can help you talk about and cope with feelings of depression before they become overwhelming. They can help you sort through your reactions to your limitations and understand any initial difficulties in performing the physical and occupational therapy tasks that are part of your rehabilitation program.

For example, is your wheelchair mobility training bogged down because of weakness in your arms, because you don't really understand the therapist's directions, or because every time you get into the wheelchair you are filled with feelings of humiliation and inadequacy? Are you refusing the occupational therapist's offer of specialized splints for writing because you don't want to pay your own bills and write your own letters, or because wearing the splints puts the disability "in your face" and makes you feel ugly, different, and depressed? Are you asking for help with dressing yourself because you haven't yet mastered the techniques for independent dressing, or because you're too depressed to put forth the energy, or because you can't express your need for social contact except by asking for this type of assistance?

One factor that contributes to depression is loss of control. When you feel that your disability is an externally imposed event, something you cannot affect through your own behavior, you are more likely to feel depressed. The hospital staff may unwittingly contribute to this feeling by providing you with equipment or developing treatment goals without asking for your input, feelings, and preferences. Remind yourself that you do have choices, that you can take some control of your situation. Some things that depress you can be changed. When *you* initiate even minor changes, you are likely to feel less depressed and more accepting of your limitations.

Joan (whose story is in Chapter 4) hated her heavy leather splints and worked with her occupational therapist to try various alternatives. They eventually developed a model for clear plastic splints and had them custom made by an orthopedic supply house. The splints proved just as effective and more esthetically pleasing. Bonnie, who has paraplegia, was disgusted with the way the outline of her long leg braces showed through her sweat pants, and she didn't want to wear sweats other than in therapy. She decided to alter her jeans to fit loosely over the braces, creating a bell-bottom effect. This made her feel presentable to visitors and more in charge of her appearance.

Making decisions about your goals, equipment, and appearance can help you avoid helplessness and depression. Understanding that even normal feelings of sadness can affect your physical progress may encourage you to get support from friends and family and to recognize your accomplishments. Making choices, asking for change when possible, and getting support help you focus more clearly and objectively on your practical and physical needs.

Anger

Another common, though not universal, feeling in response to spinal cord injury is anger, particularly for those injured in an accident or by violent crime. If your disability was caused by your own behavior, such as a one-car accident or diving into a shallow pool, you may be furious with yourself. If your injury is due to a tumor or disease over which you have no control, you may direct your anger at fate or at God. Or you may look for a cosmic reason for your injury, searching for the meaning of your survival rather than raging at destiny.

Your anger about how your injury occurred may last only a brief period, but you will be coming to terms with losses for a longer time. Anger is a normal response to losing something precious and to the frustration and dependence that you face daily as you struggle to perform what were once automatic and easy tasks.

Andrew, age thirteen, had paraplegia from a gunshot wound (see Chapter 7). When he first came home from rehab, his moods were erratic. His mother, Jane, struggled to figure out which emotional outbursts were due to his disability and which ones were normal for a budding teenager. Sometimes Andrew got so angry and frustrated, he would bang his wheelchair into the wall.

Unfortunately, many adults consider anger an unacceptable, dangerous, or immature emotion. You may fear that anger will alienate the very people whose help you depend on. You may be concerned that anger is a sign of immaturity or weakness and be worried about having a childish "temper tantrum." Or you may worry that your anger, because it feels so intense, will get out of control and become destructive.

Tom broke his neck in an industrial accident. He was angry not only at the careless co-worker directly responsible for his injury but also at the entire company for not better policing the plant. Tom was generally a friendly, easygoing man, and anger was an unusual emotion for him. He wished he could be forgiving. He felt guilty about his anger and thought his angry feelings made him a mean or bad person.

Tom held in his anger for a long time, trying to pretend he didn't feel it. This intensified his tendency to be depressed over his losses, increased his passivity and lack of initiative, and actually worsened his fear of losing control. He ini-tially performed well in therapy, and the staff involved in his care had high hopes for his return to work, school, and social life. But Tom's continuing inabil-ity to acknowledge and express his anger soon led to a deterioration in his prog-ress. He became extremely passive and apathetic and was unable to make important decisions. He couldn't act on his own behalf to apply for financial assistance or stand up for himself in personal relationships.

Tom's biggest fear was that his anger would lead to aggression. Indeed, he harbored vicious fantasies of revenge against the person responsible for his accident. But he eventually saw that he was turning this aggression on himself by giving up control of his life, that he was undermining his own recovery, and that he was being emotionally abused by other people. Tom sought help from a counselor, who validated his feelings of anger and rage and helped him find ways to turn this anger into constructive rather than destructive action.

Tom gradually began to act more on his own behalf. He got in touch with his family, who lived out of state, and asked for their support. They responded with more frequent phone calls to his hospital room and praise for his progress. He called social service agencies and filled out applications for Medicaid, housing aid, and other benefits that he would need after discharge. He talked to his law-yer about suing his employer for damages. He thought about his vocational plans in terms of what interested him, rather than what his counselor thought would be good for him. And he appropriately expressed his anger toward sev-eral people who had taken advantage of him or hurt his feelings during his most dependent and needy times.

Tom felt a renewed sense of self-reliance and empowerment. He learned that anger turned into positive action and self-expression was not dangerous. In fact, his revenge fantasies subsided as he felt better about his own life. Get-ting the anger out in the open had helped him avoid depression, regain control, and direct his energy toward helping himself, and had prevented bitterness from setting in.

Disabling anger is common, but it can be avoided by expecting and recognizing anger as a normal response to spinal cord injury and by ver-balizing it openly, perhaps with other patients in informal gripe sessions. Anger is better expressed in words than by acting it out through hostility, withdrawal, or rebellion against the rehabilitation program.

In the rehabilitation hospital, you can also get help in expressing your anger through therapy with a psychologist, social worker, or psychiatrist. Many spinal cord injury programs provide group therapy in which you can openly share feelings with other patients. Pastoral counselors may be helpful in dealing with anger at God. When possible, physical activity such as socking a punching bag, smashing a piece of clay, or bouncing a ball can be an outlet for anger. Physically demanding wheelchair sports are another constructive outlet for feelings of frustration, as Andrew, who played wheelchair tennis, soon discovered. And like Tom, you can find ways to take control of your situation and turn your anger into positive action. You may need to call insurance companies and employers to obtain or maintain benefits. You may need to write to foundations for financial help or apply for vocational services. Acting on your own behalf to get the help you deserve is another way to transform your anger into constructive behavior.

Anxiety

Posttraumatic Stress

In the first few months after spinal cord injury, a high degree of stress or anxiety is common. Some of the anxiety stems from the situation that caused the disability—for example, a car accident, shooting, or war injury. In the heat of a life-threatening emergency, and even during acute hospitalization, the body is stimulated by adrenaline and energy is focused on survival. Anxiety is automatically blocked from mental awareness in an adaptive physiological response that allows one to cope with the crisis at hand.

Once the immediate danger is over and you are settled into a safe, albeit difficult routine, you may find yourself flooded with anxiety, replaying the trauma in your mind (in flashbacks) or having nightmares with terrifying experiences of helplessness, impending disaster, and loss of control. These symptoms of posttraumatic stress are common after any emotionally overwhelming situation.

Again, talking it out helps. Research on the treatment of people with severe posttraumatic stress reactions suggests that the sooner they talk about the experience and associated fears, and the more detail they are able to give, the less anxiety they are likely to experience in the future.

Patty became paraplegic following a bullet wound to her spine. She was at her niece's home, their children playing together, when the niece's estranged boyfriend barged into the house and shot both women. Her niece was killed and Patty was seriously injured.

Patty suffered extreme pain and emotional distress while waiting for emergency assistance to arrive. At the hospital, she was mourning the loss of her niece, confronting her own disability, and worrying about the emotional effects of the event on her child. However, after emergency treatment and medical stabilization, her healing progressed nicely and her spirits were remarkably good.

Once in rehabilitation, Patty surprised the staff by talking frequently and in great detail about the circumstances of her injury, her niece's bloody death, and her pain and terror while waiting to be rescued. She told the story to anyone who would listen, to the point that some staff questioned the normalcy of her preoccupation. Yet Patty seemed immune from the anxiety that many expected of her. She was able to focus on information about her recovery, participate actively in her therapies, and maintain supportive relationships with friends and family. She was eager to learn how to use the wheelchair, to get well, and to get on with her life.

Patty was doing spontaneously what most therapists would encourage any victim of a trauma to do—managing and mastering the anxiety by talking about the trauma and the feelings it evoked. Talking not only "gets it out" but also elicits support and validation from others. Thus Patty, more than many patients, was able to make new friends in the rehabilitation hospital. Other patients and staff members saw her as courageous and determined. This reinforced Patty's sense of self-worth and diminished her anxiety about using a wheelchair, learning bladder care, and becoming independent. She left the hospital with some realistic anxiety about returning to work and parenting with a disability and, indeed, real social and physical challenges lay ahead. But Patty was not overwhelmed or disabled by the anxiety itself.

Dependence and Control

Sometimes anxiety stems from the loss of control and the extreme dependence on others imposed by the disability, regardless of how the injury occurred. Spinal cord injury caused by a vascular problem or spinal tumor (rather than an accident) may not cause posttraumatic stress, but it nevertheless results in a major loss of independent function. Basic biological functions and the simplest tasks of daily living may suddenly require the assistance of another person.

When you are no longer able-bodied, you must depend on others to take you to the bathroom, get you dressed, or help you dial the phone. You are suddenly confronted with a host of uncertainties. Will the nurse answer your call-bell in time, or will you wet the bed? Will you get help to make a call home before your wife leaves for work, or will you have to wait until visiting hours to talk to her? What if the staff doesn't like you? What if your injury is repulsive to others? Will you still get the help you need? These uncertainties produce anxiety and feelings of helplessness in the rehabilitation hospital and often afterward, when problems become even more complex. Will my office or school be wheelchair accessible? How will I reach the files? Can I use the bathroom independently at my favorite restaurant?

Just as when you were a small child, you have to depend on the care and assistance of others for many of your basic needs. At first you may expect the hospital to take care of all your needs, but you'll inevitably be disappointed. You'll learn that there aren't enough nurses, or that other patients' needs are more urgent, or that priority is given to biological over social needs, even though the latter may be just as important to your sense of well-being.

You may feel frustrated and angry about not getting help. You may also be quite anxious and afraid—that you will never get help, that others will forget about or abandon you, or that something terrible will happen to you because you are helpless and alone (you will fall, stop breathing, or lose your sanity). This type of anxiety, if left unchecked, can lead to disabling panic attacks, requiring medication or other treatment. But more often, this anxiety is experienced as a humiliating return to an infantile state of fear, frustration, and irritability, a loss of control over oneself and one's environment, which is at best unsettling and at worst an assault on one's dignity.

Learning to manage anxiety is an important task for every person, regardless of circumstances. Most people need some predictability and some sense of control over their bodies, their behavior, and their environment in order to feel secure and confident. We all learn ways to manage anxiety about new situations: by learning about what to expect (knowledge), developing skills to meet the new demands (mastery), gradually imposing some regularity or predictability (control), and allowing for periods of rest or "down time" when we temporarily set aside the new demands (pacing). These strategies are also helpful in coping with the anxiety generated by disability and dependence.

Although information about your disability may be overwhelming at first, you need to learn as much as possible about your body's new demands and functions. Ask your doctor or nurse for information about your injury and about aspects of your function that trouble you the most—whether it is sexuality, bowel and bladder control, or use of a wheelchair. Concentrate on developing new skills. Take an active role in setting daily, weekly, or long-term goals. By discussing *your* goals with the therapists, you can more fully participate in your rehabilitation and more quickly master the skills necessary to alleviate your anxieties.

Working closely with your nurses and therapists in developing a predictable routine is important. It may be helpful to involve a spouse or family member in this process. Ask the staff to give you realistic expectations about the availability of care. Waiting for things to happen is easier when you know you'll have to wait and don't experience constant anticipation and frustration.

Through communication about your needs, you and your caregivers (or family members) may be able to reach workable compromises: using the telephone at a prearranged time, changing your therapy schedule to accommodate care needs or family visits, and so forth. Expressing your wishes about seemingly small personal preferences can also be important in reestablishing a sense of control. Don't hesitate to ask for your favorite soap, cosmetics, clothes, plants, or pictures to be brought to the hospital or rehabilitation facility. Make sure you have a reliable method for controlling the television, lights, and call-bell in your room or arrange for regular assistance to do so.

Finally, try to pace your day so that you get some respite from the demands of your disability. Some people do this by becoming a couch potato at the end of the day—watching television, reading, or doing crosswords. Some build in a short period each day when someone else attends to their needs so that they can rest from the effort of doing everything for themselves. Another idea is to arrange for a psychological break from the hospital atmosphere, such as getting a special meal brought in, having a party in your room, or getting some quiet time with a spouse.

These activities can break the single-minded focus on recovery, provide relaxation and rest, and remind you of the rewards of life beyond the hospital, thus giving meaning and purpose to your daily struggles with rehabilitation.

GETTING AROUND: WHEELCHAIRS AND OTHER EQUIPMENT

Mobility, or getting yourself around, is one of the first and primary tasks in rehabilitation. For most people with a spinal cord injury, this need for assisted mobility is the most obvious change from their pre-injury status. To participate in almost any activity, you must be able to get out of bed and either walk (perhaps with a walker or crutches and braces) or use a wheelchair to move around your room, around the hospital, and ultimately around your home and community.

The rehabilitation program teaches the injured person how to transfer (move from wheelchair to bed or toilet, and so forth) and how to use the wheelchair to travel from place to place. Those with very limited arm function may need an electric wheelchair with hand, head, or mouth controls. Those with paraplegia or tetraplegia with good arm strength can learn to propel a manual wheelchair with gradually increasing speed and accurate steering and navigation. Physical therapy includes practice in these wheelchair skills, working toward self-sufficiency.

Persons with incomplete paraplegia may be candidates for leg braces, crutches, canes, or some combination of these. In this case, you may have the option of walking at times—for short distances or up a few steps—but still using your wheelchair for longer distances when walking would be too slow or fatiguing.

You may have to make some important choices about how much therapy time to spend on learning to walk versus increasing your wheelchair mobility skills. While some people have little choice because of the severity of their injuries, many individuals with spinal cord injury make personal and lifestyle choices about how to move around and which devices to use under which circumstances. Don't hesitate to discuss your options and wishes with your physical therapist and your physician. Together you can come to the best solutions for *your* needs and preferences. Even those with severely limited mobility (high-level tetraplegia) may have life circumstances and emotional needs that determine the choice between using a mouth- or breath-controlled electric wheelchair or letting a family member or attendant move them around in a manual wheelchair. For people with tetraplegia who are employed or require independent mobility for other reasons, power wheelchairs are often considered a "must." Others, who enjoy the challenge or exercise of wheeling themselves or have someone who can help them get around, may prefer a manual chair. One choice is not necessarily better than another. Each person has different priorities, values, and goals.

The need for a wheelchair to get around is often a source of psychological and social distress for the new user. Many people associate wheelchairs with illness, frailty, old age, or total dependence on others. They may feel embarrassed or humiliated by the wheelchair. They may feel trapped in the chair, or see it as a symbol of giving up, or feel that it makes them a "hopeless case." Braces or crutches may inspire similar feelings of embarrassment, hopelessness, frustration, or being "different."

It's important to talk about these feelings with your therapists and doctors and with other patients, especially if you're depressed or reluctant to learn how to get around by yourself. If you find that trying to walk (or just fantasizing about it) has become an obsession and is requiring inordinate amounts of physical or mental energy with little useful results, it is probably time for you to examine some of your assumptions, expectations, and negative feelings about wheelchair use. On the other hand, wanting to have your wheelchair pushed everywhere by someone else, resisting the exercises necessary to increase your strength for independent wheelchair mobility, or frequently asking to be waited on suggests the need for help in uncovering and working through your emotions.

Many rehabilitation programs provide recreational therapy in addition to physical and occupational therapies. Recreational therapy is geared toward helping you take part in recreational, leisure, and daily living activities. These activities might include going to a sports event, learning to paint or do crafts, shopping, or going to a restaurant or other public place. Recreational therapists may also teach patients how to participate in sports (such as swimming or wheelchair basketball) or pursue hobbies with adaptive equipment.

In many hospitals, recreational therapists provide opportunities for patients to practice their mobility skills in the community before going home, through trips to malls, restaurants, ball games, movie theaters, and so on. These trips provide opportunities to use adapted transportation (such as a specially equipped bus, van, or car) and to use a wheelchair in varied environments (flat surfaces, curbs, elevators, special seating areas, restrooms). Such excursions provide firsthand experience of the obstacles wheelchair users will regularly need to face as well as the rewards of getting around to do what one wants to do. They also provide exposure to further feelings and reactions associated with disability and "coming out" in a wheelchair.

HOW DO I LOOK TO OTHERS?

A spinal cord injury is a very visible disability. Unlike a person with diabetes or heart disease, you cannot hide your condition. A wheelchair or crutches, and any changes in physical appearance, are immediately apparent to others. The ease or difficulty of adjusting to disability depends not only on your own emotions and actions but on other people's reactions to your changed appearance.

How you look to others is likely to be on your mind from the early days of rehabilitation. And how you cope with social responses to your disability is important to your success in living with a spinal cord injury.

Stigma

People with visible disabilities are sometimes stigmatized by cultural beliefs and language and treated as if their disabilities were a mark of disgrace, social inferiority, or moral or mental abnormality. Such prejudice generally arises from fear or anxiety. To ward off their own feelings of vulnerability, many people use stigma to separate themselves from "those disabled people" and thus to feel protected and secure, certain that they could never be "one of *them*."

Unfortunately, this prejudice is manifest as discrimination in jobs, education, and socialization, as will become more apparent when you leave the hospital and attempt to reenter the "real world." But even during your inpatient rehabilitation, you need to understand that fears of social rejection and concern about how you look to others are based as much in social reality as on your own anxieties and altered self-esteem.

Even if *you* feel great about yourself, some people (not all) may be awkward, uncomfortable, or frightened by your disability.

Appearance: Looking Different

Our culture puts a premium on conformity and physical attractiveness, and children soon learn the social value of fitting in and being pretty or handsome. Spinal cord injury makes someone different, no matter how much of a conformist he or she was before. The injury is often accompanied by muscular atrophy or limb contracture or by "appendages" (urine collection bag, leg braces, corset) that can make a person feel unnatural and unattractive.

Self-conscious about physical appearance, an individual may withdraw from social opportunities—turning down offers of visits from friends or co-workers, choosing not to participate in recreational or social activities in the hospital, or avoiding contact with family. And this behavior may even extend toward the rehabilitation staff, with concerns about appearance hindering progress in physical therapy or making people hesitant to ask for needed help if it means greater exposure of their body to others.

You'll be confronted with a range of responses from your visitors and family, some of which may be difficult to manage. They may be curious and ask embarrassing personal questions about your bodily functions. They may be awkward or anxious, not knowing what to say to you. They may feel frightened, guilty, or repulsed by your disability. They may treat you like a child by being bossy, loud, or overly solicitous. They may feel inadequate and awed by your efforts at managing the disability, or they may be angry, blaming you and avoiding you like the plague. Still others will continue to see the essential you, undaunted by your physical changes.

Managing the Reactions of Others

Differentiating your own fears about how you look from the actual reactions of other people can be quite confusing. Try comparing how you viewed people with disabilities before your injury and how you now feel about yourself. Think about how you react to other patients whose injuries are comparable to, or worse than, your own.

Ask yourself a few questions. What frightens you or "turns you off"? This may help you to understand the reactions of others and not take their responses so personally. What makes a person seem attractive or approachable? You might try modeling these positive aspects of self-presentation. What makes you feel good about your own appearance? Although you may need to wear casual clothing for physical therapy, you can still dress up for visiting hours. Developing strategies to help others see beyond the disability to the "real you" also helps you see yourself as a whole person, not a collection of physical flaws.

One way of gaining a greater sense of control over social situations is to anticipate reactions to your different appearance by commenting on it or even drawing attention to it. You can use humor—making a joke about yourself—or simply comment on the facts of your situation ("You can see I need crutches now. It's because my spinal cord was damaged and my legs are weak").

You can also put your own creative stamp on your crutches, walker, or wheelchair. This can elicit a positive response from others and help them focus on your choice of embellishments—that is, on an aspect of your personality—rather than on your impairment or "sickness." Many wheelchairs and walkers are now available in a variety of colors, and you may be able to make a choice about this when you go home. Wheelchair backpacks, tote bags for walkers, and related items can also be used to individualize your equipment.

Finally, you can put your friend or family member at ease by preempting negative comments. By saying something like "I really hate this brace. It's the ugliest thing I've ever seen. I wish I didn't need it, but I guess I'll have to get used to it," you are giving the other person permission to think that the brace is ugly and thus to feel less guilty or awkward. At the same time, this also focuses the negative perception on the brace and away from you. The brace may indeed be ugly, but *you* are not!

SOCIAL ISOLATION

In the rehabilitation hospital you will most likely be separated from your family and friends for much of the time. With the busy schedule of physical and occupational therapy, visiting hours may be limited to evenings and weekends. Spouses who have worked all day will be tired at night. They may also be overwhelmed by their own reaction to your disability and losses. And given the lack of privacy, you may find it next to impossible to share intimate or personal feelings with your spouse or relatives. Though your family and friends may try hard to be supportive and available, you may still experience a loss of support, comfort, and closeness just when you could use it the most.

> *During his stay in the rehabilitation hospital, Jim found the separation from his wife and his work very stressful. His self-esteem largely depended on his role as a competent, responsible, and creative worker and as a good provider and supportive husband for his wife. Jim felt abandoned when his co-workers didn't call or visit him but felt jealous, inadequate, and embarrassed when they did. Even though his disability was no fault of his own, he felt guilty about being "less" than he was before. He feared that his wife would reject him, yet he pushed her away because it was too hard to admit his new dependence on her. Perceiving that he was angry with her, his wife felt she was failing to be sufficiently supportive. Afraid to express her feelings and having little opportunity for uninterrupted time with Jim in the hospital, she began to withdraw, too. Soon Jim felt miserably isolated from his wife and his work buddies.*
>
> *Jim didn't resolve these relationship problems until after he left the hospital, but he did find a way to compensate for his loneliness. He found friendship with another patient. Tony, a teenager with spinal cord injury, was scared and lonely and clearly admired Jim for his strength and progress. Jim spent a lot of free time talking to Tony and cheering him up. Because of their shared circumstances, they quickly became close friends. As Jim felt needed and valued by Tony, he was more motivated to go on with his own rehabilitation, even when he felt unsupported by his wife and "outside" friends.*
>
> *Reflecting on this experience later, Jim saw how his relationship with Tony had given him a sense of purpose and meaning during the hardest part of his initial rehabilitation. Knowing that he was not alone with his disability, and that others might be even more needy, continued to motivate Jim throughout his recovery.*

Like Jim, you may find talking with other patients and forming supportive and friendly relationships helpful during your hospital stay. Many hospitals have formal programs to encourage interactions among patients, but you can initiate relationships informally with your roommate, the person next to you in physical therapy, or someone you meet at mealtimes. Other patients understand what you are going through. Furthermore, they are available and can often serve as stand-ins for physically or emotionally distant family members during the hectic and stressful period of early rehabilitation.

WHO CAN HELP YOU COPE?

We've talked about a variety of difficult social and emotional issues that people with spinal cord injury might confront during the inpatient phase of rehabilitation. We've discussed some reactions to the changes in what you can do, how you get around, how you feel, and how you look to others. And we've looked at what physical, occupational, respiratory, and recreational therapists can do for you, and at some strategies that people have found helpful in coping with their injuries and resolving painful emotions. So far, we've mentioned mental health professionals only in passing (in our discussion of depression), for a couple of reasons.

Not every rehabilitation hospital includes psychological or psychiatric services as a routine part of its program, though most provide at least some access to mental health services. And while screening for psychological difficulties after spinal cord injury is helpful, not every patient needs psychological or psychiatric intervention (in contrast to physical therapy, which is a must for every patient).

As we have suggested, however, mental health professionals can help not only with depression but with issues of grieving, sadness, anxiety, anger, and relationship problems. It is helpful to know something about the different types of mental health professionals so that you can get the most effective care and treatment.

Psychiatrists

Psychiatrists are physicians (medical school graduates) who have received residency training in the diagnosis and treatment of mental illnesses. As medical doctors, they are able to prescribe medications. They admit patients to psychiatric hospitals when necessary, and they have specialized knowledge of the relationship between medical illnesses, brain function, and behavior. They may have additional training in psychotherapy or some other aspect of medicine.

Evaluation by a psychiatrist is useful when clinical depression is suspected or when a person has suicidal thoughts, and also for those with overwhelming anxiety or panic or with anger that explodes into aggression toward others. Psychiatric evaluation may also be helpful for people with a mild head injury or for those who develop confusion, disorientation, or distorted thinking for any reason.

If you were receiving psychiatric treatment before your injury or are taking psychiatric medication (for example, an antidepressant) when you're admitted for rehabilitation, make sure to tell your doctor. He or she can arrange for a psychiatrist to work with you so that you receive continuous care and have any necessary adjustments in your medication.

Medication can often reduce symptoms of depression or anxiety to manageable levels. This allows an injured person to continue with rehabilitation and enhances his or her ability to communicate feelings and needs to family or friends. A combination of medication with psychotherapy, or "talking therapy," is the most effective method for treating clinical depression.

Psychologists

Licensed psychologists are experts in mental health and human behavior. They usually have a doctoral degree (Ph.D.) in psychology, with at least three years of graduate school training in psychology, at least one year of internship training in counseling or psychotherapy, and research training that culminated in an independent research or theoretical dissertation. Some psychologists have additional specialty training, for example, in neuropsychology (a branch of psychology that focuses on the relation between brain function and behavior), rehabilitation psychology (psychology that concentrates on the psychosocial aspects of physical disability and rehabilitation), or health psychology (psychology that deals with the relation of behavior and emotions to physical illness and health). In some states, people with a master's degree (M.A. or M.S.) in psychology are also called psychologists within the hospital setting. They may provide psychological testing, psychotherapy, or other psychological services. In some settings, they are called psychology associates or psychology technicians. They may require supervision by a Ph.D. psychologist and may have more limited duties. Psychologists are not physicians and do not prescribe medications, except in a few states, where they may prescribe some medications after completing special training.

Psychologists specialize in understanding human behavior and emotions and the relationship between social and environmental factors and a person's internal experiences and outward behaviors. In the rehabilitation setting, psychologists can help you sort through your complicated feelings and work through grief, anger, and loss of control. They can also help you change behaviors that are troubling to you or interfere with your progress. They can help with issues of pain control, sexuality, and family relationships. Psychologists can also assess your personality style, former coping mechanisms, and learning abilities, then share this information with other staff members to assist them in teaching you new skills, motivating you, and understanding your individual needs. Psychologists may be asked to help evaluate cognitive problems related to mild head injury or past learning disabilities. They might also lead family therapy or group psychotherapy sessions for people with spinal cord injuries.

Social Workers

Hospital social workers generally have a bachelor's degree (B.S.W.) or a master's degree (M.S.W.) in social work. Few people with a doctorate in social work (D.S.W.) work in hospitals. Social workers have special training in evaluating people's needs for social and human services such as assistance with housing, welfare, medical care, or mental health services. Some social workers also have specialized training in providing clinical mental health services such as family counseling or individual psychotherapy. Some states license M.S.W.'s as licensed clinical social workers (LCSWs). These professionals can work in any social service or mental health agency or maintain a private practice in psychotherapy.

Communication with family, friends, co-workers, and others close to you is essential as you integrate new limitations, needs, and emotions with old roles and relationships. You also need good rapport with your spouse or family to ensure competent and loving care or assistance when you return home. Social workers can help with this communication by talking regularly with your spouse or family about your progress, your concerns, and your discharge plans.

All hospital-based rehabilitation programs have social workers on staff. Depending on the facility, their role may be weighted more toward patient and family counseling or more toward solving the practical problems associated with returning home—arranging for in-home therapies, transportation to work, disability payments and insurance, and so forth. The social worker is the primary person involved in securing placement in a nursing home, another hospital, an outpatient rehabilitation program, or a home care program, when necessary. He or she helps to coordinate any care or equipment needs before your discharge and makes sure that appropriate aftercare is set up with the doctor, mental health professional, or nurse practitioner.

Your social worker often acts as your advocate, helping you identify and solve practical problems, obtain assistance and training, and get information on community services. He or she also provides (or makes sure that you get) help with emotional or psychosocial problems. The social worker will, when necessary, help communicate your needs to your doctor, family, employer, or school.

SOME OVERLAP IS USUAL IN THE ROLES AND ACTIVITIES of the various mental health professionals. Although this can be somewhat confusing, it also ensures that in most rehabilitation settings you can turn to more than one person for guidance in coping with social and emotional issues. Even if you don't need psychological treatment, these professionals are helpful in providing information, support, and a sounding board for your concerns, ideas, and questions. They can help you understand yourself better and enhance your adjustment by helping you build on your personal strengths and existing social supports.

Other Helpers

You may encounter a few other types of professionals in the rehabilitation hospital, depending on the type of facility. Some programs employ certified rehabilitation counselors (CRCs), who are trained to counsel people with disabilities on a variety of adjustment issues. They receive their credentials from a national board, and some are licensed or certified by their state. CRCs can play a significant role in the transition back to work. They make sure that all elements of the return to employment are in place, including the disabled client's readiness and ability to do the job in question, the employer's awareness of the client's abilities and special needs, and the physical accessibility of the work site. CRCs often help prepare management and co-workers for the entry or return to work of a person with spinal cord injury.

Vocational rehabilitation counselors, who are sometimes also CRCs, are usually employed by state governments to help injured workers return to the workforce. Their role is to help people with spinal cord injuries return to their jobs or receive college or technical training. A vocational rehabilitation counselor can be instrumental in finding employment opportunities for clients by evaluating skills and aptitudes and advising them about training opportunities or new types of work for which they may be qualified.

Increasingly, case managers may play a role in planning for discharge from the hospital and successful reentry to independent living and return to work. Hired by third-party payers or hospitals, case managers assist individuals with spinal cord injury in making decisions about their medical, rehabilitation, and vocational needs. Most case managers have a background as helping professionals; they are often nurses or rehabilitation counselors. Case managers assigned by private or workers' compensation insurance often continue to work with clients after their discharge from the hospital, ensuring the coordination of outpatient care and a smooth transition to home and work life. People who have benefited from the skills of a case manager say that this relationship was crucial to their success at independent living.

THE NEXT STEP

As you approach the midpoint in your rehabilitation, you may feel a sense of accomplishment. You've survived your injury and progressed in mobility, self-care, and daily living skills. While you may be more stable medically and emotionally, much physical and psychological work lies ahead. Coping with changes in self-image and identity, finding meaning in your injury, and discovering a purpose for recovery are challenges that we explore in the following chapter.

As Jim reached the midpoint of his rehabilitation, he remained hopeful for recovery but still felt lost and confused. He had found a friend who shared his feelings and eased his loneliness, but his relationship with his wife was strained. He agonized over when and how to discuss his sexual dysfunction and fear of infertility. His self-image and identity were up for grabs. He knew he wasn't the old macho worker he'd been before the accident, but he wasn't sure who the "new" Jim was or could become. While throwing himself wholeheartedly into the "good patient" role, Jim knew he wouldn't be a patient forever. He could already see his discharge date looming on the horizon.

Jim wondered how he would make sense of his injury, find a new role, and live as a different person outside the hospital. His marriage, his relationship with his family, and his career and goals would all be changed in some ways by his disability. The challenge of reshaping the future seemed daunting, and he knew that he'd have to travel a different road now. The next step in his journey would require a different road map. And despite his fear, Jim was ready to read it.

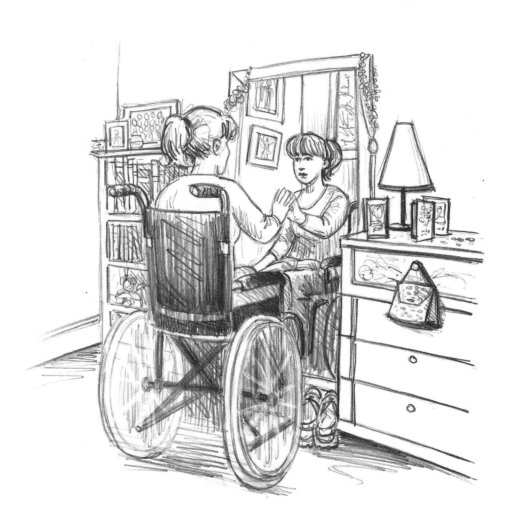

3

Reading the Map
Pathways to Adjustment

Vanessa worked as a waitress while attending community college part-time. Her family was financially comfortable but not wealthy; Vanessa had always known she would have to make her own way in the world and support herself after high school. She was an attractive, hard-working young woman with a good sense of humor. She had many friends and enjoyed going out to bars and parties, and liked to take boating trips near her bayside town. Although she had dated in high school, Vanessa had not had a serious romance. She hoped to get married and have a family, but not until she had finished college and found the "right" man.

Vanessa prided herself on her independence, her loyalty to her family (she lived in an apartment with her sister and visited her parents and grandparents often), and her physical fitness (she regularly went bike riding and swimming and could handle a small sailboat). Her career goals were still somewhat hazy. She enjoyed her business classes and thought about going into accounting or possibly law, then building a business or practice in her small hometown.

On a beautiful sunny day in the summer she turned twenty-one, Vanessa was out on the bay in a cabin cruiser owned by the father of a friend. A group of friends had planned the outing: a picnic, some beer, and dance music on the boat. Sometime after lunch, Vanessa became aware that several of the young men had had too many beers and were becoming reckless. The man steering the boat was going much too fast and swerving dangerously close to the shore-line. Most of the group was caught up in merrymaking, many below deck, and didn't seem to notice the danger.

Vanessa called out to the man at the helm to slow down, but he didn't respond. She started to walk up the deck to confront him when, suddenly, the boat careened into a piling on the shore. The back of the boat jerked up and Vanessa was bounced up into the air. She landed hard on her back on the deck and felt a jolt of pain. Minutes later a friend tried to help her up, but Vanessa could not stand up.

Vanessa had sustained a spinal fracture that required fusion surgery and resulted in incomplete paraplegia. After two months in a rehabilitation hospital, she could walk with crutches for moderate distances. Although she was building strength and endurance, uneven muscle strength gave her a gait that, though functional, was clearly abnormal. She managed her bowel and bladder care. She had no "accidents" (incontinence) and had mastered the use of catheterization kits that could be stored in her purse or pocket. Her doctors expected her to get stronger and more proficient with the crutches, and even to progress to the use of canes. But they thought it unlikely that Vanessa would ever walk without an assistive device.

Vanessa's humor, independent spirit, and supportive family helped her through her initial recovery and the emotional roller coaster of early rehabilitation. Initially she had been very angry about the accident—at herself for misjudging her friends and at the driver of the boat for his recklessness. She had been sad about her injuries, though not clinically depressed. She knew that waitressing and most sports would no longer be possible, but she was eager to get on with college and hoped to find an office job. After talking to her physical therapist about sports, she found that swimming and riding a stationary bike were still possible. She would be able to get in and out of her apartment without difficulty and drive a car with hand controls. Overall, her recovery went more smoothly than she could have imagined that first day in the ER.

Yet as Vanessa's discharge date approached, she became increasingly anxious about facing the world. A casual comment from a friend—"I'm sure you'll get rid of the crutches if you keep working at it"—set off an explosion of questions and concerns. Vanessa worried about her appearance and acceptability to others. As she stood before the mirror, she wasn't sure she looked the same as before the accident. Did the crutches make her ugly? Was her unusual gait "gimpy" and repulsive? Was she working hard enough for recovery, or was she wimping out? Would her friends want to be seen with her at parties? Had she changed inside because of the accident? Was she the same person as before?

She had just started to feel good about her recovery, but now the road ahead looked very scary. For the first time, Vanessa asked herself if she could manage life, especially her social life, with her disability. She knew it was not enough to be physically independent. She would have to confront her changed appearance, self-image, and identity in order to reenter the world of her peers.

After a spinal cord injury, a person's concern with appearance can be triggered by a friend's remark, as it was for Vanessa, but more often it arises spontaneously early in rehabilitation or soon after going home and resuming social activities. A variety of visible changes can accompany a spinal cord injury, and these changes can affect one's self-image and identity. And, like all people with disabilities, individuals with spinal cord injury may encounter mixed reactions to their appearance.

HOW DO I SEE MYSELF?

Appearance and Self-Image

Following spinal cord injury, the most likely physical change that is readily visible to others is in the way you move. Our image of ourselves, as well as other people's perception of us, is shaped not only by facial features and physique but by expressions, gestures, and characteristic patterns of body movement. "The way you wear your hat, the way you sip your tea . . . they can't take that away from me"—these old song lyrics express just how much our image of others, and even what we love or cherish about them, is related to movement. These changes in the capacity for movement or in the way of moving after the injury may affect not only how you appear to others but how you see yourself.

In some cases, when injuries occur high in the cervical spine, all movement below the neck is lost. Although facial expressions, voice quality, and unique speech patterns are preserved, people with high-level tetraplegia lose their characteristic hand gestures, body movements, and defining grace or clumsiness. They may feel that their head or mind is disconnected from their body, or feel trapped in their body, wanting to move but unable to do so. Or they may see their body as a burden to be dragged around. In cases like Vanessa's or Jim's (whose story we told in Chapter 2), mobility may be largely restored, but uneven or awkward gait patterns look different from normal walking and draw attention to one's altered function. In other cases, spasms can lead to uncontrolled shaking or jerking of the arms and legs, another highly visible alteration of normal movement.

Another physical change accompanying many spinal cord injuries is muscular atrophy. When muscles are not used, muscle mass decreases, resulting in the skinny appearance of normally large muscles such as the quadriceps (the front of the thigh). Weakened abdominal muscles can result in a flabby appearance even in a thin person. Contracted or flaccid muscles can create gnarly hands, lopsided trunks, or limp, lifeless-looking limbs. (See Chapter 8 for information on therapies to help maintain muscle mass after spinal cord injury.)

The impact of these physical changes on overall appearance, as well as the difficulty of integrating them into one's self-image, is compounded by the presence of "appendages," the many assistive devices needed for living with a spinal cord injury. Braces, wheelchairs, crutches or canes, ventilators, and other adaptive devices are visible, tangible signs of disability or differentness. On the other hand, these assistive devices are essential to the injured person's process of reintegration because they allow more varied motor activities (braces, crutches, or wheelchair) or self-care and feeding (adaptive splints or utensils). As their benefits become increasingly apparent and begin to outweigh concerns about appearance, these devices often become completely incorporated into one's self-image, inseparable from one's identity.

Body Image and Sensation

Body image refers to the psychological experience of the body. This includes feelings and attitudes about one's body, its parts, and its functions, as well as awareness of bodily boundaries (what's inside and outside the body), where the body is located in space, and the relationship of the body to the environment. Body image is a part of overall self-image, and this may be disrupted or altered by the effects of spinal cord injury on sensation.

In complete spinal cord injuries, sensory as well as motor function is lost below the level of the injury. In incomplete injuries, partial loss of sensation is common. So accompanying the changes in how the body *looks* are dramatic changes in how the body *feels*. These changes run the gamut from complete loss of all bodily sensation below the level of the injury, to diminished sensation for touch, temperature, pain, or position, to distorted or "phantom" sensations of pain, tingling, or position (that is, having the sensation that part of your body is in a position other than the one it's actually in).

If you have diminished or distorted sensation, you have to rely on visual cues and memory to maintain a cohesive body image. Visual feedback can be essential for incorporating changes in the way your body functions. You may need to look at your leg to know whether it is properly placed on the bed or chair. Similarly, if you have a visibly altered gait or use a wheelchair, others will respond to you on the basis of these visual cues. Perhaps in part to counter these cues (still generally perceived as negative), people with spinal cord injuries often pay more attention to their personal appearance and to looking as attractive as possible than they did before the injury. This creates visual and sensory feedback that helps restore an accurate body image, and it focuses positive attention on oneself, further improving self-esteem and promoting social encounters.

Loss of tactile (touch) and kinesthetic (movement) sensation has obvious practical implications, too. Without normal pain and pressure sensations, you are more vulnerable to accidental injuries such as burns and to pressure sores (decubitus ulcers) on your skin (see Chapter 1). Instead of relying on pain sensation to tell you when your body is threatened, you need to anticipate your body's needs. For example, doing pressure releases on a schedule will prevent pressure sores, and testing (or asking someone else to test) the temperature of water, cookware, and so forth will protect you from burns on body parts that can't feel heat or pain. You may need to examine your skin for signs of accidental bruising, cuts, infection, and so on. Similarly, if you cannot feel pressure in your bladder or bowel, you must schedule regular catheterization and a bowel program to avoid bladder infections or bowel impaction.

Diminished or absent pelvic and genital sensation, in addition to its effects on sexual function, can play havoc with body image and sense of self. While it is only one part of total sexuality, genital sensation is, for most adults, an important part of feeling feminine or masculine. Until you have had the opportunity to explore other aspects of sexuality or sexual experience and to discover other erogenous zones, the loss of genital sensation may be disorienting. Your sense of self as a sexual being may seem to be irreparably damaged.

The extent of permanent changes in mobility, appearance, and sensation after spinal cord injury varies widely, depending on the level of injury and degree of recovery. These changes inevitably have some effect on self-perception, body image, and self-image, but their effect on overall psychological adjustment is not necessarily devastating. The extent of the impact often depends more on attitudes, social context, and the psychological meaning of particular changes than on the extent of the actual alterations in mobility and sensation.

Jim's sensation was largely intact after his injury, and he could walk efficiently with a single cane. But because the physical condition of his body had been a major source of his self-esteem, and because he viewed acceptance of the cane as wimping out or giving up on himself, his changed appearance had a negative effect on his self-perception for many months after injury.

The situation for Melinda was somewhat different. Melinda was a young woman with tetraplegia resulting from spinal injury in a car accident. She had major sensory loss below the level of her injury. Melinda had grown up with a sister who had cerebral palsy, and she had learned at a young age that physical appearance does not reflect a person's true abilities or character. Although saddened by her lost abilities, Melinda did not feel "less than" other people because of her injury. She played up her positive attributes and continued to see herself as attractive and capable.

Image and Identity

As the inpatient rehabilitation stay draws to a close, or perhaps in the period just after leaving the hospital, the overall changes in your image may lead to questions about personality and identity. How can you incorporate new self-perceptions, images, and feelings into the sense of yourself as a unique person? Will your past personality and identity endure, or will this experience change who you are?

For many people, psychological adjustment involves two seemingly contradictory processes: on the one hand, developing an identity that includes having a spinal cord injury, and on the other, separating the physical consequences of injury from one's true, or core, self. Put another way, adjustment requires making a distinction between the losses associated with the injury and the positive aspects of your personality. In finding a way to "repackage" yourself to incorporate both limitations and strengths, you may also discover some unexpected, positive consequences of the changes brought about by your injury.

The end of inpatient rehabilitation signals the resumption of "real life." The future must be faced. Like Vanessa, you may wonder who you are now and who you may become. At first your identity may seem to be in limbo, and you may feel anxious and unsure about how your identity will change. You may need to focus for a time on losses, either by grieving or by simply acknowledging them. By this point it's probably clear, at least on an intellectual level, that some functions, sensations, or images are permanently lost or changed.

Some people find it helpful to cement the reality of these changes with some sort of practical or ritual action. The sale of a previously prized bicycle that you'll never ride again, or the move from your "dream house" that has three unmanageable flights of stairs, can become metaphors for saying goodbye to lost abilities. Well-meaning friends or family may urge you to hold on to these possessions longer, "just in case." But selling the bike or making the move can be both an acknowledgment and a letting go of loss. This type of action can help you move on to new and different activities, to forge a new image based on what you *can* do rather than what you *can't*. Putting your energy into discovering, reviving, or developing your individual strengths and interests will help you develop a new identity, a healthy sense of self-worth and self-esteem, and an attitude of self-acceptance.

In Chapter 2 we discussed the concept of stigma, the process by which society excludes, invalidates, and suppresses people with disabilities. Early in your recovery, you may see the changes in yourself as invalidating, unacceptable, or repulsive—you may, in effect, stigmatize yourself. Your early social encounters may reveal social strain, physical distance, intrusiveness, or outright prejudice. Physical and social barriers will loom large in your adjustment to living with a disability. You may begin to feel that you're on the outside looking in; you've become one of "them."

You may be shocked to realize that by virtue of your injury, you've joined a minority group. Like any marginalized group in society, people with spinal cord injuries are often denied access to many avenues of mainstream life, including acceptance in social and personal relationships. Even your own family members may initially look at you as alien. Their emotional acceptance may not come as quickly or completely as you'd like.

Many people find it helpful, particularly in the early stages of adaptation, to associate with other people who have similar injuries. The positive side of minority or "out-group" status is joining a new group of peers with whom you can identify and from whom you'll get support and acceptance. Identifying yourself as part of a group with unique characteristics, needs, and accomplishments can become a source of pride and strength. However, not all people with disabilities find this identification necessary, and many discover other ways of viewing themselves that are equally helpful.

The growing disability rights movement generally subscribes to a minority group model for understanding the life experiences of people with disabilities. According to this model, the social and environmental barriers to integration in society have a greater impact on adjustment and successful living than do an individual's psychological or medical factors. While disability per se reflects the functional difficulties the person has because of a medical condition, handicap (disadvantages experienced as a result of a disability) results from the interaction between a person and the environment. The crucial point is that the attitudes of other people and the physical/environmental barriers to mobility are problems separate from the physical or mental adjustment of the person with a disability. This perspective can be psychologically liberating. It makes clear that your capacity for emotional or psychological strength is not the only relevant factor in adjustment. This eases the pressure you may have put on yourself and helps you direct more of your energy to solving the problems caused by external obstacles, whether physical, attitudinal, or economic.

The development of a peer group identity is particularly important for adolescents and young adults. As teenagers struggle to differentiate themselves from parents and adult authorities, to gain self-sufficiency, and to "find" themselves, identifying with and fitting in with a peer group is of paramount concern. Defining oneself as "different" (from adults) paradoxically requires a definition as "same" (as peers). Teenagers of every generation develop styles of clothing, music, and language that distinguish them from adults—and then demand from other teens a strict adherence to these new group norms!

While teenagers may struggle at times with the pressure of having to fit in, they nevertheless gain a great deal of support and self-esteem from identifying with their peer group. Teenagers with spinal cord injury often can develop a positive self-image by interacting with other teenagers with disabilities. A young adult with spinal cord injury can mentor a teenager to help him or her cope with changes in appearance, self-image, and identity. Some hospitals have special support or therapy groups for younger adults and teenagers with spinal cord injuries, or they may be able to arrange peer counseling for a teenager who is getting ready to leave the hospital. After going home, teens can get acquainted with peers who also have spinal cord injuries—for example, by becoming involved in wheelchair athletics or camping trips for teenagers with disabilities. Some of these groups and activities are included in the Resources section at the end of this book.

Part of the shift in group identity after spinal cord injury, for teens and adults alike, occurs through the adoption of new language and new labels. You and other patients, perhaps without thinking about it, may have begun referring to yourselves as "paras" or "quads." Vanessa found herself adopting the medical lingo and introducing herself to new hospital interns as "a T12." Some people with spinal cord injury refer to themselves as "crips" or "gimps," turning these previously stigmatizing labels into expressions of unique identity and pride, in much the same way that some gay people use "queer" or teens use "grungy" and "raunchy" as positive descriptors. You may also find yourself adopting a new slang vocabulary for the equipment that is so much a part of your life—vents, chairs, caths, TEDs, and a host of other medical abbreviations and acronyms that describe your injury and its functional consequences. Finally, you may discover from your new "in group" a language that describes non-disabled people in "out-group" terms, such as "walkies" or "a.b.'s" (able-bodied). These shifts in language are all part of the process of differentiating oneself and integrating the new variables of disability and acquired minority status into one's personal identity.

Along with these changes in self-labeling or self-identification may come changes in your perception of specific aspects or consequences of your disability. In the initial period after spinal cord injury, especially if the injury was traumatic and the disability sudden, changes in bodily appearance, function, and mobility are typically seen as symptoms of illness, needing to be cured or fixed. Like a broken arm or a stomach virus, the initial effects of spinal cord injury are often viewed as alien, not part of oneself, temporary, and erasable. Indeed, in many cases, partial recovery of function does occur over time and some symptoms disappear totally. But for most people with spinal cord injury, some degree of disability is permanent, and many patients leave the rehabilitation hospital with significant impairments.

As you become increasingly aware that some impairments or limitations may not be fixable, you may find it harder to maintain a separation between your "real" or "normal" self and your disability. The psychological challenge at this point is to make the transition from seeing the disability as alien, not the "real me," something to be overcome, to seeing the disability as "part of me," an aspect or characteristic of the self, something that does not *have* to be eradicated.

Alicia, a young woman with tetraplegia since the age of fifteen, described the reaction when she and her boyfriend announced their engagement. Her future mother-in-law said, "We like *you,* but we don't like your circumstances." Alicia replied, *"I am* the circumstances." As shown by her simple but eloquent reply, she had incorporated spinal cord injury into her personal identity. In effect she was saying, "If you like *me,* then like my disability—because it's part of me and I'm part of it." This process appears to be one of incorporating or integrating the disability as a characteristic of oneself, while simultaneously relinquishing the perception of the disability as a symptom or illness. Put another way, it is the transition from being a patient (sick, damaged, broken, dependent) to being a person (with the variety of attributes, strengths, and weaknesses that all humans have).

WHO AM I NOW?

A week before she was discharged, Vanessa's anxiety spurred her into action. She asked her best friend to visit for an "image consultation," and together they planned Vanessa's makeover. She had her hair styled and her nails done in the hospital beauty parlor. She agonized with her physical therapist about color choices for her crutches, eventually choosing teal blue. She gave her friend a shopping list: brand-name athletic shoes, stretch jeans, a long skirt, some V-neck tops. She was ready to ditch the baggy sweats that had been her hospital uniform.

That night, after showering, Vanessa stood naked before the bathroom mirror—the first time she'd really looked at herself since the injury. She was surprised to see that despite the changes in her mobility and sensation, her figure was barely changed and still attractive. The physical therapy and crutch-walking had made her upper arms more muscular, and she approved of their sculpted appearance. Her legs were thinner than before, not as toned, but the changes were subtle. She considered the crutches held against her naked skin. They didn't look too bad—as long as she was standing still. Though overall she felt more confident, Vanessa still worried how her altered mobility would affect her life outside the hospital.

Vanessa returned to her apartment just before Thanksgiving. Her sister surprised her with a welcome home party attended by good friends and family members. Vanessa spent Thanksgiving weekend at her parents' home surrounded by relatives. Everyone expressed delight at her progress and encouraged her to "keep working on it." During the holiday season, she busied herself with shopping and seeing girlfriends. She went to physical therapy several times a week, working to increase her strength and improve her gait. She returned to the health club where she'd worked out before the injury, this time with a personal trainer to help her strengthen and tone her body. She registered for classes at the community college, to begin in February, and she started looking for a part-time job.

Eventually, Vanessa started going out with groups of friends, and before she knew it, she had a date. She was very excited, but also nervous about how to present her disability. In group settings she had already "passed" as able-bodied by telling people that she'd hurt her leg in an accident, implying that she'd be better soon. At other times she'd answered questions about her injury by telling the whole story from the boat trip to the ER to the details of her treatment. To her disappointment, this seemed to overwhelm and alienate people rather than create the intimacy she'd hoped for.

When the question did, inevitably, come up, Vanessa told her date what she'd been rehearsing—that she'd hurt her back in a boating accident and had some neurological damage that made it hard to walk. She thought this was an *honest answer, but not overly detailed or too personal. And it allowed her to be matter of fact about the disability rather than making it the central focus. Suddenly Vanessa felt weary of constantly thinking about physical therapy and her weakened legs. She wanted to focus on her strengths again—her humor, independence, and outgoing nature. The date became a symbolic turning point: she decided to be herself, not a "para," first. She surprised herself with her ability to kid around, laugh, and talk about her interests and ideas. She had a wonderful time.*

As your recovery progresses, you are likely to experience a variety of self-identifications, self-presentations, and self-labels. As people, with or without disability, mature and enter new stages of personal or professional development, they shed some aspects of their identity and take on others. Your "adjustment" to disability is an ongoing process that begins in the hospital and continues as new relationships, environments, and activities pose challenges to your physical and emotional coping skills. Self-acceptance depends not only on making peace with the physical limitations of having a spinal cord injury, but also on developing and expressing your intellect, emotions, creativity, and personality. By maintaining or redefining your unique sense of meaning and purpose, you will be better able to live successfully and keep your disability in perspective.

WHAT DOES MY INJURY MEAN?

A spinal cord injury is almost always a life-changing event, a critical moment that forever divides a person's history into "before" and "after." The injury often results from disease or random accident, though it may be the consequence of violence, unusual risk-taking, or self-destructive behavior. Coming to terms with the reason (or lack of reason) for the injury can be an important part of emotional recovery. Not everyone finds it necessary or productive to grapple with the questions, "Why *me?* What is the meaning of the injury for *my* life?" But many people find that their answers to these questions shape their outlook on the future and help them live productively and meaningfully after the injury.

People make sense of their experience of spinal cord injury in many ways. Three common pathways to understanding are the rational (cognitive), the emotional, and the spiritual. Many people tend to zero in on one of these aspects, while others draw insights from all three. Each path provides ways of interpreting the experience that can lead to guilt, bitterness, cynicism, and despair, but also to opportunities for personal growth and change, hopefulness, spiritual renewal, and joy.

Each person finds an individual path to adjustment. You may find your path through work, relationships, creativity, or simply "tincture of time" and gradual resumption of life's daily tasks and rhythms. Our discussion of rational, emotional, and spiritual aspects of understanding spinal cord injury is offered simply as a framework to help guide your exploration. In no way is it meant to limit or define your individual experience.

Rational Paths to Recovery

Some might say that the only rational understanding of an accidental spinal cord injury is that it is irrational! There is no logical reason why a particular car is rear-ended on a particular day with a particular person inside. Much of life is serendipitous, chaotic, or random. Yet the human proclivity for imposing sense or order sometimes helps us cope with unexpected and disruptive life events.

Psychologists have studied the impact of attribution of responsibility on psychosocial adjustment following spinal cord injury. This dimension of cognitive processing (intellectual understanding through reasoning) of the injury refers to whether the injured person believes he or she was or was not responsible for causing the injury. One study found that patients who believed they were responsible for the injury were not as well adjusted emotionally during inpatient rehabilitation as those who believed they were not responsible. The degree of adjustment was not related to the medical staff's ratings of patients as either responsible or not responsible, even though medical professionals are presumably more objective than patients. This suggests that a belief that one caused the injury is more important in adjustment than are the objective facts of situation.

The same study found that by one year after injury, many people had changed their attribution of responsibility for the injury, and the researchers no longer saw any difference in adjustment between the groups with different beliefs. This suggests that as recovery progresses and the injured person moves out of the hospital environment, other factors become more important in overall adjustment than how responsibility is attributed. However, for those in the early phase of rehabilitation, accepting random events at face value, rather than imposing personal responsibility, may be psychologically helpful. If you are able to see your injury as neither victimization nor self-induced but simply a random event, you may be better able to put your energy into living with your injury and be less preoccupied with anger or guilt.

Viewing an accidental injury as a chance or random event may help you avoid irrational self-blame, guilt, or unresolvable anger. Yet the perception that, in general, you can control events in your life may be beneficial to your recovery. If you see your own behavior as a factor contributing to your *injury* (as it sometimes is—driving while drunk or participating in a risky sport without proper safety equipment, for example), you may also believe that your behavior can influence your *recovery*.

A related concept in psychology is locus of control, which refers to the extent to which an individual believes that changes in events and in the environment (good or bad outcomes, rewards or punishments) are either internally (self) or externally (other or chance) controlled. "Internals," believing their behavior and actions can affect their life circumstances, tend to be more active in their approach to problematic situations. "Externals," believing that life events are not under their control but brought about by fate, luck, or powerful external forces, are more passive and less likely to spend energy on problem-solving.

Again, the critical issue is one of cognition. What matters is not the objective fact of having control but the belief or expectation that your behavior can affect the outcome of events. For example, consider a woman with tetraplegia who is an "internal." She has a high degree of expectancy of control and can use her mental and emotional energies to make her life more satisfying. Now consider a woman with paraplegia with far fewer physical limitations and, viewed objectively, more control over her immediate environment who is an "external." She is passive and emotionally helpless, assuming that any effort will have little effect on circumstances that are beyond her control.

Rehabilitation, in the broadest sense, combines physical, emotional, cognitive, and spiritual changes. But hospital rehabilitation is primarily a learning process. Alterations or limitations in one's ability to perform once-mastered tasks—dressing, walking, eating, socializing—require the learning of new ways. Adopting a student's approach to rehabilitation can help you view each "problem" or "loss" as a mystery to be worked out or a blank page to be filled with your own imagination and ingenuity. Observing, trying new approaches, and getting positive results is a rewarding process. Not only does it keep you from dwelling on pain or loss, but it focuses your attention on the creative process of rebuilding your life.

Journalist John Hockenberry's description of his own encounter with rehabilitation emphasizes the intellectual challenge of problem-solving: "my body now presented an intriguing puzzle of great depth and texture . . . The future seemed like an adventure on some frontier of physical possibilities. Each problem—getting up, rolling over, balancing in a chair, getting from here to there—needed a new solution. I was physically an infant endowed with the mind of an adult . . . Solving each problem offered a personal authorship to experience that had never before seemed possible."

The benefits of an individualized problem-solving model in rehabilitation have been described by physiatrists (specialists in physical medicine and rehabilitation). Through independent thinking, self-directed behavior, and experimentation, persons with spinal cord injury can regain a healthy sense of personal effectiveness and develop solutions that are tailor-made to their environment, activity preferences, and other individual needs.

A rational approach to recovery shifts your focus away from the question of "Why?" toward the issue of "How?" It helps you to limit your handicaps by finding ways of changing the environment or making use of devices that compensate for your impairments. When you ask yourself, first, "What do I want/need to do?" and then, "How can I get it done?" you'll find practical solutions specific to your situation. Setting goals and inventing or discovering ways to meet them gives a sense of direction, purpose, and personal effectiveness. The ends become more important than the different means by which you achieve them. "Please don't say that I'm . . . 'confined to a wheelchair,'" says Ralf Hotchkiss, a designer of wheelchairs who has paraplegia. "I've been liberated by a wheelchair." This sentiment applies equally well to other assistive devices, to personal care assistants, to structural or organizational modifications at your workplace, and so on. As you gain a rational understanding of your spinal cord injury, meaning and purpose will emerge: you discover what works for you, what makes you more functional, and what lets you reach your goals.

Emotional Paths to Recovery

One way of coming to grips with the "reason" for a spinal cord injury is to search for the emotional meaning of the injury. Emotional pathways to understanding are, by definition, unique to your life. The psychological impact and meaning of the injury depend on your individual characteristics and your age and stage of life. As your emotional landscape changes over time, so will your insights into the emotional meaning of your disability. Given the uniqueness of emotional experience, the emotional impact and meaning of spinal cord injury have countless personal nuances. However, several processes or tasks are common in people grappling with the emotional meaning of an injury: life review, development of emotional priorities, and resolution of past internal and interpersonal conflicts. As is evident in the examples that follow, these three tasks often occur simultaneously or overlap.

Life Review and Emotional Priorities

Life review is a process of examining our life experience, taking stock of where we've been, examining what is happening to us now, and deciding where we might set our sights for the future. This process often happens almost automatically at certain milestones, such as a fortieth or fiftieth birthday, marriage, retirement, or becoming a parent or grandparent. We naturally try to give meaning to these events, to understand their emotional impact within the context of our own experience. This process is also useful in coping with the emotional impact of a spinal cord injury.

In developing our emotional priorities, we sort out the relationships, activities, and values that are most important to our emotional well-being and disengage ourselves from those that are less important. We all go through this process from time to time, and it can be particularly helpful when a change in life circumstances limits our energies or creates new demands.

In Chapter 2 we talked about the variety of strong emotions possible soon after spinal cord injury—anger, sadness, frustration, and isolation, all common, normal reactions. Yet *your* particular combination of feelings is unique and depends in large part on the kind of person you have been and the experiences you had before your injury. You are still the same person after a spinal cord injury; your basic personality is not likely to change. But the injury is likely to slow you down, at least for a while. Yet at the same time it can act as a catalyst, stimulating you to review and reexamine your experiences, values, and accomplishments. This in turn can lead to important changes in your approach to life, to a new appreciation for yourself and an experience of more positive emotions.

Peter developed paraplegia in his sixties as a result of a spinal hemorrhage. He was semi-retired from his job in real estate sales, but he still served as choirmaster for his church. A lengthy hospitalization, recovery from surgery, and inpatient rehabilitation gave him plenty of time to examine his life, a process he continued after going home. As he took stock of his life, Peter felt a growing sense of pride in his past accomplishments. He had a successful career, a stable marriage, and two grown children with good jobs and families of their own. And he had a passion for singing that had been nurtured and expressed through years of leading a choir.

Although he was initially frustrated and anxious about his disability, Peter found emotional strength in assessing his life and distilling its essence—singing. On a leave from the rehabilitation hospital, he went back to his church and after that, he recalls, "Getting depressed was not an option. I had to get back to the singing." Peter realized how much the people in his choir and his church community cared for him and depended on his leadership. He felt an increased sense of purpose and a renewed commitment to giving his time and energies to others. At the same time, he decided to quit his real estate job because it no longer seemed important to him or to reflect his values. His emotional priorities had changed.

As a result of his life review and reassessment of emotional priorities, Peter gave more energy to the activities and relationships that were truly meaningful to him and set aside those that were not. He put his disability into perspective as a practical obstacle he could generally get around with some ingenuity and adaptation. The spinal cord injury was the worst thing that had ever happened to him, but in looking to the future he felt more relaxed because he was "on the other side of tragedy." Although Peter's injury was not something he would have wished for, it became the impetus for developing his unique talents, broadening his commitment to others, and learning to set aside the things he found unfulfilling.

Resolution of Emotional Conflicts

The crisis of dependency created by a spinal cord injury can lead to emotional regression and the resurgence of old internal and interpersonal conflicts. A young adult who has to return to the family home after a spinal cord injury may reexperience conflicts with parents that were not fully resolved during adolescence. An older person, previously self-sufficient but requiring a period of nursing home care after injury, may regress to a state of childlike emotional dependence or may reexperience grief over previous losses never fully mourned. A middle-aged person may find that changes in marital roles following disability revive old control issues with a spouse and internal conflicts about career choices and self-esteem.

Like any crisis, spinal cord injury may cause psychological conflicts and dysfunctions to worsen, but it may also provide an opportunity to rework past conflicts and develop more mature and satisfying solutions.

David was forty years old. He lived with Myra, his fiancée, had a job that he loved, and was looking forward to buying a new home before the wedding. One winter morning as he was working in the garage, part of the roof gave way under the weight of recent heavy snow and David's spine was crushed. The damage caused paraplegia. David was strong and energetic and had a positive outlook. He left the rehabilitation center, having made substantial progress. But he couldn't drive, and there were many household tasks that he couldn't yet handle without help. While he was recuperating at home and attending outpatient physical therapy several times a week, Myra had to continue working full-time. David's sisters took over the jobs of transporting him to therapy and doctors' appointments, helping with his personal care, and doing chores around the house.

Myra was thrown into conflict. She wanted the increased intimacy of caring for David, yet could not give up her work commitments at a time when David was not bringing in a paycheck. She thought he'd be "all hers" in the evening, but more often than not his sisters were still at the house when she got home.

Myra felt useless and displaced, and she began to feel jealous and resentful of the sisters' involvement with David. She thought they were taking over and that she was getting pushed aside.

David was the only son in a family of three children. His mother and sisters had always doted on him and been overly protective. He had responded by trying to please them, not just by living up to their expectations for success but by returning their affection and allowing himself to be their "pet." Even before his injury, David's engagement to Myra had disrupted the balance in his relationship with his sisters, creating a triangle in which David often felt pulled in several directions by conflicting loyalties.

On one level, David wished he could lean more on Myra, but he was afraid of seeming weak or unmanly. At the same time, his increased vulnerability made him fearful of rocking the boat with his sisters, whose help was essential to his recovery. He rationalized his increased dependence on his sisters as a way of protecting Myra from overwork. It was hard for him to empathize with Myra's emotional needs and to see that his attempts to be independent of her were creating more distance between them. He felt helpless in the face of the power struggle developing between Myra and his sisters. Unable to face his own fears, David could not take an active role in resolving this family conflict. Eventually, he and Myra separated, and David entered a period of intense dependency on his sisters that was reminiscent of childhood.

David was in outpatient physical therapy for eight months, during which he learned to become completely self-sufficient. As his physical dependence on his sisters lessened, he was finally able to risk hurting their feelings or making them angry by pulling away emotionally. He and Myra had kept in touch during their separation and, after four months, they got back together. David set better limits with his family and committed more of his emotional energy to his relationship with Myra. Myra sought professional counseling to cope with her anxiety about David's injury and soon felt stronger emotionally and more sure of her commitment to him. David began to challenge the overprotectiveness of his family, and he surprised them with his new mobility skills and the ease with which he returned to work.

David's injury had pushed him to resolve both internal and relationship conflicts in a way that ultimately led to a better balance in his emotional life. A year and a half after his spinal cord injury, he had an unrelated, serious medical problem that required surgery. His sisters were very upset. He remembers them saying, "Here we go again," and expecting him to be more distressed and depen-

dent. But David was able to keep his cool and make some difficult choices among various treatment options. This time, no struggle for control of David's fate was necessary—he took charge of his own care. Now he feels comfortable making decisions for himself, taking reasonable risks, and seeking Myra's emotional support without suffering a loss of self-esteem.

Spiritual Paths to Recovery

Spirituality is an important aspect of living for many people. Organized religious rituals and prayers, self-help groups that appeal to a higher power, and individual experiences of connection with a supernatural entity, life force, or collective consciousness—all are pathways for spiritual experience.

Spirituality refers to the experience of connection with a force or spirit that gives meaning to all of life's events, including the "bad" ones. Carolyn Vash, psychologist and author of *Personality and Adversity,* believes that all adversity, including spinal cord injury, has intrinsic spiritual significance—the "nonverbal universe" is telling you something. The search for meaning, purpose, and connection is a psycho-spiritual journey that is stimulated by the struggle to cope with dramatically altered and difficult life circumstances:

> Adversity serves as a catalyst to psycho-spiritual growth. Much to our dismay, it jars us from comfortable complacency and makes life scary enough, enraging enough, or depressing enough to either kill us or get our attention. Once we pay attention to the crude communication efforts of a nonverbal universe to tell us that there is more here than meets the eye, or that we could be moving in a more fruitful direction, the battle is half won. The other half, however, can occupy the remainder of our lives . . . It is an inner war, the struggle between the spiritually lazy or scared or "stuck" aspects of our personalities against aspects of our souls that long to grow, evolve, understand, love and rejoice.

People's spiritual orientation and experience are likely to influence their early understanding of spinal cord injury. Disability is sometimes viewed as a punishment for transgression or a divine retribution for sin, regardless of the circumstances of the injury. This belief may stem from interpretations of biblical references linking disability with moral weakness. It is also reinforced by societal fear and stigma that have more to do with disability as a symbol of emotional losses than with religious conviction. That is, people fear disability not because it is a sign of moral weakness but because it represents their own emotional vulnerability.

Those whose injury is a result of risk-taking behavior may be particularly vulnerable to viewing the disability as penance, blaming themselves not just for the accident but for perceived moral or personal failures leading up to it. This view can lead to shame and self-loathing or to overinvestment in the "sick role." If someone views continued suffering as the only way to assuage guilt feelings or to obtain absolution for sins, then being disabled itself becomes a means for maintaining spiritual equilibrium. People with this view may not allow themselves to make physical or psychological progress.

The outcome may be similar if the injury was the result of street violence or war. In such cases, people may see themselves as heroes or martyrs rather than sinners, yet their suffering may take on religious significance. This can be culturally reinforced by specific political or religious circumstances. Hockenberry, writing about a young Palestinian with a spinal cord injury incurred in the violence of the Intifada, notes that for this young man's "existence as a paraplegic to make sense among his peers he would have to become a martyr." Rather than encouraging this young man's recovery and independence, his peers and family imposed on him the role of religious martyr and symbol of the collective sacrifice of their community. Religious interpretations of disability, as well as religious means for healing, may also be more prevalent when medical and rehabilitation resources are scarce, as was the case for the Palestinian youth. His family's "idea of rehabilitation was to pray for their child to walk again some day." This was consistent with their religious beliefs but reinforced by a lack of medical resources and ignorance about the possibilities of rehabilitation.

Although some religious teachings emphasize punishment for transgression, others stress tolerance for differences and imperfections, forgiveness, and compassion for oneself and others. Even if believing an injury was caused by God because of "bad" behavior, an injured person can see this as an opportunity to change, perhaps by getting more in touch with the sanctity of life and reconnecting with his or her own capacity for goodness. Religious rituals for spiritual cleansing, admission of mistakes, atonement, and repentance (such as the Catholic practice of confession or the Jewish practice of ritual bathing) may help someone to move from guilt or self-recrimination to feelings of self-worth and constructive engagement with the community.

Some religious traditions, such as those of some Native American tribes, meld physical healing with sacred or spiritual rites so that healing and worship experiences are intertwined. Body, mind, and spirit must be in harmony for true wellness to exist. Along with physical rehabilitation, a person must understand the disability or illness in spiritual terms. A process of spiritual change can restore harmony by changing attitudes and responses to the disability, even if the disability itself remains constant.

Writer Hugh Gregory Gallagher expresses a similar notion with the biblical metaphor of Job. The "reality of disability wins . . . and yet somehow . . . the self prevails . . . In the great infinite miracle that is life, pain and suffering is trivial . . . What matters is that I am, and it is enough." This spiritual understanding allows the soul or spirit to live harmoniously inside (to "accept") an imperfect physical body, while transcending its limitations.

Vash points out that the assumption, shared by various religious traditions, that we "summon to ourselves everything that befalls us" or, put another way, that we are responsible for all aspects of our wellness, does not necessarily imply spiritual deficiency or moral transgression as the cause of adversity. "The soul of a saint may be as likely to summon disability as that of a sinner. For example, my disability may have been summoned . . . to expose me to needed life experiences that I could not access in other ways." In this view, the disability has a spiritual reason, not necessarily as punishment but as an opportunity for psychological or spiritual development and change.

A variant of this interpretation sees disability as part of a divine plan: God has chosen an individual to bear adversity (disability) for a particular cosmic purpose. Some people with spinal cord injury have expressed this view in statements such as "It was meant to be," "God works in mysterious ways," or "God did this to me for a reason." Finding the reason becomes a soul search, in which the person can renew or discover a unique sense of purpose or conviction. Sometimes this leads to a special mission to develop one's own potential more fully, to find a way to help other people, or to revitalize connections with family, community, or religious institutions.

Spirituality comes naturally to some people. But even those intimately involved with organized religion need to discover their own path to a personal relationship with the divine. For Peter, the act of singing was a way to connect with God, a means of expressing what Vash has called the "aspects of our souls that long to grow, evolve, understand, love and rejoice." Peter believes that God does not interfere with day-to-day events, and he has never asked what he did wrong to cause the injury. Yet he needed to reconnect with God before he could heal psychologically and spiritually.

Elliott (whose story is in Chapter 6) had rejected organized religion before his injury and continues to be "turned off" by it years afterward. But immediately after his injury, he was angry with God. Unlike Peter, he wondered why God had done this to him. He saw some of the other patients "dive right into religion" after being injured, sometimes with helpful results. For Elliott the process of spiritual reconnection took longer. "When you get older," he says, "you realize that this stuff [injury] just happens. I believe in God, and I have a basic set of beliefs, rules I live by. I try to treat people the way that I'd like to be treated." Though he does not go to church, Elliott now sees himself as a spiritually aware person who has become more connected to God and more accepting and tolerant of other people.

Art, who has incomplete tetraplegia, is, like Elliott, skeptical of religion as an "answer." He rejects the notion of religious "zealots" that faith can cure paralysis. For Art, spirituality entails a belief in the soul and a higher power. His connection with this power has helped forge a strong sense of purpose in his life with spinal cord injury and has inspired his efforts to help other people with similar injuries.

Recent studies of coping and health suggest that spirituality is one of several dimensions of wellness. Some studies have looked at styles of "religious problem-solving," the relationship of prayer to life satisfaction, and the role of spirituality in coping with loss and grief. Greater spirituality may be associated with less depression and better coping soon after spinal cord injury, perhaps because of the connection between faith and hope. Not much research exists on the role of spirituality in long-term adjustment to spinal cord injury, but many personal accounts suggest that, as one dimension of coping, spirituality can be an important strength.

Spinal cord injury clearly presents an opportunity to reexamine your philosophy of life in the aftermath of loss, suffering, and survival. Rediscovering or reinforcing your capacity for spiritual connection is one possible pathway to greater personal fortitude. Some people do not need or desire a spiritual path to recovery, but use other means to cope with their experience.

> *After the success of her first date since the accident, Vanessa became increasingly comfortable with having a disability and a social life. She was more willing to try new things and test the limits of her physical abilities. As time went on and she continued to use crutches, Vanessa told her new friends about the real cause of her disability. Most of them were surprised, because they associated spinal cord injury with total dependence. But rather than rejecting her, many expressed their admiration for her self-sufficiency.*
>
> *Vanessa developed a short "rap" about her disability, which she could use to answer new acquaintances' questions about her use of crutches. She found that, once explained to others, her disability quickly faded into the background and her relationships seemed more relaxed and natural. At the same time, she was more comfortable telling people what she needed in the way of physical accessibility or assistance with particular activities.*
>
> *Vanessa started going to church again with her family. She was uplifted by the support of her pastor and congregation, and she found in praying an outlet for her joy in being alive and a way of expressing her fears and hopes. She found a part-time office job in a friend's insurance business. It wasn't a job she wanted forever, but it was a start. Vanessa was ready to accept the challenges that lay ahead: living independently, developing an intimate relationship, and forging a career.*

In this chapter we've explored several questions that a person with spinal cord injury might ask: How do I see myself? Who am I now? What does it mean to be me? What does my injury mean? Most people with spinal cord injury experience some changes in self-image and self-understanding as they grapple with changed physical abilities. How you experience these changes and how they affect your function in the world is an individual discovery, guided by past experiences and new explorations into your thoughts, feelings, and sense of life's meaning. Many health care providers, social workers, clergy, and support groups are available to help you in this process of discovery and to prepare you for your entry into "life after rehabilitation."

PART II

THE CHALLENGES
OF READJUSTMENT

While you are still in the hospital or rehabilitation center following a spinal cord injury, the world may seem to revolve around your needs. You are in the spotlight. A great deal of concentrated energy is focused on you, your injury, healing that injury as fully as possible, and helping you with rehabilitation. But the time in this medical setting comes to an end. Life goes on.

On your return home, the spotlight expands to include the changing roles and needs of family members. The family begins to balance your needs with its own and may devote less attention to your individual needs. And the responsibility for finding and evaluating the services you need, once taken care of by the hospital or rehabilitation center, shifts to you and your family. While relying on your own resources can be intimidating, it can also be empowering.

In Part II we explore the move from the medical system back into your own world. Chapter 4 looks at the issue of the move home itself, including the adjustment to new family roles, expectations, and contributions. Other matters you may need to deal with include further defining and adjusting to your physical limits, working with personal care attendants, creating new goals or realigning old ones, and improving communication and intimacy skills.

Chapter 5 is addressed to the families of persons with spinal cord injury. We discuss the consequences of the injury for family members, including emotional reactions, relationship stresses, and role changes, as well as the problems and needs of family caregivers.

Sexuality is the focus of Chapter 6. We explore how you might renew your relationship with your old partner or find a new partner; how you can learn about sexual function and dysfunction and the treatments and techniques available to manage problems; and issues of fertility and pregnancy.

Finally, in Chapter 7, we address the basics of independent living with a physical disability: housing and transportation, vocational and economic support, adaptations for work, possible changes in career, and access to education. Beyond all these we examine the need for you to become an advocate for yourself, and we outline how the Americans with Disabilities Act and other legislation legitimize your right to get what you need.

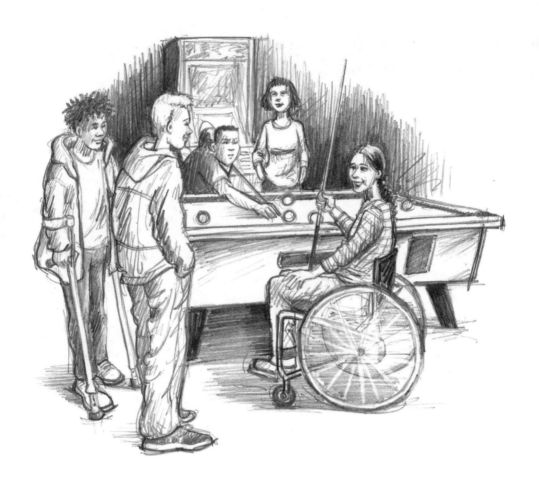

Going Home
Old Territory in a New Light

In 1984, while a sophomore at a prestigious southern university, Joan fell from a third-floor dormitory balcony where she had been sunbathing with her room-mates. Recent heavy rains had softened the earth and she survived the fall, but she had an incomplete C6 spinal cord injury. Joan had tetraplegia. She had no movement below the level of injury but some sensation—for instance, she couldn't feel touch but could sense the deep pain of a pressure sore and she got a "funny sensation" in her head when her catheter was kinked or she had been sitting too long.

Joan spent a month in the hospital, two months in an intermediate care facility, and then about six months in a rehabilitation facility (this length of stay was common in the 1980s). Although she had planned to return to the univer-sity after her discharge, she knew, as the day neared, that she was not at all prepared to go back to school. Furthermore, her roommates were having a dif-ficult time finding a wheelchair-accessible apartment. Joan and her family decided that she would go to her parents' home and return to school the follow-ing September.

Just before Joan's release in February 1985, the rehabilitation center dis-patched a team to evaluate the family home for physical accessibility. Prepar-ing the house for her return was quite simple, says Joan. First she was given the family room on the first floor. It was only one step up from the backyard, and her father built a ramp over the step. The room was just off the kitchen, near the social center of the family. Her father provided privacy for her by installing shut-ters between the rooms. Because Joan preferred bed baths (she didn't like to take showers because of the time involved), a roll-in shower wasn't necessary. The only structural change in the bathroom was installation of a sink under which Joan could push her wheelchair. The rehabilitation center sent two wheelchairs—one electric, the other manual—for her use at home, along with an electric bed and a shower chair in case she should need it. Her father purchased a "very simple" Volkswagen van, the only van on the market at that time that didn't require roof or floor modifications to accommodate the wheelchair. He unbolted a seat and put in a plywood board with bolts to secure Joan's chair. (She now has a new van with all the latest electronic gadgetry, but she has kept the VW van as a backup.)

With home now accessible, Joan made two visits before she left the rehabilitation center for good. She recalls, "It was a funny time. In the rehab center you want out yet it is very secure. Everyone in there is like you. They understand what you're going through. You can laugh and joke. The feeling of leaving that security is quite scary. For me, it was, like, there are all these myths and stereotypes of disability and going back . . . I'm social. Would my old social life still be available to me on the outside? Would people want to have me around? Would they treat me differently? My big anxiety, the most awkward thing, was seeing people the first time and having to deal with what they were going through. It was awkward. People don't know how to handle it, how to help you. They're sad and they're glad you're there." Before going home, Joan found the anticipation nerve-wracking. While Joan was still in the rehabilitation center, her family found a personal care attendant. Although her mother also helped her, Joan realized that her mother felt too much of her daughter's pain. Joan also noticed that she was more likely to "moan and groan" when getting care from her mother. She thought an attendant would have more emotional distance. The attendant came each morning to help Joan with bathing, bowel and bladder care, and personal appearance.

Joan doesn't remember very much about being home that winter, although she does recall finding the following summer boring. Her role in the family hadn't changed, primarily because she was independent and didn't allow it to change. Her parents, once they found out what she could do, expected that of her. They knew she would go back to school and then get a job. "I got grief if I sat in front of the TV; they didn't put up with whining or feeling sorry. After a while, it sucked, yes, but this is it. It's all about choices, you can dwell or get on with it. It's not a fair world. There is always someone worse off or better off than you."

Joan refused to use the electric wheelchair. She found it ugly and she felt "gimpy and disabled" using it. She preferred the cooler, jazzier, manual sports chair and used it for two years before deciding that the electric wheelchair gave her more mobility and control over her life. "When I couldn't get wherever I wanted to, that's when I switched."

Her real adjustment came in September when she began her junior year at the university. "I was very apprehensive about going back to school. If I hadn't told my roommates I was coming back and felt I couldn't back out, I would not have returned. Would they accept me? What if I had a problem? How would I get around? Luckily I had these roommates who adored me. They pushed me to classes and then classmates pushed me to the next class."

In college, a different personal care attendant arrived each weekend. Joan had to talk each new attendant through her routine. Having someone help her go to the bathroom and get dressed was a humiliating experience, and having to teach a new person every week was daunting.

It was hard for her family to see her move out, to take the risk. "But," says Joan, "moving out was the best thing I ever did for my mental health."

The moves from hospital to rehabilitation center and from rehabilitation center to home are major transitions for the person with spinal cord injury. All transitions—all changes—are experienced physically, mentally, emotionally, and spiritually, and the most emotionally laden passage in this case is that to the home front. Although eagerly and joyfully anticipated by the injured person and the family, the return may also be feared or dreaded because of the unknown. What challenges, dilemmas, and problems lie ahead?

As a person with a spinal cord injury, your expectations and concerns may differ from those of your family. Perhaps family members are fearful about the changes in your physical abilities or about your ability to cope emotionally—or perhaps they have few or no concerns, feeling confident that they'll be able to handle whatever develops or find the resources to deal with any problems.

Joan's story demonstrates one family's journey. It illustrates the complicated dynamics and interactions of the injured person, the family, and friends and the multiplicity of needs that have to be addressed in the Big Switch from rehabilitation facility to home or school.

Returning home, in fact, "brings home" the reality of these needs.

Physical needs normally arise first, followed by emotional needs and then social needs. Each issue must be dealt with before you can progress to the next. As one issue is addressed, at least at an elementary level, energy is released to go forward to tackle the next. This pattern of devoting energy to one target then moving on to another is a useful strategy, not only in rehabilitation but in all aspects of your life.

PHYSICAL, EMOTIONAL, AND SOCIAL CHANGES ON THE RETURN HOME

The Physical Return

Those of you who have already made the transition from medical institution to home probably remember many details of this event, from the preparation all the way through the move itself. Like Joan, you may have visited home before you were discharged from the rehabilitation center. Such visits, which are not as possible today due to the health insurance system, allow a gradual shift in gears to the tempo of home life and provide brief insights into how your physical needs and abilities have changed. Some rehabilitation hospitals arrange for a brief visit home with the physical therapist so that he or she can evaluate the home's accessibility and recommend any needed modifications or equipment prior to discharge from the hospital.

With the architecture of your home and the psychological makeup of your family in full view, you can assess whether either or both of these need some adjustment before you come home.

As the discharge date approaches, most injured persons find their minds occupied by basic questions about changes in their physical abilities and energy levels—the extra time required to accomplish tasks and how to do the things they used to do in new and different ways. A preoccupation with these hurdles as the day nears is to be expected.

When the day comes, you may transfer to the car along the sliding board, then wait while someone stows your wheelchair in the trunk; you may arrive at your home with its newly erected ramp. Having someone push you along the front walk and up the ramp into the house signals a dramatic shift in physical control in your life. Or you may return home in a lift-equipped van and use a power-driven wheelchair to navigate yourself into the house.

If your spinal cord injury resulted from a gunshot wound, you may feel a mixture of fear, anger, emotional numbness, and distrust of the safety of your neighborhood on arriving home, moving quickly from van to front door. If you are returning to your parents' home at a time in life when, like Joan, you'd expected to be on your own, you may feel as if you were going backwards and becoming like a child again.

If you use a cane or crutches for walking when you arrive home, family and friends may perceive you as a person with a "lesser" spinal cord injury, as having a less drastic disability. This is not necessarily so. You still feel the difference between your "old" and "new" lives—needing more time for even simple tasks, getting tired more quickly, and having new routines, such as catheterization and physical exercises, that require a reformatting of the daily schedule.

Regardless of the particular circumstances, the first days at home can be both comforting and challenging. You may be presented with new roles and changed expectations about your contributions to the family. Your world may seem to be in a state of constant, accelerating change. The key to survival in this world is adaptation. Given that you need to restructure your life, how will you choose to do so?

Once you are within the safe confines of home, the need for more changes in the physical environment may become apparent. You may need devices such as an electric-powered lift to help you into bed or assist you in shifting positions. Structural changes, such as carving out room for the wheelchair under sinks and widening doorways, may have to be accomplished. A roll-in shower that can accommodate a portable shower chair, and a hand-held shower nozzle and easily accessible water controls, might make your bathroom more usable.

Other technological aids are available: speakerphones, which can be used without hands; computers that respond to voice commands; and central switches to control the environment, including heating, air conditioning, lighting, or a central speaker system. Information on these technological advances is available in magazines and journals published for persons with disabilities, from organizations serving persons with disabilities, from medical and orthopedic supply houses, and from architects who practice accessible design (see the Resources section at the end of this book).

The Emotional Return

After the physical transition to home, the really hard work begins: the psychological readjustment to living in the real world. You will be faced with the reality of disability on a personal level. At home, your focus will need to shift from "me" to "we," which requires recognizing and dealing with other people's feelings and reactions as you move around your community.

While facing these new situations, you may not feel ready to be home. One reality of the present world of managed health care is that you may return home at a much earlier stage of your rehabilitation and recovery than did those who preceded you. For instance, Joan stayed in the rehabilitation center for six months, going on excursions into the community and having overnight stays at home to prepare her for her return. Compare that rehabilitation and preparation time to the present norm, which may be as short as one to two months in some states.

How might this shorter stay in the hospital affect you? You may be less physically, emotionally, and socially adjusted to your newly acquired disability than were your predecessors, because you have had less time to "get the hang of" it or to "deal with" it. You've had less opportunity to incorporate the disability into your picture of who you are, less time to process and "gel" your new reality. All of this may result in shaky self-confidence, insufficient physical skill training and development, and less readiness to be at home.

Once home you may experience a variety of emotions, all of which are normal reactions to an abnormal situation. Sadness, resentment, anger, frustration, and anxiety, among many other psychological reactions, are common. These may become apparent only after the initial return-home euphoria has dissipated and the hard physical reality of using the sliding board to move from bed to chair becomes a constant reminder of your physical status.

One normal reaction is to compare what was and what is, the old world and the new. Many people feel a need to mourn what they've lost so as to feel ready to move into the future. (This feeling of loss may arise again from time to time as you pass into new stages of life and face different challenges. The feeling will probably be less intense each time you experience it.)

The old question "Why me?" may loom as you compare your use of a wheelchair with your brother's ability to run to catch the train. You may begin to resent not being able to do what others do. If you have these feelings, find someone to share them with so that you can sort through them and hear them spoken aloud. For all of us, being aware of what we are feeling is important, so that we don't "stuff" it or ignore it. Attempts to bury feelings often lead to their erupting in inappropriate, angry outbursts that may have no connection with the specific situation—confusing you and those around you.

Occasional feelings of sadness are different from depression (as we discussed in Chapter 2). Some hallmarks of serious, clinical depression are persistent sadness, decreased interest in the world, chronic fatigue, sleep disturbance, lack of or ballooning of appetite, and inability to concentrate. If these signs persist or if you begin to feel that life is not worth living, call a mental health professional to get some help.

Frustration may be a key issue as you try to solve many problems at the same time. Patience, creativity, and the ability for thoughtful problem-solving wane as energy is exhausted and frustration sets in. For example, Patricia, who has paraplegia, has driven to an appointment with her obstetrician, and she finds an illegal occupant in the only wheelchair-designated parking space. One other space is available, but it has too little room to open the driver's door, pull the wheelchair from the back seat, and move across the sliding board into the wheelchair. What can she do? First, she might give herself time to vent her anger. Then she can tackle some problem-solving strategies. If she has a cell phone, she can call the police to report the illegal parking. Or she can ask a passerby to go into the office to ask the driver of the illegally parked car to move it. Or, if she has given herself extra time before the appointment, she can wait for a wider opening for her car. The point is that Patricia has behavioral options from which to choose.

Feeling anxiety during this transitional time is not unexpected. On many occasions you'll confront situations you have never dealt with and for which you have no road map. For instance, a work colleague has asked you and your spouse to dinner at her home. You feel anxious, wondering about the accessibility of the house. Are there steps to the front door or steps inside the house? Are the hallways and doorways wide enough for your wheelchair? Will you be able to get in and out of the bathroom? For all of us, anxiety is often a response to a situation in which we have insufficient information, feel unprepared, or feel we have little control. The best solution is to get information—in this case, about your colleague's home—so that you can figure out a solution. Perhaps the home can be made accessible with a portable ramp, which you happen to own. However, if the architectural hurdles are too formidable, perhaps you can meet in a local restaurant for dinner.

The key to dealing with all such emotional reactions is to name them, to express your feelings, and then to tackle a creative response.

The Social Return

Life is social. It is an interdependent give and take, relying on others and taking responsibility for others. It asks for a balancing of the needs of all—the shift from "me" to "we."

Cecily, at thirteen years old, was newly released from a rehabilitation program after sustaining a T7 break in a sledding accident. She found the move home difficult. Her younger brother was constantly playing with her wheelchair. Her older sister was angry because Cecily took up so much of their mother's time that she couldn't attend the sister's basketball games. For her part, Cecily, accustomed to constant attention in the hospital and rehabilitation center, expected that attention to continue at home. She was angry with her siblings because they wouldn't "get with the program." Her mother felt guilty that she was not filling the needs of all her children.

Cecily's father began to assume some responsibility for household chores to relieve his wife, giving her time to attend the sister's games. Both parents began to integrate Cecily into the family, assigning her chores such as filling the dishwasher and dusting furniture. Although she was angry at first, Cecily grew to feel pride in her contribution to the family.

As Joan observes, in the rehabilitation setting, everyone is concentrated on the same goal: your regaining as much physical prowess as possible. At home, while this is still a goal, the many competing goals of other individuals have to be considered.

In some ways, the social return home can be the most daunting because of the expectations both you and others have about your new situation. You may feel unsure and anxious about reactions. Some may react as if the disability is overwhelming, defining you, while others will find it irrelevant: you are who you have always been. Although you are physically different from your pre-injury self, you are still the same person.

So not all people will have negative reactions. For instance, one husband didn't think to tell business associates that his wife used a wheelchair when he brought them home for dinner, because he didn't see her disability as an essential or defining characteristic. His concept of his wife spread to his associates' views of her so that the wheelchair became part of the background in their socializing.

Interestingly, some acquaintances may see this as a chance to get to know you better. For example, Bob's friend from church, a girl he had always admired, became a close friend after his accident, and finally, his girlfriend.

The key here is: YOU. If you expect others to see you as "less than," they just might perceive you that way. On the other hand, if you expect to be treated on an even playing field, that will be the way you are treated. Sounds too simple, doesn't it? Indeed, it is more complicated. You will be combating negative stereotyping, getting past the wheelchair or crutches or limp or slowness as the foreground that defines you, to refocus the picture so your assistive devices become just a part of the background.

To make this transition, you may need to learn some techniques, such as talking up for yourself, using "self talk" to think through what you want to say, or finding a buddy or "coach" who can work on problematic situations with you.

Of course, there are always people who have problems of their own that they may put on your shoulders and then see your disability as overwhelming. Their own problems predispose them to see anything different as threatening. Remember, though, that you aren't responsible for other people's reactions and don't have to incorporate their reactions into your self-image.

Moving into the Community

Getting together with friends who have not seen you since your injury may be another source of distress, depending on how you feel when you see them and how they feel about disability. Each encounter will be different. Go easy on yourself. Don't expect to handle every meeting with grace or humor. Each outcome will depend on your emotional reservoir and what is going on in your life at the moment.

Nora (whose story you will read in Chapter 7) remembers shopping in a department store, using her wheelchair, when she met a friend who had not heard about Nora's recent paraplegia. The friend was stunned, not able to speak, and fled. This was a very unpleasant situation for Nora. However, she and her friend began to talk by phone. Once the friend got over her initial surprise, she became very comfortable and accepting.

As you "move on" you'll find that reentry into the life of your neighborhood or community requires some extra time and planning if you use a wheelchair or other devices for mobility. For instance, checking accessibility of restaurants and theaters—even doctors' offices!—before you begin your journey may eliminate lots of frustration and loss of time. And even with advance preparation, things may still go awry. One woman using a wheelchair remembers calling a restaurant to ask if it were wheelchair accessible. Yes indeed, she was assured! She arrived to find that there were three substantial steps leading to the door. When she called the restaurant to complain, she was told that there were three waiters who would have been delighted to carry her in; thus they claimed barrier-free entry.

Sports venues can be challenges. A woman on crutches found a major worldwide event, held in the United States, was accessible in the interior of the stadium but not on the exterior. Sporting, dance, drama, and other theatrical events require advance booking for wheelchair-accessible seating. Obtaining accessible seating becomes more competitive as our population ages and there is a greater pool of people needing it.

There are some benefits. In some theaters, if you buy a ticket for a wheelchair space, the person who is attending with you may get a discount on her ticket; make sure you inquire when purchasing tickets.

Getting into friends' homes is one of the barriers people using wheelchairs report as most distressing. The normal "dropping in" on a friend, or taking chicken soup to a friend with a cold, or just "hanging out" is no longer possible unless your friend's home is a "visitable home," or you are using an iBOT (a wheelchair that climbs stairs), or you have some strong friends who are able to pull you up and take you down the stairs.

This means that in most instances, you meet at your own home or you go out to restaurants, bars, or other places people gather to socialize. If there are small steps into a friend's home, however, you may be able to use one of the lightweight ramps that can be stowed in the trunk of a car.

CHANGING ROLES, EXPECTATIONS, AND CONTRIBUTIONS
New Roles

What are some new roles and skills you may have to learn after returning home?

1. How to be psychologically independent while being physically dependent
2. How to improve communication skills to get what you need
3. How to become the manager of your life
4. How to manage your mental well-being in new ways

Many people with spinal cord injury need to learn how to be physically dependent, that is, how to rely on someone else for certain aspects of daily needs. Because our society values independence and self-reliance, dependence on others may be perceived as a sign of weakness or laziness, even when it is unavoidable. The ability to physically depend on others, while maintaining confidence in one's ability to be psychologically self-reliant, has to be learned. This skill-building begins in the hospital and rehabilitation center. In the institutional setting, dependency seems more natural, with professionals available and paid to deal with your needs. At the same time, you may be offered opportunities to make choices and decisions about your schedule, care, and activities. These choices will not as a rule be impacted by the choices or needs of others in the hospital. After returning home, however, you need the family to do things for you, or you may have a personal care attendant. The key to dealing with this dependency is to realize that, as social animals, we are all dependent on each other to some degree. Although the needs of a person with a disability may be magnified, this increased dependency is limited to the physical. You still are in charge of the direction of your life.

Although physically dependent on others, a person with a spinal cord injury is not psychologically dependent. Each person, injured or not, is a distinct entity with his or her own personality, needs, and dreams. Understanding this will be most useful as you work with helpers, whether members of the family or professionals. You have a right to assert your needs and to see that they are met, as does every other person.

While communicating your needs to caregivers, remind yourself that this is a two-way street: their needs have to be considered also. Joan, for instance, knew that she was dependent on the hospital staff for her rehabilitation. She became aware of their needs and time pressures, and she knew that sometimes she would have to wait for help.

Getting needs met requires that the needs be communicated. Clarity in communication is essential when you have a specific need, for example, if your catheter is kinked or your eating utensils are not in the proper place for you to pick them up. You need to translate your situation and your needs into spoken language. For those who are not particularly articulate, this may be a challenge. And those who are shy or question their self-worth may have difficulty asking for their needs to be filled. Bear in mind that only you know what your needs are. Others cannot read your mind or feel your body's sensations. You are your own spokesperson.

Seeing yourself as the manager of your own existence is at once exciting and intimidating. The present medical system demands that you become educated about your situation and advocate for your own needs. Passivity will not work. You must be informed about medications, treatments, equipment, medical and rehabilitation personnel, and the latest findings in research. You must be an active partner in your care and the planning of your life. Joan is someone who decides what it is she wants. For example, she decided she would use a manual chair at first, then changed her mind later when she found the motorized chair gave her more mobility. Elliott (whose story you'll read in Chapter 6) decided to stop taking medication for spasms because it made him groggy. He learned to control the spasms by applying pressure to his legs, and even to use the spasms for assistance with dressing and pressure releases. After going home from the hospital and realizing that his bowel care regimen kept him "tethered" to home, Bob, a socially active teen, decided to have an ACE stoma procedure. This allowed him to manage his bowels independently and thus be free to travel with his friends. With proper information, you can make these decisions for yourself.

One of the most challenging new roles is managing your emotional well-being, for instance, finding ways to release frustrations. Many able-bodied people release anger, frustrations, worry, and concerns through physical activity. If that avenue is not available after a spinal cord injury, how do you vent? Some people do this destructively through critical comments, angry outbursts, blaming, or letting their own physical condition deteriorate. Others find they can release pent-up feelings by changing their situation or how they think about their situation. Some find talking with a friend or peer counselor helpful. Refocusing energies by listening to music, reading, or taking up a new hobby can also help.

Expectations

Expectations are essential for orienting one's life course. You must make sure that they are *your* expectations, not those of family, friends, or others. For example, Joan's family wanted her to return home to live, but she knew that she had to live independently, like any other person of her age. Although this was difficult for her family, they were able to draw back and allow her the "space" to risk going back to school to live with her roommates.

Because they also had respect for Joan, her family did not let her submerge herself in self-pity during her early days at home. They urged her to become involved in activities, to prepare for an independent future. Expectations of family members feed off one another and can help to build self-confidence and healthy egos. For teens and young adults, the family's expectation of participation in age-appropriate social activities as well as responsibilities is particularly important in promoting healthy development. When Bob came home from rehab, his younger brother, Jeff, willingly became his "unofficial manservant" and gofer. After the novelty wore off, thirteen-year-old Jeff states, "I learned what a paraplegic is . . . you need to help him [Bob] at first, but you should try to get him to do things on his own . . . [He's] still the same person even if he's in a wheelchair." Similarly, when twelve-year-old Andrew was in rehab after a shooting left him with paraplegia, his mother encouraged him to continue preparations for his bar mitzvah (a Jewish religious ceremony for thirteen-year-olds as they "come of age"), and she supported his desire to become a wheelchair tennis player and travel with a team.

Some people, however, try to please others and fulfill their expectations rather than their own, often unaware that this is happening. Trying to reach goals set by other people, and failing, can produce depression, anxiety, or anger. Try the following exercise. Close your eyes. Ask yourself whose goal it is that you study law, or leave school, or move in with the family, or retire from your job. Whose face appears? This little exercise often reveals that you're following a certain course because it pleases Dad or Mom or your children, not yourself.

Perhaps the goal is your own, but reaching it is next to impossible. Goals and expectations that seem excessively high may indeed be possible, and you need not dismiss your goals or dreams because of a spinal cord injury. You will need to examine how your goals mesh with your resources, including not only your physical ability but your social supports and financial resources. Failure to meet high expectations can create depression for people who are accustomed to being high achievers. These individuals may need to reorient their goals and create some more realistic expectations, so that they will not continually feel they are letting themselves down.

Will your expectations change after a spinal cord injury? The answer depends on what you expected before the injury. For instance, Joan always knew she would make a living by using her brain. The only change she needed was to retool with the equipment necessary to do her artwork. But for a person who was totally immersed in physical activities—on the job and off—expectations may need to change after spinal cord injury. Consider, for example, a young man who is injured in a motorcycle accident. He is a bricklayer. He has never been an avid student. Certainly his expectations differ drastically from those of another young man who, before a spinal cord injury, had planned to be a computer programmer.

It is sometimes helpful to erase, temporarily, your old accomplishments and prior goals and concentrate on where you are now, so that you do not constantly contrast "now" and "then." Rejoice in being able to pick up a spoon with your new splint—you couldn't do that last week. Or revel in doing a wheelie or in walking twenty feet using the walker. The energy and determination you once used in schussing down a ski slope can be applied just as appropriately on the physical therapy mat. Having cemented your self-image with your new physical reality, you can reconnect with your old history to reintegrate yourself as a whole person. This may mean finding a new vocational goal or hobby (see Chapter 9).

Contributions

At first, everyone is thrilled that you are home. They may treat you as a guest with special privileges—until they realize that you're still you, a member of the family. It is at that point, fairly soon after your return, that you need to begin fitting into the family organization. This means bearing normal family privileges and responsibilities.

You need to assess what contributions you can make to the family. If you can no longer do your usual chores—washing windows, mowing the lawn, taking out the trash—be creative in finding new ways to contribute. Some people shift to doing computer planning of meals for the family, reading to and supervising children, cooking, planning the family's social life, or taking telephone messages. Of course, family members must be open to accepting your help and be willing to ask for it.

Ted had tetraplegia following a skiing accident. He took over the household budget and bill-paying on the computer, a chore his companion, Dan, had always tackled before the accident. Dan, in turn, became a gourmet cook, Ted's former role. Sometimes the realignment in responsibilities reveals undiscovered talents.

TESTING AND EXPLORING PHYSICAL LIMITS

Much as a little child begins to explore her or his world, you may be starting anew, trying to do things differently or testing the limits of what you can do. After they return home, many people with spinal cord injury begin to test their abilities and to learn the fine art of balancing risk and safety.

Brushing your teeth with an adaptive hand device, pushing yourself up a steep ramp, testing crutches on a rain-slicked sidewalk, or bending to pick up a ball for the first time—all these activities allow you to assess both your potential and your limits. Although this exploring and problem-solving is lifelong, the most intense period is soon after your arrival home. Testing also includes finding ways around obstacles to reach your goals. Joan's "ways around" included using a computer for her artwork and learning to hold and manipulate a paintbrush in her mouth. Later, an arm implant gave her use of her left thumb (see Chapter 8, where we discuss technology).

Creativity is a key component in testing and exploring. What if you can't lean over far enough from your wheelchair to pick up the newspaper from the grass? Does that mean you can't retrieve the morning paper? Not at all. What about using long tongs—"reachers" or "grabbers"—to pick it up? These are advertised in many orthopedic supply catalogs. Or maybe you want to get a trained companion dog that will retrieve things for you. Another option is to notify the newspaper delivery person that you need your paper placed on the waist-high ledge by the front door. We don't want to belabor the point, but creativity and seeing the possibilities of many different options have a most beneficial effect on the direction and quality of your life.

On the other hand, brick walls do exist, and you will come up against them. At times you can get over, under, or around them, but sometimes they are too formidable, too high, or too wide. After giving your best efforts, a time comes when you're better off recognizing that perhaps your energies would be more fruitfully directed toward another venture. Give yourself some time to mourn the loss of reaching your original goal. You will then be able to recoup energy and move on to a new, attainable target.

THE REAL—AND LATER—RETURN HOME

At some point after you arrive home, the honeymoon will end. With the onset of this new phase, life will suddenly feel real again. It is time to return to work or retrain for new work; to return to school; to renew housekeeping chores or tend the children. You are expected to pick up the reins of your life and its responsibilities. As family and friends begin to see that you are not fragile and not to be feared, their expectations of you increase and they begin to express their true thoughts and feelings.

Before this next phase, you may have felt that you were not allowed to "be real," to reveal your feelings and frustrations, and that you were expected to be upbeat all the time, to keep everyone else's spirits up. Family members may have felt a similar burden. Maintaining a constantly positive atmosphere takes a huge amount of energy on each person's part, and eventually the reservoirs of energy are depleted. At this point, everyone begins to have normal ups and downs. And everyone's feelings will not move in concert. You may be feeling depressed while your spouse is on top of the world. The following day your moods may be reversed. Letting each other know where you are will help you help each other.

Family Reactions to the Return Home

As we have noted, family members may experience a wide variety of emotional reactions to the return home. They may be afraid of dealing with the intricacies of the physical care or may find it difficult to face the psychological reactions of the injured loved one, not to mention their own feelings.

Family expectations about the future may need to change as well. Imagine that a teenager is riding his dirt bike on a nearby hilly course. He hits a muddy area, slides out of control down a hill, and injures his spine. Until then, his parents had always "known" that he'd get a basketball scholarship to college, perhaps go on to play in the NBA. Now that their son is home from the rehabilitation center, the time has come for the parents to reevaluate. One of their roles may be to help their son see himself as an athlete who just happens to use a wheelchair.

Some of the psychological reactions of family members that we addressed in chapters 1 and 2 can arise again in transition periods such as the injured person's return home. Feelings of guilt, grief, loss, anger, and frustration often resurface. The difference this time is that the feelings probably will not be quite so painful. Having survived the first awareness of the loss, family members know the techniques that helped then and can be used again. Some helpful techniques are releasing feelings through talking or tears or writing; using meditation or religious supports; taking a few minutes for an activity that is completely diverting; or getting medical and psychological help. Another boost is to connect with other families that have a member with spinal cord injury or to take advantage of advice available from national caregiver associations (see the Resources section at the end of this book). They can be a great source of support and information.

As a family member and caregiver, feeling the weight of responsibility for the physical well-being and existence of a loved one with spinal cord injury can be more complicated when friction or unresolved issues exist. It may be helpful to find an outsider or a professional therapist to help you when you have this "double whammy."

> *Sylvia felt guilty that she'd allowed her daughter Laura to go out on the date during which she'd fallen from her bicycle while going round a bend too fast. Laura's fall resulted in paraplegia and she had to use a wheelchair. Sylvia focused all her energy on Laura in the hospital but was very apprehensive about her ability to care for her daughter at home. Another mother of a young person with spinal cord injury called to talk with Sylvia about her guilt and anxiety. But this did little to relieve Sylvia's feelings, and her physician recommended psychological counseling. After some time in counseling, Sylvia understood that she had no control over the situation in which the injury occurred. Laura was eighteen and responsible for her own decisions. Sylvia was able to let go of her guilt, thus giving Laura the freedom to make the transition to adulthood, making some good decisions, some bad.*

> *Andrew's mom, Jane, also struggled with guilt, although she knew that she was not to blame for her son's spinal cord injury. Although Jane tends to see "the negative side" of life, she "understood that guilt was not going to help my son . . . There is a myth that you can protect your children. We [parents] see ourselves as protectors. But you can't really—you can't protect them against their feelings and against physical danger." Instead of dwelling on her anxieties about Andrew, Jane put her energy into supporting his efforts to have a successful adolescence and achieve his life goals.*

Setting Goals Together

Although this can be a rocky time, it is also an opportunity for enhancing communication and intimacy. The first step is listening to and accepting the feelings of each member of the family or group with honesty, empathy, and creativity.

From a foundation of inclusion and trust, the family can begin to solve the new dilemmas that arise. Mom used to do the wash; who will be responsible for that now? The teenager formerly mowed the lawn; who will do it this summer? Dad made a living for the family as a truck driver; will Mom have to go out to work, or will Dad go back to school to learn a new trade?

Establishing a structured forum in which the family can discuss and debate possible courses of action unites the family, empowers individual members, and helps everyone through the rough times. Getting this system in place early is extremely helpful. Some families schedule weekly meetings to discuss problems and work on new ideas and plans for solving them. Others prefer to meet as needed, whenever one family member calls for a discussion. And some families use a daily event, such as dinnertime, as an opportunity for shared problem-solving.

Caring for Caregivers

A common phenomenon when a person with spinal cord injury returns home is the physical and emotional overextension of family members. They feel totally responsible for the well-being of their loved one and may have high expectations for themselves. They may not be informed about the resources available to them or their right to receive them. And they may not be aware when they need care themselves.

When the injured person or any other family member sees the family caregiver in need of relief, this should be brought to the attention of the caregiver. Here are some signs of caregiver "burnout":

1. Withdrawing from favorite activities
2. Paying less attention to appearance
3. Seeming fatigued much of the time
4. Having difficulty concentrating on his or her own goals
5. Being in a highly emotional or apathetic state

Often the caregiver will be unaware of having any of these problems. Other family members then need to gently persuade the caregiver to take a break or make arrangements for help in caregiving.

What are some possible solutions? One answer might be to arrange for attendant care, at least part of the time, so the fatigued family member can renew his or her energies. Another avenue is to suggest someone with whom the caregiver can talk, such as a minister, friend, psychologist, or physician. Encourage the caregiver to participate in whatever activity is most restorative, whether "time outs" for lunch with a friend, taking a class, attending a religious service, or taking a walk.

Finding out what is most helpful to the person with spinal cord injury is sometimes beneficial to the caregiver also. Sometimes too much caregiving can actually get in the way of the progress of the loved one, who would benefit from more responsibility or more chances to take risks. Caregivers can inadvertently overprotect or "baby" the person with a spinal cord injury, stifling the injured person's attempts to gain independence. Seeing a loved one take risks, become fatigued, or take additional time in caring for his or her own needs can be frustrating or hurtful to a family member. The caregiver may think, "It would be so much easier and faster for me to do the ironing," then step in to take over the chore. But this may not be what the person with the disability wants or really needs.

> *Andrew's mom recalls having this feeling the first time she watched him put gas in his car at the self-serve station. He had to take his wheelchair out of the car, transfer into it, pump the gas, and reverse the whole process. She empathized with "what a pain" this was for Andrew, while for Andrew, his ability to drive and pump his own gas were proud reminders of his new adolescent privileges.*

Periodic consultation with a doctor or physical therapist can help family members clarify the actual capabilities of the person with spinal cord injury and adjust their caregiving behaviors to these changing needs and capabilities. Sometimes, family counseling is necessary to help caregivers let go of tasks they no longer need to perform for their family member, or to help the person with spinal cord injury assert his or her capabilities and take more risk and responsibility within the family system.

Communication and Intimacy

Communication is a basic human need, although some people seem to require it more than others. When you have a disability, communication is a tool you'll need to hone in order to get your needs met. The more extensive your disability, the greater the necessity for you to describe what you need and how you would like it to be delivered.

Step one, then, is getting across what you need. Step two is delivering your message in a way that makes the other person want to respond to your request. Being sensitive to the way you come across helps to alleviate family tensions or feelings that you are "demanding." If you regard your family or attendants as equals, your relationship will be more resilient and longer lasting.

Having a disability may require putting more energy and attention into communicating and explaining oneself to others. Because you may rely on a wheelchair, companion dog, or walker, you'll encounter questions, comments, or looks that you didn't get before your disability. Should you react to them or ignore them? Your decision will probably be determined by your energy level and mood at the time. Although it is "nice" to respond to overtures from others, especially from children, don't hold yourself to the impossible standard of *always* having a positive response.

You may be particularly apprehensive about arriving home if you are in an intimate relationship (this is addressed more fully in Chapter 6). You and your partner will need to confront your feelings and expectations about being together. Both of you are probably feeling some trepidation about how your physical intimacy will change. You might want to talk with other couples, read some of the excellent books available on sexuality and spinal cord injury, or talk with a counselor experienced in disability and sexuality. As in other areas, avoid having impossible expectations for yourselves. Talk with your partner about what feels good and what works. This can be a time for fun and experimentation. The expression of caring comes in many forms, and all couples work out their own ways of showing they care.

Working with a Personal Care Attendant

Some people need more extensive care than their families can provide. Unusually demanding care can stress family energies and resources, creating animosity and resentment. If your family is unable to provide for your needs, or if you want to be independent of your family, you can hire a personal care attendant (PCA). Locating and securing a PCA is a core challenge for people with higher-level spinal cord injuries, who may need continuous care.

A personal care attendant is qualified to assist you with whatever personal care you are not able to manage yourself. This care can include help with bathing; bowel and bladder care; hair washing and styling; food preparation and feeding; writing checks; movement in and out of bed or chairs; getting to and from work; shopping for or with you; and setting up tools for you to use—anything, in short, that allows you to maintain your activities of daily living. Some PCAs come into the home for a few hours a day or visit in the morning and evening. Others live in, providing round-the-clock assistance.

Attendants come from a variety of backgrounds. Some have been formally trained and others have not. Some are trained practical nurses, others have taken weekend training in becoming a PCA. Organizations such as Easter Seals occasionally offer training.

You may need to make arrangements for a PCA before your return home. Rehabilitation hospitals often have lists of PCAs or agencies that provide home care. The rehabilitation social worker may give you this information and help you find an attendant or agency that fits your needs and budget. Independent living centers may have lists of resources as well. You can also find agencies that send out nurses and attendants. Most agency PCAs have been trained to work with elderly people and may require more specific instructions or training in spinal cord injury care. Veteran PCA users say that the best referrals are from other people who use attendants. Some nurses, wanting a change from the hospital setting, agree to become an attendant for a patient who has been released from the hospital. People with spinal cord injury sometimes advertise in disability-related publications or in a mainstream newspaper's "help wanted" section. A PCA can also be a friend or acquaintance who is hired and trained by you and your family to manage your care needs.

Schedule face-to-face interviews with the applicants for the PCA position. Make sure you include other members of your household so that you all have the opportunity to ask questions and find out whether you feel comfortable with the person. What questions should you ask in an interview? First, you must determine whether the applicant has experience performing the tasks you need him or her to perform. You should also ask about the person's education. A high school education and basic nurse's aide training are the recommended minimum requirements. And remember to ask for personal references and then follow up with phone calls—this is essential.

The relationship with a PCA is a delicate one, because you are simultaneously in a very intimate situation *and* an employer. You must be very clear about what is expected, when it is to be accomplished, and what the payment will be. Balancing your needs with your PCA's needs is crucial. Of utmost importance is establishing a communication system that ensures you are never left stranded because your PCA doesn't report for work. Joan recalls a weekend at home in bed with no relief because she and her PCA miscommunicated and Joan had no phone by her bedside. That is a horror story not to be repeated. A safety factor is to have a list of backup PCAs and/or agencies that can provide a PCA on short notice. If several PCAs become sick during a flu epidemic, having a long enough list ensures that you won't be left stranded. Taking good care of your attendants will also keep your list full, because they will enjoy working for you.

Fitting the PCA into your living situation when you return home requires some fine-tuning, especially if you live with a spouse or other intimate companion. Preparing and positioning for sexual intimacy require trust and clear communication. Some people find that asking the PCA to attend to necessary preparations, such as removing a catheter or inserting a contraceptive diaphragm, allows the subsequent interaction with their partner to feel more spontaneous and romantic. Others may prefer to train their spouse or partner to make these preparations, to avoid involving the PCA at intimate moments.

Joan asserts that the key to being a "happy quad" is good attendant care, and she has devoted much thought to hiring and maintaining good attendants. Her observations may help you. For instance, she has made it a rule to hire only attendants who have been mothers. She has found that they are more responsible, caring, and considerate, and less squeamish. She treats her attendants like members of the family and feels that this makes a huge difference. Although many training programs advise users of PCAs to maintain a strict employer-employee relationship, Joan says that, for her, the relationship is too close and intimate for that distancing to be possible.

Joan advocates paying attendants somewhat more than the going rate, if you can afford it. Along with providing good remuneration, Joan doesn't get demanding. "You have to realize they are people, too." On the other hand, she doesn't allow the PCAs to "walk all over her." Her one stipulation is that when her attendants are working, they keep busy. Joan is a hard worker and expects the same of her attendants. Obviously, her guidelines have worked for her because she has retained the same weekday attendant for eleven years and the same weekend attendant for five years.

In Joan's high-rise condominium complex, two women have instituted an attendant care cooperative. (Several people in Joan's complex need PCA care.) They have hired a full-time attendant to live in the building, providing her with an apartment and paying her electricity and phone bills. For some people she is the primary help; for others she is a backup. For instance, Joan needs her only when her regular attendant is sick. The group attendant wears a beeper to respond to calls for assistance. This project, established on a grant from a local independent living center, became a model for five other locations in the United States.

There are several state and federal programs to assist people in obtaining funding for personal care attendants. Medicare, the federal health insurance program for elderly people and those receiving Social Security Disability, has a new pilot program called The Money Follows the Person. People who qualify for this program can use funds that would ordinarily pay for nursing home care to hire PCAs instead. Medicaid (or Medical Assistance), the federal health insurance program for people with low incomes, has the Medicaid Waiver Program, which provides some individuals, who would otherwise require nursing home care, with funds for PCAs. A person who needs a PCA must fill out a special application for a waiver. The program typically has a long waiting list. In some instances, a family member can assume the role of PCA and receive payment for her or his services under the waiver program.

State agencies for children with disabilities go by various names; even when these names include the words "developmental disability" the agencies may provide services for people with spinal cord injury if they were injured before twenty-one years of age. These agencies often supply funds for personal care assistance, along with other services.

THE RETURN HOME IS A COMPLEX, gradual process. With the passage of time it brings increasing levels of comfort, self-confrontation, and "being yourself." As we've emphasized, coming home is experienced on the physical, psychological, and social levels, and your needs will probably be addressed in that order. And coming home, as in Joan's case, may be two-tiered: an initial adjustment at home, then a next step to school or another setting that offers more independence and self-reliance.

Returning home is a time of risk assessment that leads to risk-taking. It is a time of relearning in order to release yourself to do old tasks in new and innovative ways. It is a time of fatigue, self-doubt, and conflicting emotions, and a time of soaring joy in accomplishments that you and others thought you might never achieve. You'll find reservoirs of strength and abilities of which you were completely unaware. And your spotlight will broaden, defining your old territory—and *you*—in a new light.

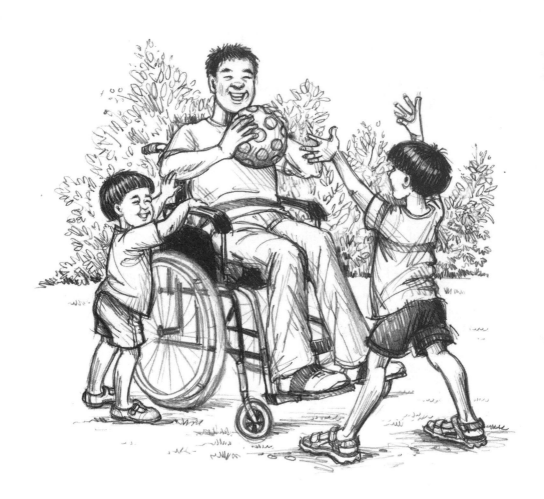

5

Focus on the Family

ONE FAMILY'S EXPERIENCE

Trauma

Susanna and Flip had gone to the movies, something they'd not done in a long time. Their older son, Bob, sixteen, had driven his dad's pride and joy, the new VW Beetle, to band practice and had promised to be home by 9:00. His brother Jeff, thirteen, was spending the night at a friend's home.

As the parents were leaving the theater a bit after nine, Susanna tried Bob's cell phone; there was no answer. When she repeated the call a few minutes later, a message from the state police said Bob had been in an accident. He had been flown to a specialized trauma unit in a nearby city; he was awake and conscious.

It was February, cold and icy. Bob had dropped a friend off after band prac-tice and headed home. He hit a stretch of black ice; the Beetle flipped on its side and slid into a telephone pole, the only thing standing in a wide area. That pole had lodged between Bob and the seat; the steering wheel broke at the site where Bob's back was fractured, at T11. It was a bloodless accident. Although he hit his head, he was conscious, giving rescuers his parents' telephone numbers but saying he was fifteen rather than sixteen years old. Paramedics were amazed he had survived. One of them rescued Bob's beloved musical equipment from the wrecked car.

Susanna and Flip arrived at the trauma unit about 11:00 p.m. Bob couldn't feel his legs; the x-ray revealed a broken spine. Surgery would be performed in the morning. "You hold out hope something will pop up, that it won't be so bad," says Susanna. Flip kept hoping there would be some magical way the doctors could fix his son.

They spent most of the night at the hospital but left early in the morning to catch an hour or so of sleep and then pick up Jeff at church. Friends at church were tearful; Susanna and Flip broke down for the first time in the midst of their friends' support.

Jeff remembers the quiet of the church as Susanna told him his brother had broken his spine and it would take "lots of bolts" to put it back together.

That Sunday morning Bob's spine was fused. Bob says he has no recollection of the events surrounding the accident or the rescue, although he had been awake and capable of giving information at the scene. He "woke up" a few days later, while he was still in the trauma unit.

Jeff was not allowed to visit Bob until he was "awake" in the ICU. Jeff entered the room, laid his head on Bob, and told him he would be his slave. (And he was for six weeks, until Bob returned to his normal big brother role—"he can be so mean," Jeff says—and Jeff was not so inclined to be at his beck and call).

Rehabilitation

Bob remained in the trauma unit nine days and then was transferred to a nearby rehabilitation hospital. "We chose the rehab facility because it offered hope," says Susanna. "A euphoria went with me for six months"; she was so thankful to have "her boy": there was no profound brain damage, he was recognizable, and he could talk with them.

During rehabilitation, Susanna struggled to find where she fit into the recovery process. Everything was new to her, but she wanted to learn. How could she hone the skills necessary to meet Bob's needs at home? She wanted to know which signs and symptoms to note, and when she learned and saw them, she reported them to the staff. She felt that some on the staff saw "the mother" as peripheral and preferred that she stay on the sidelines and let them do their jobs. In one instance she reported cloudy urine to the nurse for three days but her reports were discounted; it turned out that Bob had a serious infection.

Her only breakdown occurred near the end of Bob's stay, when the nurse told Susanna she needed to learn Bob's bowel program. "I can't do this to him," she said. She learned, however, to reorient her thinking, to put this task into a new type of "normal." Bob eased the situation for her by emotionally detaching himself from the potentially embarrassing, intrusive procedure.

Flip visited his son in the hospital and rehab center every day. Doing so brought him to the stark realization of what had happened and what would be *entailed. He liked the nurses and doctors who cared for his son. Flip had some understanding of hospitals and the medical system, as he had experienced a heart attack and three strokes in the few years preceding Bob's injury. His own recovery resulted in an optimistic and hopeful outlook on Bob's prognosis and trust in the medical system. "We live in hope and pray that some magic or solution medically created may be made available to do the trick for Bob."*

For Jeff, his brother's time in rehabilitation "was weird. I spent lots of time thinking how life would be different. I thought he'd need everyone's help." Jeff attended a siblings' workshop at the rehab hospital but found it was not useful to him because the other siblings had brothers or sisters with brain injuries.

Meanwhile Bob was reluctantly waking at 5:00 a.m. to take medication; he felt isolated—he was the only person his age at the rehab center who did not have a brain injury. A friend from school and church orchestrated weekly visits by seven to ten other high school friends to the rehab center. Bob and the girl who arranged the gatherings became a couple and dated for many months.

Outpatient Rehab and Medical Complications

Released in May from rehabilitation, Bob got home in time to see his friends coming out of school. He returned to school the following day. However, he developed some common medical complications, requiring additional treatment at home.

For Susanna, the return home was positive; she was delighted to watch Bob meet his friends as school let out. And she learned to deal with medical needs as they arose. Soon after the homecoming, Bob developed an open wound, requiring a two-hour cleaning and changing of dressings every day. Susanna added that to the daily regimen; later there were also bladder infections to contend with. Susanna missed having other mothers in the same situation to call for support and guidance. "I felt alone trying to figure things out." She wished there were nurses available to respond to problems on the telephone: " 'When he has a cold, do this . . .' so he won't get pneumonia." She also felt that guidelines for parents were limited. For example, no one told her to watch for swelling in Bob's legs; he developed a deep vein thrombosis, for which she was unprepared. "I've learned through his complications. I wish it were not necessary."

Further outpatient rehab included travel to another city to work on a bowel program and walking. Bob liked the standing frame, saying it was nice to be upright, not having to look up at everyone, but at the same time he was still in a "contraption," and this one had no wheels. Still later he returned to his original rehab center for twice weekly therapies. The family's remote rural setting had few resources, resulting in a lot of driving to rehabilitation facilities and anxiety. "I was all alone trying to figure things out," Susanna says. After a long search, they finally located a water therapy program in a town not too far from their home.

Adaptations and Adjustments

As for Bob's initial reaction to the injury, he says it "didn't hit me as abnormal. I can't walk . . . but . . . whatever. Mom describes my reaction as peace of mind. I don't get fed up with anything. I'm blasé." But he does admit that about a year post-injury, he did feel down when he had difficulty participating in a post-prom party in the woods with his friends. His friends assisted him in getting into the woods, but they started leaving and he had to tell them in no uncertain terms to come back and get him to the party.

The week after this event, Bob became depressed, in part due to the party incident and in part because he couldn't join his girlfriend on a graduation trip to the Caribbean. Bob's mother was still doing his bowel care, which left him feeling "tethered; I can't go anywhere."

Because of this realization, Bob elected to get an ACE stoma operation, allowing him to manage his bowels independently. This freed him to come and go when he pleased, without needing his mother's daily care.

As a parent, Susanna had always felt it was her job to solve all of Bob's problems. She had fought for services for his learning disability, dyslexia, when he was young; in fact, she had home-schooled him one year. Now Bob was striving for independence and didn't want Susanna to help him with his care or to ask for special services for him even though he was entitled to them. He wanted to make it on his own. This was a difficult transition for Susanna, as it is for all parents.

Community Living

Bob has become fully integrated into community life. He drives the family car, which has been adapted for him. He plays in two bands. On most school trips his friends haul him up the bus steps; when that isn't possible, he follows behind the school bus in his car. In his senior year he is a full-time dual-enrollment stu-

dent at the local college and has a 3.7 GPA. Next year he will be off to a four-year university with flat terrain not too far from home. He plans on a computer major.

Susannah says she has found a "new normality" in life. It involves activities never entered into before, new routines, and a sense of anticipation. "Bob has been extraordinary for us. He is a normal kid. He can be a lazybones when he doesn't want to do something for himself, like using the washer/dryer. And then he turns around and pushes for dual enrollment at high school and college and wants to go traveling."

As for Bob's future, Susannah says, "His trajectory is going to the same place. It will just be a little different."

The needs and feelings of family members are often overlooked in the books and articles on adjustment to spinal cord injury and in the clinical practice of rehabilitation. Families report that they often feel "out of the loop" of information and decision-making, with many of their questions and concerns unanswered, as Susanna articulates. This is partly because, in the early stages of hospitalization and rehabilitation, doctors, nurses, technicians, and other medical staff members must concentrate primarily on sustaining the life, limiting the extent of the injury, and maximizing the remaining physical abilities of the patient. Thus medical care providers have little time for the concerns of the patient's family. Family members may also feel alienated because they are unsure what questions to ask or what rights they have within the medical system. And, emotionally overwhelmed, they often can't put their thoughts and feelings into words.

Think what happens when the media do a story on spinal cord injury. Newspaper headlines spotlight the injured person. Feature stories describe the heroism and fortitude of someone surviving with a spinal cord injury. Television specials feature famous people who have sustained spinal cord injuries. While these stories are inspiring, they tend to focus almost exclusively on the person who has been injured, and it may seem as if the injured persons deal with their disability in a vacuum—as if a stone dropped into a pond has no effect on the surrounding body of water. Yet we know there is a ripple effect and that family members also go through emotional upheavals and adjustments in coming to terms with spinal cord injury. The trauma enters their lives too. They, like the injured person, enter a new world, unprepared for their new roles and the new demands on their energies and resources. This strange world of medical care and rehabilitation runs on different time schedules, speaks a different language, and offers limited understanding or education for family members.

In this chapter, we directly address families who have a loved one with spinal cord injury. Experiences differ for each family member, of course. Parents must deal with the emotions that arise whenever their child is hurt. For brothers and sisters, already existing emotional issues or conflicts with their sibling may be complicated by the trauma. When a parent is injured, children must deal with a heightened sense of vulnerability and a loss of trust. And the spinal cord injury of a husband or wife or other intimate companion raises issues of sexuality and interdependence.

While everyone in the family experiences strong emotional reactions, these seldom occur at the same time for each family member. For instance, the injured person may be deep into depression, while Mom is still in denial, Dad is angry, and younger sister still believes her sibling will be "healed." These differences add to the challenge of coordinating care. And they make communication both more difficult and more important. Supporting each other and acknowledging feelings will help clarify where each family member is on the emotional roller coaster.

We present here the stories of various family members—mother, wife, sibling, and other relatives—of persons with spinal cord injury, all of whom have struggled to come to terms with the injury and its aftermath. We discuss some ways in which families can reduce the impact of spinal cord injury on family functioning and improve communication and mutual support. We suggest ways to connect with other families and professionals who can help you cope with the emotional turmoil, physical exhaustion, and financial hardship that may follow a family member's spinal cord injury.

FIRST THINGS FIRST

Finding Support

A severe physical injury is always emotionally stressful, and sometimes emotionally traumatic, for the family of the injured person. Spinal cord injury, often caused by automobile accidents or shooting incidents, may not be the only injury the person suffers—significant injuries to the head, limbs, or internal organs may also have occurred. These conditions and complications can be life-threatening, requiring a period of intensive care in which the survival of the injured person is uncertain. For the family this means a period of vicarious suffering, feelings of sadness and loss over the damage to their loved one, and fear that the injured person will die. Even when the risk of death is past, family members may be uncertain about the extent and permanence of the injury and confused about the long-term effects. They may be frightened by medical interventions and rehabilitation techniques in which they witness the pain or helplessness of their loved one.

As a family member of a person with spinal cord injury, you may initially have great difficulty processing the information you receive about the patient's condition and prognosis. This may be an overwhelming time, a time when you need support from the hospital social worker, a pastoral counselor (available by request in many hospitals), and friends or extended family members who are more emotionally removed from the patient. You need to express your pain, fear, or despair. Doing this will help you clear your head for the next phase, rehabilitation, when you will need to keep track of information, ask questions, and support the person with the injury.

Increasing contact with other family members—perhaps temporarily leaning more on siblings or adult children for support and encouragement—can ease your loneliness and anxiety. Friends and neighbors can also provide companionship. This is not a time to "tough it out" or "go it alone." Social support is essential to your well-being, and it will help you to help your injured loved one. Family, friends, and neighbors are often incredibly responsive to a crisis such as spinal cord injury, and they will usually give support if asked.

We should also note here the effect of spinal cord injury on the broader family. Many extended family members experience a sense of loss, even if their lives are not directly affected by their relative's disability. Grandparents of an injured teenager, or adults who live miles away from their injured sibling, or aunts, uncles, and cousins—all feel the impact of the trauma and disability as the ripples from the stone in the pond form ever-widening circles.

If, as the spouse, child, parent, or sibling of a person with spinal cord injury, you look to these extended family members for support, remember that they, too, are experiencing loss, though perhaps less intensely than you are. When they seem sad or angry, you may feel like screaming, "It's not about you! This is *my* problem. Help me!" But acknowledging your shared loss may encourage your relatives to be more emotionally involved and supportive. It also helps you to recognize that comments that appear unsupportive or disapproving may arise from their unsettled emotions. Try to bear with them. Give them accurate information, ask for their support, and tell them how they can get more information and help for themselves as well. However, if their neediness overwhelms your ability to cope, distance yourself from them until you have met your own psychological needs.

Coping with Loss of Control

One reaction to spinal cord injury shared by many families is the feeling of loss of control as the person hospitalized with the injury is "snatched" away from them. The family may feel that its influence over the patient's life has been usurped by the hospital or rehabilitation staff, as Susanna did at first. The life of the family itself is severely disrupted by the injury and the prolonged absence of an important member; this may lead to feelings of helplessness or anxiety. And families may be frustrated by their inability to heal or help their loved one.

Lark (whose story is told in Chapter 8) became tetraplegic after a diving accident. She recalls that her father suffered terribly because he couldn't "fix" her. He was a successful businessman and a good father who had always done everything possible to help his children. Now he felt powerless and defeated. With these kinds of feelings, combined with the knowledge that the injury represents a long-term disability, families may think that none of their efforts can make a difference to the patient, and some family members may withdraw.

These feelings are to be expected during the initial phase of adjustment, but there are several ways to regain a feeling of control. First, you can influence what goes on in the hospital by talking with the treatment team regularly, reading about your family member's condition, asking questions or requesting consultations, and asking the injured person to discuss his concerns, ideas, and plans with you. Second, you can tell your injured loved one what's on your mind. Obviously, you'll want to avoid burdening your "patient" with difficult family problems while he is in intensive care or dealing with a medical crisis. But there is no reason why you can't talk about everyday problems, just as you did before the injury. Asking for your loved one's help with decisions about household budgeting, parenting, or your job will help you maintain the emotional support you need. It also shows the person with the injury that you still value his role in the family.

As your family member enters rehabilitation, you will no doubt have many additional concerns about the effect of the spinal cord injury on you and your family. Talking about your fears and anxieties with your injured loved one helps you develop an honest and open relationship. Often families are afraid that their emotional "weakness" or fear will upset the injured person or "put negative ideas in her head." This is unlikely. The patient shares the same fears and may in fact be waiting for your "permission" to talk about them! You do need to be sensitive to her reaction to what you are saying, of course, and stop if she gives you signals that she wants you to stop. Together, you can face your anxieties more easily and begin to plan solutions to anticipated problems.

A PARENT'S PERSPECTIVE

The Trauma and the Separation

Lamar had just started a new job, when her ex-husband, Michael, called from overseas. Their daughter, Bella, had been in an accident in Europe, where she lived with her husband. Could Lamar get there immediately? "Will she live?" asked Lamar. "I don't know," was Michael's reply.

On her arrival, Lamar was picked up by Michael and her daughter's husband at the airport. They told her that Bella was in grave danger because her spine had been broken at a high level. Initially, Lamar was angry at her son-in-law, believing he had caused the accident. At the same time, she felt compassion for him and reached out to touch his arm.

Seeing Bella in the hospital room, Lamar didn't recognize her. Bella's face and body were so swollen "she looked like a float in New York's Thanksgiving Day parade." Lamar had to use her imagination to see that the person before her was actually her daughter. Bella said, "Mom, help me," but Lamar didn't know how she could help. Bella just kept saying, "Help me." Although she couldn't touch Bella, Lamar put her arms in the air around her and assured her that she would make things better. Coming out of the hospital room, Lamar fell apart, screaming and sobbing. "Once I started, I couldn't stop." She was helped onto a bed in another room.

She knew that Bella was in trouble, and she didn't want to lose her. She also felt that God would have to play a role in this. "It would have to be God's will that Bella would live." Lamar approached a priest, asking "Why? Why did this happen to my daughter?" He had no answer. (More of Bella's story is told in Chapter 9.)

Lamar's experience of having to travel back and forth across the ocean to see her injured daughter is unusual, but some degree of geographic separation is not uncommon. People with spinal cord injury are frequently treated at regional rehabilitation centers rather than local hospitals, far away from family members. This can create physical and financial stress as families commute long distances or take a leave of absence from work to live near the person who is hospitalized. Consider the situation when fifteen-year-old Hannah became paraplegic after a car accident. The rehabilitation hospital where she spent many months was three hundred miles from her family's home. Family life was disrupted by frequent trips back and forth to the rehabilitation center.

If you have a long journey to visit your loved one, you may feel uninformed or confused about his care, and perhaps feel emotionally cut off from him, missing him more because you cannot be there all the time. Separation from a spouse can be acutely painful, even if you live in the same town and visit daily, especially for a couple that has rarely spent a night apart. The forced separation may result in the able-bodied spouse feeling disoriented, anxious, or lonely on returning to an empty house after a day at the hospital. Separation for the night, or for a week or a month, is made more difficult by worry about the loved one's condition.

If you cannot visit the hospital daily, you can arrange for regular communication by telephone both with your family member and with someone on the hospital staff. The unit social worker sometimes initiates contact with the patient's physically distant family members and provides weekly updates. However, you can request information from the social worker or doctor—you don't have to wait to be called. Your family member's nurse can also give you information about her care and relay any concerns you have to the doctor. And you can arrange to hold a meeting with the staff during your next visit.

Desperation and Bargaining

There was a small chapel on the grounds of the Catholic hospital where Bella was being treated. Though she is not a Catholic, Lamar sought out the mother superior to tell her of the recent events and of her worries. The mother superior replied, "You know, Madame, I think you need a little espresso." Lamar was grateful for the small comfort of coffee and a friendly ear. As they sat together, Lamar heard the nuns singing in the chapel. She asked the mother superior if the community would pray for Bella. The mother superior invited Lamar to speak to the nuns. They walked to the front of the chapel and Lamar told the nuns briefly about her daughter. The nuns recited in unison a prayer to a female saint, perhaps Saint Teresa. Lamar was touched by the beauty of the prayer and felt hopeful again.

Lamar recalls another touching moment. She was staying at a boarding house near the hospital. Each morning she went into a common room for breakfast with the other guests. She became friendly with another couple, and their son brought holy water from Lourdes for Bella. Before Bella's injury, Lamar would never have put her faith in holy water. But she found herself excited by the possibility of a cure for Bella. "I was so grateful for the holy water. I snuck it into the Intensive Care Unit where Bella was on a respirator." She wanted to put it on Bella's feet.

"What are you doing, Mom?" Lamar at first replied that she wasn't doing anything, but finally admitted her intentions. Bella protested, reminding her mother that they weren't Catholic and didn't believe in such things. Lamar recalls feeling "panic," wanting some connection to God and being afraid to let go of the holy water.

The doctors were skeptical about Bella's prospects for survival. Bella's mother-in-law, Marie, came to the hospital to ask Lamar for some of Bella's clothing. Marie said she had heard about a witch who thought she could help Bella (and who was "highly recommended"), and Marie needed to provide the witch with some of Bella's clothing. Lamar gave Marie the clothing.

Bella did survive, and Lamar was not sure whom to thank: God? The holy water? Saint Teresa? The witch?

As the family member of a person with spinal cord injury, your feelings of powerlessness and fear may sometimes make you desperate. Whether concerned with the very survival of your injured loved one or with his ability to walk, you may feel so driven to find a cure that you're willing to suspend your usual judgment. Like Lamar, you may be tempted to try anything from holy water to witchcraft, regardless of your previous belief system or that of your loved one. Following the initial emotional shock and numbness, you may experience a period of heightened energy, even a mild euphoria. During this time you may be tempted to pursue a frantic search for a cure. You may experience a kind of tunnel vision, recognizing only the hoped-for goal and blocking out the reality of your loved one's disability.

"Bargaining" with God for the complete recovery of your family member may be a part of your search. Bargaining can include participating in religious or superstitious rituals not necessarily related to your usual belief system, making resolutions or personal sacrifices "in exchange" for your loved one's healing, or dedicating all your time and energy to the care of the injured person, with the hope that your "righteousness" will be rewarded with a cure. Bargaining sometimes seems to work, temporarily, and initial improvements in your loved one may encourage false hopes or a denial of reality. But in most cases, the hoped-for miracle does not occur and no further bargains can be struck. When your injured family member begins rehabilitation or leaves rehabilitation still using a wheelchair, the reality of the situation begins to sink in. This can precipitate a "crash" in which depression and anger are the dominant feelings.

Depression and Hopefulness

After spending a month in Europe with Bella, Lamar returned to the United States to resume the job she had started shortly before the accident. But because of her need to go back and forth to Europe to tend to her daughter, Lamar was unable to keep the new job. She then alternated between months working at temporary jobs in the United States and trips to Europe to be with Bella. She was exhausted and "hard hit" financially.

Every time Lamar saw her daughter in the ICU, the doctor would say, "Madame, your daughter will never see the blue sky again." But Lamar became determined that Bella would see the blue sky again; she would live and get bet-

ter. Lamar challenged Michael to find a good hospital for their daughter. She felt that they had to take the risks necessary to move Bella into a first-rate rehabilitation facility. Bella was refused admission to several European hospitals, but finally she was flown to London, where she was taken by helicopter to a specialist rehabilitation hospital.

Lamar flew to see Bella at the London hospital. She was upset to see the pressure sores on Bella's back, which had developed during her first hospitalization because of prolonged bed rest and immobility. (Bella eventually had skin grafts to heal these deep pressure sores.) But Lamar never lost hope for improvement. She was encouraged by small changes in Bella's function during her rehabilitation. For example, one day she thought she saw movement in Bella's wrist. The physical therapist had said this was impossible, but Bella did gain some ability to move her wrist.

At this stage, Lamar had shifted from desperation and bargaining to constructive action. She and her ex-husband had found a rehabilitation program for Bella, and Lamar had consulted with a specialist and spent time at the hospital learning about Bella's care and planning for the future. Once her daughter's survival was no longer an issue, Lamar was cautiously optimistic, encouraged by small improvements, and hopeful for the future. She did not deny the severity of Bella's impairments, but neither did she give up. Lamar's use of any and all available supports during the initial crisis, and her determination to leave no stone unturned in her efforts to keep Bella alive, helped to give her strength to face the long road ahead.

Your experience might be very different from Lamar's. Some families do "crash" at this point, when the crisis is over and they must watch their loved one begin the slow, hard work of rehabilitation and living with the daily impact of a disability. At this stage, the realization that your own life will be significantly and permanently affected may compound the sadness you feel for the injured person. Admitting that you are depressed can be difficult when you're concerned about supporting and protecting your "patient." But as with any other mutual loss, sharing your feelings openly is usually validating for others and creates greater closeness and support for everyone. Trying to hide your sadness is usually not effective. Your injured family member can often read between the lines. David, for example (introduced in Chapter 3), was sure that his mother and sisters went home and "had their little cries." That they didn't cry in front of him was more of a burden to him, because he felt that he, too, had to "be strong" and protect them from his feelings.

You may also find it useful to get additional support and help from a mental health professional or counselor, especially if depression makes you unable to take part in making decisions or solving problems related to the effect of the injury on your family life. Ask for a meeting with a psychologist or social worker in the rehabilitation facility. He or she can either help you directly or refer you to an outside therapist.

Guilt

Bella was finally able to travel to live in the same city as Lamar. (By this time, Bella's husband had returned to his home country, as related in Chapter 9.) But Lamar was not sure whether Bella should live with her or live separately—after all, they were two grown women with different lifestyles. At the same time she felt she should be doing everything for her daughter, that she should be at her beck and call. Lamar talked to another mother of a person with spinal cord injury and to a woman who herself had a spinal cord injury. Both strongly suggested that Bella live independently and that Lamar needed a life of her own.

Mother and daughter opted for separate residences. Bella bought a one-level home that was modified for her needs. But Lamar was still on call when attendants didn't arrive for work. Bella would say, "I'm being abandoned by the attendants." Once, when an attendant didn't show up, Lamar had to perform Bella's bladder catheterization. She was terribly nervous and afraid she would hurt her daughter. Bella started to get angry at the way her mother was performing this chore. And Lamar, for the first time, was able to respond to Bella's anger: "You may not scream at me or you will not have your bladder drained." In the hospital, Lamar had accepted Bella's anger, frequently directed at her, because she thought Bella had had "such a raw deal; she was dealt terrible cards." So how could Lamar protest?

Feelings of guilt can cloud the picture of an injured loved one and strain relationships for many family members. Parents and siblings often feel that, somehow, they could have prevented the injury, even when that was clearly impossible. Some parents feel they hadn't adequately prepared their child to avoid risky behaviors, such as driving while intoxicated. And siblings may experience survivor guilt, asking, "Why him?

Why not me?" Confronting feelings of guilt is important so that these feelings don't cause depression or cause you to avoid the injured person or in some way hinder her recovery and return to independence.

David's fiancée, Myra (see Chapter 3), felt guilty that she couldn't stay home with David during his recovery, although he was well cared for by other family members when she was at work. Myra felt increasingly anxious, angry, and emotionally isolated from her fiancé, eventually seeking psychotherapy to help her cope more effectively.

Guilt sometimes leads family members to feel they have to make up for the losses their loved one has suffered through spinal cord injury. David's sisters "spoiled" him by providing much more assistance with daily tasks than he actually needed. Eventually, David had to refuse their help and let them know he could function on his own.

Similarly, Lamar talks about how she felt guilty and made great sacrifices to help her daughter, sometimes getting no appreciation in return. She felt that Bella had suffered so much that she had no right to demand her daughter's respect and appreciation. A friend eventually helped Lamar to see that she needed to stand up for herself, not to accept this behavior from her daughter. Lamar realized she would be a more effective helper if she demanded respect from her daughter and stopped "martyring" herself. It was also healthier for her daughter to begin accepting responsibility for her behavior and resuming adult roles with her mother and other caregivers.

In Lark's case (see Chapter 8), her mother also became overprotective for a time. Her mother dealt effectively with the period of crisis following the injury, but couldn't shift out of crisis mode. Finally, Lark had to tell her, "Mom, I don't need that anymore. Do for others in the family." As Lark felt ready to manage her own life, she no longer needed someone speaking for her. Her mother was relieved to be "released" by Lark and to resume her varied roles and activities.

Support from Friends

Lamar was sad that her family had not come together as a unit in this time of crisis. She felt alone. "Through all these years, what I feel is most important for a family with a major tragedy is to come together and be supportive as a unit

for the injured person and the caretakers. I didn't have it. It made it more diffi-
cult." She felt even more isolated when she underwent a major operation for a
serious health problem of her own. She was angry that she was alone. She
began a new job a week after surgery. "No one was helping me."

For Lamar, excellent support from friends was crucial in dealing with
her situation. Lamar advises the friends of someone in a similar situation to do "whatever is necessary." This may mean just being there or
taking the person out to dinner. She urges them to do whatever brings
comfort to the family member of the injured person.

Reclaiming One's Life

Lamar hoped to start dating again. Before doing so, she sought psychological
counseling to help her deal with the complicated emotions surrounding her
and Bella's lives. Lamar found that her involvement with her daughter's care
made dating difficult. For instance, one potential date told the friend who
wanted to introduce him to Lamar that he didn't want to go because he didn't
want to confront Lamar's "situation."

Lamar began to feel that no man would want to have her in his life. She felt
like a "victim, crushed." But as she examined her feelings, her personal emphasis
began to change. She realized that any man she dated would have to accept
her daughter along with her. Her friends and therapist reinforced her innate
drive to be positive, helped shift her perceptions about her self-worth, and bol-
stered her ability to assert her needs. "When I took charge, it was no longer an
issue." As a result of her experiences, Lamar, like Jane (introduced in Chapter 7),
stresses the importance of psychological support from a professional, even if
that person has no personal experience with spinal cord injury.

Lamar says that she no longer seeks religious support. She believes that God
has some role but she doesn't know what it is. "Now I don't look for the answer
to 'Why?' It is a part of life, haphazard. It is just no longer a question for me."

Lamar's experience illustrates how the passage of time, new experiences, and connections with others can help convert our perceptions of
loss to an understanding and acceptance of who we are and the strengths
we possess. It is this transition that will enable you to reclaim your life
and point it in the direction that you want to take.

Parenting an Adult Child with Spinal Cord Injury

Parents of an adult child with spinal cord injury are often exposed to the same social stigma that their child experiences. Lamar's potential date, for example, could not deal with the fact that she had a daughter with a severe disability. At first Lamar accepted this with resignation, assuming that no man would ever be interested in her. Later, as she achieved a more stable, enjoyable relationship with her daughter and gained more confidence in herself, she could shrug off social rejection or stereotyping. She was able to restructure her thinking and adopt the view of herself as someone whom any man would be fortunate to know.

Other parents face similar difficulties maintaining confidence in themselves and their choices in the face of social disapproval or even ridicule.

> Steve was a single man who had always lived with his parents. In his thirties he was shot in a robbery attempt and sustained C4 tetraplegia. His mother, a youthful and extremely energetic woman, eagerly welcomed him back to the family home after his rehabilitation and happily assumed all of his attendant care. Steve's father took him out every weekend, and the family enjoyed a close relationship with many mutual interests.
>
> But Steve's mother faced disapproval on two fronts. The rehabilitation staff thought she should "get a life." And some of her friends implied that her providing Steve's personal care was "perverse" and that she was letting Steve take advantage of her by caring for him at home. In fact, Steve's family was simply continuing the kind of relationship they had before his injury. He had always lived at home and had never intended to marry or move out. He had always gone out with Dad on weekends, and Mom had always taken care of him by fixing his meals, cleaning his room, and so forth. Steve's parents valued him and the relationship as much after his injury as before. As their lives at home resumed a stable routine, Steve's mother felt sure she was doing the right thing. When her friends and Steve's doctors saw how well he was doing after several months at home, they developed a new respect for his mother's exceptional competence as a caregiver and for the easy rapport between mother and son. The critical remarks soon disappeared.

Not all parents choose the role Steve's parents did. When an adult child has been living independently for some time before the spinal cord injury, parents may not want to care for her in their home.

> As a twenty-two-year-old graduate student, Sonia was injured in a motor-cycle accident, resulting in C6 tetraplegia. Her parents lived in another state, but temporarily moved to the city where she was hospitalized. After returning home, they decided that they did not want Sonia to live with them. Since starting college at seventeen, Sonia had lived away from her parents. During that time her mother had resumed a career and her father had been promoted to a demanding job in his company. Sonia had always been an independent person and her parents did not want to make her "feel like a baby" by assuming her care. Nor did they wish to give up their own independence and career advancement to care for her. Sonia's parents decided not to bring her home temporarily after her discharge, only to uproot her again later. Instead, they asked Sonia to begin looking for an independent living situation in the city where she'd been in school.
>
> Sonia's parents, whose decision was the opposite of Steve's parents, also faced social disapproval. Many of their friends thought their decision was heartless and cold, and some of the rehabilitation staff saw them as rigid and uncooperative. The couple lost many nights of sleep in soul-searching and second-guessing themselves, but they stuck by their decision despite social pressure.
>
> The social worker at the rehabilitation center helped Sonia find an accessible apartment and apply for Social Security Disability Income. Her parents offered to help pay for her attendant care expenses while she finished graduate school. They kept in touch with her by phone and visited periodically, sometimes offering advice or helping manage a problem with the personal care attendant. When their friends learned that Sonia was successfully living on her own and nearing graduation, their criticisms turned to congratulations. Sonia's parents, far from lacking compassion, had done what was right for their family—fostering Sonia's independence and academic success.

As these examples clearly illustrate, there is no universal road map for parenting an adult child with spinal cord injury. And no matter what choices you make, at times you'll hear criticisms and doubts. For a child with a severe disability and without a spouse or committed partner, parents have to make choices about their role based on financial resources, the accessibility or adaptability of their home, whether they are employed or retired, their own physical health, and so forth. But perhaps the most important factor is choosing a role that is consistent with the relationship you've shared in the past. Compromises may be required, as in any time of crisis, but maintaining the emotional integrity of your relationship with your child is more important than trying to fit into social expectations of self-sacrifice and devotion or rugged independence.

As Lamar's experience shows, the parent of an adult child with spinal cord injury is affected emotionally, socially, financially, and spiritually. In some cases, the family as a whole will come together to support the parent(s) and injured child. In other cases, family or social bonds are severed, and parents must make difficult choices and decisions without much support.

The parents of an injured person come and go from the hospital or rehabilitation center—they are not physically damaged. But they do not escape the emotional and social consequences of spinal cord injury.

A SIBLING'S PERSPECTIVE

Bailey's sister Joan was four years his senior. Despite normal sibling teasing and competition, she'd always "looked out" for him. He admired Joan. She was a good athlete and artist, and Bailey and his family never doubted that when she graduated from college she'd be successful in every way.

Bailey arrived home one day during his sophomore year of high school to find his parents in their room, weeping. A suitcase was sitting on the bed. Bailey had never seen his father cry before, and his first thought was that Joan had died. His parents told him that Joan had fallen from her dormitory balcony and was in the hospital, unconscious. (Joan's story is told in Chapter 4.)

What followed was so tangled in intense emotion that it is somewhat jumbled in Bailey's memory. Not knowing exactly what had occurred, Bailey had only the notion that it was something terrible. He was startled by his parents' rare display of emotion and unsettled by the discovery of their vulnerability. Bailey recalls that being a brother helped him to be tougher. He remembers thinking, "We'll get through this."

His parents went without him for the initial trip to the hospital, but told Bailey everything they had learned about Joan's injury, which had resulted in incomplete tetraplegia. They didn't "sugar coat" it for Bailey, and their ability to face events squarely gave him confidence. He describes the whole family as having an unspoken understanding that they would be strong and get through the crisis, and that the accident wouldn't change them.

Sibling relationships, which endure over a greater span of time than any other family relationship, are important developmentally, emotionally, and socially. They can be important sources of support and companionship. And although they can be strained by competition and jealousy, sibling relationships are strengthened by shared experiences, intimacy, and cooperation.

When a person experiences a life-changing event such as spinal cord injury, the impact on siblings is significant and lasting, as Bailey's story shows.

Sibling Rivalry

Shortly after Joan's accident, someone asked Bailey if he thought Joan would resent him because he could walk. Bailey had visited Joan by this time and knew she was not likely to walk again. But he never felt this resentment from her. Nor did he ever feel jealous that she was getting too much attention as a result of her injury.

All young siblings experience some jealousy, rivalry, or competition for attention as part of normal development, but as they get older this is usually less intense. For young siblings or those with a history of consistent competition, survivor guilt may arise when a brother or sister is injured. The uninjured siblings may feel depressed or unworthy, unable to tolerate the unfairness of being whole and healthy while their sibling is suffering. This was the case with Jeff, who coped with his brother's injury by offering to be his "manservant" until his brother regained independence in activities of daily living.

A sibling can also feel resentful, jealous, and left out when a brother or sister is severely injured and requires an extraordinary amount of parental attention and care. Parental preoccupation with the immediate crisis of the injury, months of rehabilitation, and perhaps years of caregiving can leave the uninjured sibling feeling that she is missing parental involvement. Her positive accomplishments and difficult challenges seem to pale in comparison with the overwhelming concerns of the sibling with the spinal cord injury.

Communicating these feelings is often the key to resolving them. Discuss your guilt feelings or jealousies with your injured brother or sister. This crisis can be an opportunity to forgive each other for old hurts, to improve and deepen your relationship. Providing support and becoming involved in your sibling's rehabilitation are constructive ways to deal with feelings of guilt or despair. Asserting your own needs and setting limits on your involvement will keep resentment from building and help normalize your relationship as your sibling progresses toward greater independence.

Parents of a young teenager with spinal cord injury can reduce potential conflicts between children by including the able-bodied children in planning and preparing for any changes that may be necessary. These changes might include altered sleeping arrangements or daily routines, different childcare plans, or reassignment of chores. In our experience, the less the children's routines and responsibilities are affected, the less resentful and more positive they will be.

Let your children share their opinions and be actively involved in reassigning chores, as well as visiting and talking with their injured sibling. And try to have some special time for each child. If you must be away from other children in order to care for the injured child, communicate frequently with them and let them know they are important to you. As much as possible, try to balance rehabilitation with the normal family process, so that all family members can express their feelings, be involved in planning, and experience a sense of family cohesion rather than family conflict.

Siblings' Anxieties and Coping Skills

Bailey was actively involved in his sister's recovery from the very start. He visited her frequently during her stay at the rehabilitation hospital, became involved in her physical therapy, and even learned to do everything in a wheelchair himself! He enjoyed the time that he and Joan shared in the hospital, time they wouldn't have had if she had been at college. He grew closer to Joan as he spent many hours talking with her.

People often remark that Bailey's experience must have been "unbelievable," but Bailey says it was just something he had to get through. He discovered a lot of strength in himself and his family, and he believes that we all have more strength than we realize. Bailey's ability to focus on the here and now and on solving immediate problems helped him to keep his anxieties at bay. "Our whole family is very good about saying, 'Let's fix it, correct it, and get through it.'" He didn't deny the severity or permanence of Joan's disability, but he chose to focus on the belief that she could handle it and that they would get through it together.

Just as the person with a spinal cord injury has to focus on the positive and defend against negative thoughts and feelings at certain points in the recovery, so do brothers and sisters. Most siblings are anxious about the injury. Some decrease this anxiety through intense intellectual efforts—seeking out information, thoroughly analyzing the situation, and learning what is needed to cope with various "disasters." This method of coping includes plenty of verbal communication and may allow an emotional catharsis while preventing anxiety from becoming overwhelming.

Some siblings attempt to deny the trauma by not discussing it at all. A brother or sister who deals with anxiety in this way may try to control expressions of emotion in other siblings, forbidding discussion of the injury. This is generally a maladaptive pattern. It temporarily eases anxieties but effectively blocks problem-solving, and it leads to a buildup of emotions that may eventually be released in harmful or inappropriate ways.

Bailey used a combination of methods to cope with Joan's injury. Following the family pattern, he openly confronted the reality of Joan's injury, but he decided not to analyze or dwell on his anxieties. He blocked out negative thoughts and emotions and chose to focus on positive changes in Joan's condition. This enabled him to support Joan and become involved in her recovery without feeling emotionally burdened.

Siblings as Advocates

Bailey identifies with his sister's difficulties. Initially he was worried about how she would make her way in the world, and even now, although she is success-

fully employed and living independently, he gets angry when her progress is blocked by architectural barriers, economic restrictions, or the insensitive atti- tudes and behaviors of others. Like many people who are employed after a spi- nal cord injury, Joan "falls through the cracks" economically, in that she makes too much money to qualify for government assistance programs but not enough to pay the high prices required for the best equipment. Bailey feels frus- trated: "I don't know how to change all that."

His other pet peeve is people without proper permits who park in spaces des- ignated for those with handicaps. "I'd like to be a traffic cop!" he jokes. But he sees that this is a serious source of frustration for people who really need these designated parking spots.

Bailey is also upset with medical doctors who aren't cooperative with Joan. Often he sees doctors who want to "cure everything" and urge Joan to focus just on her physical condition, rather than addressing the particular problem Joan has brought up. As an advocate for Joan, he sometimes wants to challenge her doctors but is afraid of "turning them off" and perhaps interfering with Joan's ability to get help in the future.

Adult siblings can be forceful advocates for a person with a spinal cord injury, and this is also a way for siblings to channel some of their anger and anxiety. Letter writing, political action, and legal recourse are ave- nues for dealing with architectural, social, and economic barriers to living with a disability. Responses to single incidents of disregard for the law can also be effective, such as reporting cars that are illegally parked in handicapped spaces or complaining to the Better Business Bureau or the Department of Justice, Disability Rights Section, about businesses or other public places that refuse to accommodate people using wheel- chairs.

Because of previous experiences, Bailey is extra cautious in his ap- proach to Joan's doctors. A person with spinal cord injury who goes to a hospital for treatment of medical complications may be cared for by a doctor unfamiliar with the case or even with spinal cord injury. Siblings can be a valuable source of medical information and can help the doctor understand the patient's social situation and individual needs.

Bailey was there every step of the way as Joan progressed from rehabilita- tion to college graduation to successful employment in graphic arts. Though he has been very involved in her life, he often wonders if he has helped enough. And he continues to worry about her when she has pain or other complications due to her injury.

Bailey values his relationship with Joan and admires the person she has become. He asks himself, if the accident had never occurred, would Joan have accomplished all that she has? Bailey sees Joan's spinal cord injury as part of who she is, and he knows that her accomplishments, relationships, and giving nature were shaped in part by the process of adapting to the injury.

Over the years, Bailey's view of Joan's spinal cord injury has broadened to include not only the positive aspects but an appreciation of the difficult realities that must be faced throughout life. Balancing what he can change or control with what he must simply accept is Bailey's juggling act. Like any loving sibling, Bailey shares the bad times and the good times with Joan.

TWO WIVES' PERSPECTIVES

Michaela was a young pharmacy technician on her day off; she was to meet a friend at the local military base barracks and go to the rodeo. During her search for her friend, she met Scott (who was introduced in Chapter 1). They were married not too long after.

Scott was a dedicated career Marine. Michaela was proud of him and found the role of military wife one she enjoyed. When he was deployed to Iraq, she lived on the military base, raising their children, a girl, two, and a boy, five.

One day shortly after arriving home with the children from a free carnival put on for military families, Michaela found a captain in "dress blues" and a chaplain at her front door. "On behalf of a grateful nation . . . ," the captain began. She immediately thought that Scott had been killed; she wouldn't let them leave until "they told me he was alive." (At pre-deployment she had not been warned that not only death but serious injuries also warranted these visits.) She remembered "tuning out" the Navy chaplain because the visit seemed so routine to him.

Michaela felt alone and unprepared for Scott's injury. "I was an orphan," she says. Four months earlier, her mother had died. Before that she had lost her father, whom she had cared for into his eighties as he battled Parkinson's disease. "I was completely shocked. Scott was the last person anyone expected to get hurt. He was in the armed forces for life; he had been in for nine years and *was a sergeant. He was so good." Scott was injured one day; she was notified the next. She knew that life would be different.*

Scott was flown to a naval hospital where he was in the ICU for five days. Then he was transferred to a Veterans Administration hospital for rehabilitation. She remembers the great hope they had for recovery; they were confident Scott would walk in three months. The staff were much more pessimistic; on the fourth day, a nurse told them, "You guys are on drugs." Scott's family was involved and present when he arrived home from Iraq. Michaela regretted that there was no private time for Scott and her to be alone to talk and console each other.

Emotional support came from a social worker at the hospital. They couldn't afford a babysitter so a volunteer played with the children at the hospital. It also helped that Michaela could sleep in the extra bed in Scott's room. The nurses ordered in pizza for them.

Michaela felt abandoned by some families with whom they had been friendly. When she called to tell them about Scott, some hung up on her, either in disbelief or because they were unable to process the information. Michaela, feeling the loss of old friends, had no time or energy to seek out new friends during Scott's recovery. But some people did come to their aid; especially helpful were people in his unit. The church helped, too, sending the children to camp and bringing dinners for the family.

Michaela's emotional reactions to Scott's unexpected injury ran the gamut from fear, grief, and feeling alone, to hope and confidence in Scott's recovery. Despite the fact that Scott was on active duty in a war zone, she had thought of him as invulnerable and was shocked by his serious injury. Michaela knew that life would be different, and she needed time to reconnect emotionally with Scott, to renew her feeling of intimacy with him, and to integrate his disability into their life as a couple and family. She felt stymied in this process by both a lack of privacy during Scott's rehabilitation and a lack of meaningful social support.

Michaela's experience was very different from that of Tricia, who met her husband Lee after he had been living with a spinal cord injury for some time.

Tricia had some firsthand experience in living with a person with spinal cord injury. When she was a freshman in high school, the fiancé of her older sister,

Pam, was paralyzed in a car accident. Tricia's family took in the fiancé because his family couldn't deal with the disability. The seven children in Tricia's family teased him and treated him like one of the family and certainly did not cater to his disability.

Pam and her fiancé were asked by the mother of a young man with a recent spinal cord injury to visit him in the hospital. Tricia recalls Pam's comment after the visit: "He'll do all right. He's already making adjustments." The young man was called Lee (his story is told in Chapter 10).

Following high school graduation, Tricia took her college degree in business management. Her grandmother had always advised her "not to look at boys" until she'd finished her education, and Tricia took the advice to heart. She met Lee shortly before her college graduation, and soon they started dating. Her future mother-in-law said she knew Lee was serious, because he'd never taken flowers to a girlfriend before Tricia.

Sometimes a person "marries into" disability, as did Tricia when she fell in love with someone with an existing spinal cord injury. The impact of the disability on the able-bodied spouse is different from that experienced when a husband or wife is injured after marriage. The able-bodied partner does not have to grieve for the loss of her partner's abilities or adapt to the change. Instead, her lover comes as he is. The disability is just one of many characteristics of her spouse. By marrying someone who has a spinal cord injury, she makes a choice, and this puts the disability in a different light. Acceptance of the partner includes acceptance of his disability. The injury is not seen as something that invades the relationship, and there is less feeling of loss of control than in cases of injury after marriage.

Expectations, Preconceptions, and Loss in an Extended Family

Tricia and Lee dated for a year and then became engaged. When they told Tricia's parents, her mother and father were concerned. They thought Tricia was just following in her sister's footsteps. They wanted her "to be taken care of." They asked, "Are you sure you know what you're getting into?" Their reaction was disappointing to Tricia and Lee, who had hoped her parents would share their excitement.

For the family, acceptance of the marriage may be difficult. Tricia's parents already had one son-in-law with a spinal cord injury, and they probably had fewer preconceptions about this type of injury than most prospective parents-in-law. Their apprehension was most likely not based on prejudice. They knew very well the problems and limitations that Tricia and Lee would have to manage. They may have experienced a vicarious sense of loss for what Tricia might miss by not having an able-bodied husband. They may have feared that she wasn't strong enough to manage the special problems of living with a spouse with a disability. Or they may have feared that they would be expected to provide an overwhelming amount of assistance to the couple.

Tricia's experience is not unusual. In a study of able-bodied women's perspectives on their marriage to men with spinal cord injury, about half the women reported that their own or their husband's family members objected to the marriage on the basis of the husband's disability, warned the woman against marrying, questioned the woman's motives, or expressed disappointment with her decision. These women were able to withstand their families' disapproval and go ahead with the marriage, something the authors of the study attribute to their "maturity, resiliency, and high levels of autonomy." It is not clear whether conflicts with family members were resolved later in the marriage.

We can speculate that more open communication from family members about their feelings, attitudes, and expectations, combined with a non-defensive attitude and clear explanation of the anticipated realities on the part of the able-bodied spouse, would help ease these conflicts—especially as the marriage proves strong and stable. Although Tricia's family was close knit, they tended to keep feelings to themselves and were not verbally expressive. Had they been more open with Tricia, perhaps she could have understood the fears underlying their apparent disapproval of her marriage.

Extended family members often have a variety of expectations and preconceptions about spinal cord injury—some accurate, some not—that influence their opinions and affect their feelings. Even when a spouse is injured after marriage, the extended family's expectations can cause problems if not addressed directly and openly.

Billy became paraplegic as a result of a car accident. Two years later, he was talking to his cousin Alan about Alan's recent marital problems. In the course of this discussion, Alan said, "I can't believe you're still married. I thought your wife would've left you after the accident." Billy, happily married for ten years, was shocked and hurt. But in talking further with Alan he realized that his cousin's remark reflected Alan's own insecurity and fears of inadequacy and some false assumptions about the effects of spinal cord injury. Billy explained how he and his wife had adapted to his injury and how much more important was their love for each other than were his physical limitations. He corrected some of Alan's misconceptions about paraplegia, and he helped Alan see that his own imperfections did not mean that he was unworthy or unable to repair his marriage.

Extended family members' concerns are best addressed by acknowledging the mixture of realistic and distorted ideas about spinal cord injury and providing information and discussion that can increase understanding and reduce anxiety for everyone.

Marriage, Children, and Family Life

While her parents were apprehensive about her marriage, Tricia's brothers and sisters were excited and supportive. "They knew how I loved Lee and knew we would take challenges as they came along," Tricia recalls. Friends' reactions were generally positive. Tricia lost touch with some girlfriends, but she attributes this to the fact that she no longer had lots of time for friends.

Tricia was twenty-four and Lee was twenty-six when they married. He was a third-year law student, and Tricia managed a shoe store to support them. After Lee graduated, they moved to a city where he was offered a good job by a large organization. The couple led a very active social life, including lots of travel, and they were close to their families. Both were sports oriented: Tricia was a tennis player and Lee was into wheelchair basketball.

People would ask Tricia, "What are you going to do about kids?" She felt they were asking about the physical ability to conceive, which she considered a private matter, and were questioning Lee's ability to handle the physical aspects of raising a child. But Lee and Tricia wanted a family and were determined they would find a way to work out the practical problems of parenting. Several years after they were married, Tricia became pregnant with their first child, a son.

Three years later, Tricia gave birth to triplets, a boy and two girls. Their arrival put the family into "automatic mode," says Tricia. Her mother moved in with them, and each adult tended one of the triplets. The newest son was very ill with a liver ailment and had to sleep with Tricia for the first six to eight months. After that, Lee assumed the boy's nightly care, preparing all his medications and sleeping with him. The boy had to be tube-fed and catheterized. Tricia notes that, though difficult, it was a time of bonding between father and son. The little boy underwent surgery to correct his liver ailment and responded very well.

Does their life differ from that of any other family with four children? Tricia thinks they are more like other families than not. When Lee arrives home from work, they have dinner. Then Lee spends time with the children in the basement, doing homework or playing ball. When the children were young, Tricia bathed them, Lee wrapped them in towels, dried them, and dressed them for bed. He took them on his lap in his wheelchair up the elevator to their bedrooms for a story. That was Tricia's break time. After Lee had tucked in the children, he cleaned up the kitchen, not liking clutter facing him the next morning.

Tricia keeps "open lines" for her children to express feelings. One day, after Lee had accompanied his son's class on a field trip, Tricia asked him if it bothered him that Dad used a wheelchair. He replied, "Sometimes, Mom, I wish he could run." But on another occasion he told her, "I forget Daddy uses a chair because he can do everything other dads do."

They follow the children's leads in answering questions about Lee's disability. The first question was, "Why don't Daddy's legs work?" Now when the family is out in public and a child asks why Lee is using a wheelchair, the children take responsibility for the reply: "His legs don't work." In order to desensitize the children to the disability and wheelchair, Lee has taught them how to use the wheelchair and invites their friends to play in the chair. Sometimes there are challenges from children. When Lee was an assistant coach on his son's soccer team, one boy on the team approached Lee, saying, "You're telling me how to do it, but you can't do it." Lee explained that although he couldn't actually get up and show him how to do it, he knew all the rules and plays in soccer and he could teach him, verbally, how to improve his game.

Always close to her own family, Tricia has also grown closer to Lee's parents as the years have passed. Lee's folks have always been very active in their lives, visiting often, usually once a month, helping to paint or fix a swing set. They also telephone frequently. At first, Tricia had to get accustomed to these frequent calls, which she interpreted as the parents' attempt to make Lee dependent. Her own family was very independent and stood back. She now under-

stands that his family simply has a different, very open communication style that she has come to appreciate.

Lee's parents had been excited about the marriage. His mother cried when they announced the impending arrival of the first grandchild. They were so happy that Lee was going to have a family. And they were amazed at the arrival of the triplets. Lee's father had a hard time when Lee was first hurt. He blamed himself and God and stopped going to church. He asked, "Why did God do that? What is the lesson?" However, when his grandson's liver problem was repaired surgically, Lee's father returned to church to thank God for "this miracle." He also feels now that Lee is not missing out on anything in life.

Of Lee's relationship with his mother and father, Tricia says, "I cherish Lee's relationship with his parents. In my household we kept feelings in. You'd stay mad for a couple of months. I learned how to get feelings out with Lee." Although she and Lee have been married many years, Tricia sometimes finds that she forgets he has a disability. "Recently I hit him on the leg to get his attention and was upset with him when he didn't respond!" On the other hand, her greatest fear is that Lee won't be there for her if something happens to him, like a pressure sore or a problem with his legs. "His body takes so long to heal." But Lee's greater physical vulnerability is balanced by his emotional strengths and the many contributions he makes to the marriage. As Tricia points out, when two individuals, one of whom has a disability, fall in love and choose each other as partners, their union accommodates the limitations imposed by disability. The effect of the disability is lessened by adapting the home for individual needs, delegating chores fairly, communicating feelings openly, and accepting help from extended family when necessary. These strategies are used by many successful couples, with or without a disability.

CHILDREN OF PARENTS WITH SPINAL CORD INJURY: ADJUSTING, LEARNING, COPING

Surprisingly little has been written about how a parent's spinal cord injury, or indeed any disability, affects a child psychologically or socially. As far as we know, the child suffers no ill effects in emotional, social, or intellectual development. However, research data are lacking. Most of the available literature for parents with spinal cord injury focuses on the needs of the parents themselves, such as adaptive equipment for baby and child care and sources of emotional and social support. These resources are very beneficial for new parents who have a spinal cord injury or for those who are injured while they are raising small children. One such resource is Through the Looking Glass: National Resource Center for Parents with Disabilities, which publishes a newsletter and has an Internet site for sharing information (see the Resources section at the end of this book). Other Internet sites also focus on how to parent with a disability. While this type of assistance to parents clearly benefits children, it doesn't deal directly with the *children's* perspectives or needs. Some general comments about how children adapt to crises and loss may be helpful.

Young children are very adaptable and can thrive in almost any type of family situation that meets their needs for physical care, affection, intellectual stimulation, and emotional security. One parent can take on specific physical tasks that the parent with a disability cannot perform. Except in cases of severe disability, the parent with spinal cord injury can, perhaps with special adaptations, still participate in tasks such as bathing, dressing, and carrying children. Even when physical care of the child is limited or impossible, there is no reason why the child cannot form a close relationship with that parent with affectionate bonding, learning, and play.

Nora (whose story is told in Chapter 7) raised five children after becoming paraplegic, and she is now a grandmother. Her children helped out with a variety of household chores, but not necessarily more than might have been expected in any large family. They developed normally and went on to have careers and families of their own.

Children born or adopted as infants into families in which a parent has a spinal cord injury learn about their parent's disability from day one. They adapt to it as they do to any other circumstances that might be somewhat different from those of their friends. On the other hand, when a parent acquires a spinal cord injury during a child's school years, the child is likely to experience some temporary emotional disruption. Children react to trauma in a parent primarily with anxiety and fear, sometimes in the form of nightmares, developmental regressions, or problems at school. Children may also grieve. Older children or teenagers, who have a better grasp of the implications of their parent's injury, may react with sadness, mourning, or depression.

Children need time to adjust to the changes in a parent who has a significant injury. Giving them simple but truthful answers to their questions ("Mommy's back got hurt and her legs don't work, but she can use a wheelchair"), validating their emotional responses ("I know you are scared about Dad. Mommy's scared, too"), and reassuring them ("Dad's not going to die"; "Mom will be coming home soon") will help them understand what's going on and allay their fears. If you have young children, you may want the family to meet with a social worker or psychologist for a few sessions of counseling. This can help you become comfortable talking with your children about the impact of the spinal cord injury on family roles and responsibilities and about other unavoidable disruptions such as moving to a new house, job changes, and so forth. Once children feel certain that the spinal cord injury will not prevent you from loving and caring about them, they usually make a good adjustment.

Children, like all members of society, are becoming more knowledgeable about disabilities. This has resulted in part from the mainstreaming of children with disabilities and from disability awareness programs in public schools.

Elliott (see Chapter 6), whose daughter was born after he developed incomplete tetraplegia, volunteered to speak to her class about disability, and the class enjoyed his presentation. Parents with spinal cord injury such as Lee and Elliott, who are involved in their children's school, sports, or other group activities, project a positive image for their own children and for others. They help to dispel fears and misconceptions just by being "out there."

Some children of parents with spinal cord injury will have emotional difficulties, however, despite the best efforts of parents, teachers, and community to educate and reassure them. If a child appears depressed for more than two weeks, has persistent trouble at school, or withdraws from playmates following a parent's injury or return home from the hospital, seek professional evaluation and guidance. The school guidance counselor, the school psychologist, or a community-based child psychologist can help the child cope with feelings or work with the family to help create more emotional security for the child.

PHYSICAL STRAIN, FINANCIAL STRESS, AND CAREGIVER BURNOUT

When Scott returned home after his inpatient rehabilitation, Michaela found that there were few protocols in place to help young service men and their families. Scott was one of the first American soldiers to sustain a spinal cord injury in the conflict in Iraq, and his housing and accessibility needs were not well understood by the base authorities. The initial move home (to the base) was stressful because Michaela was "scared to death" of the total responsibility for the care of Scott; there had always been a nurse at the other end of the call button. She took him for outpatient physical therapy five days a week. A home health nurse came two hours each day and a Navy corpsman who lived two doors away helped her if Scott had a medical crisis.

At first, base housing wanted to move Scott and Michaela to a two-story unit, which would have been inaccessible to Scott. Michaela felt they were saying "we were worthless, just kick them out of the service." Fortunately, the commanding general stepped in, saying, "You don't do that to my Marine." They then became the first to get accessible housing, which meant only "one floor" to the builders. They didn't understand that Scot needed entrée to and from the house, wide doors and hallways, lowered switches, and an accessible bathroom and kitchen. Michaela says, "We helped; we were the guinea pigs; we picked out things for the fifteen accessible housing units that were erected."

Once in accessible housing, Michaela felt like they were pioneers. One set of problems was solved, then another arose. She frequently had to advocate for Scott's and the family's needs. She requested that the base install curb-cuts so that Scott could move around the neighborhood in his wheelchair. When there was no reply to her request, she discovered the power of the press. Local TV featured Scott on the news, restricted by lack of curb-cuts; they were soon set in place. Scott could then walk his children to school. He could also take them to the playground, but then his wheelchair would get stuck in the sand. Michaela campaigned for wood chips so that the children would have their father near them while they played.

When Scott was away on duty, Michaela had all the time in the world. Now she was providing total care of her husband and two small children and constantly helping Scott to overcome physical and social barriers on the base. Michaela was exhausted, up every two hours at night, to care for Scott. Their once-confident five-year-old boy was now very fearful, while their two-year-old daughter was still not potty trained.

Scott decided that his family would be better served living near his parents and siblings in the Midwest, far from the coast where Michaela had grown up. While this has made it possible for Scott's family to help Michaela with Scott's care, it has been a difficult transition for her. She misses her friends and the outdoor activities of a beach community.

There has been dramatic change—and stress—in Michaela's life in the last few years. She finds that she is less patient, has a "shorter fuse," and is usually tired. She sometimes forces herself to put work down to play with the children. She has become a worrier, concerned about risks and how little things have the capacity to change your life.

Families feel the physical impact of their loved one's disability when they have to take over physically demanding chores that were once performed by the person with spinal cord injury, while at the same time providing attendant care or other physical assistance for the injured person. Homemakers like Michaela whose husbands are injured may be faced with double duty, taking on chores that were once the husband's responsibility, such as yard work, household repairs, or shoveling snow. A person working full-time whose spouse has a severe spinal cord injury might have to take on additional homemaking chores in the evening, such as cooking and cleaning, bathing the children, or shopping for groceries. A spouse may also have to help the injured person transfer in and out of a wheelchair, push the wheelchair, assist with bathing or dressing, and act as a "gofer" for items that aren't readily accessible to his or her mate. When the person with spinal cord injury develops a medical complication, for example, a decubitus ulcer (pressure sore), the spouse may temporarily have to assume all responsibility for running the home.

Spouses like Michaela may also experience emotional burnout, the combined result of excessive physical demands, lack of sleep, role changes, loss of social support, and limited opportunities for enjoyable activities or time alone. Spouses share the emotional and social impact of a new spinal cord injury. Taking on new social roles as Michaela did (such as advocating for accessibility), can be rewarding, but is often initially a source of stress and fatigue. Whether you are a spouse, parent, sibling, or other relative, living with a person with spinal cord injury frequently produces physical stress and fatigue. When you feel overtired, it's a signal that you've done too much and need a break. Sometimes family members push themselves relentlessly because they feel guilty or entirely responsible, as we discussed earlier. But pushing yourself too hard can lead to burnout. You become exhausted, depressed, resentful, and emotionally detached.

> *How is Tricia's life different from what it would have been if she'd married someone without a disability? "The burden is on me to do much of the physical." For example, she had to put the triplets in their car seats and buckle them in, because Lee could not get in the back of the van to do that. When they took the children to the doctor, she did most of the carrying. "Sometimes it seemed as if everything fell on me, especially getting in and out of the car." The physical demands of caring for and traveling with four small children were frequently exhausting. Although Lee knows when she's "out of steam" and is willing to help in any way he can, Tricia still performs a greater share of the physical chores.*

Physical stress and exhaustion are not products of your personal failure. These are common phenomena when close family members assume care for a person with a significant disability. But you can minimize this stress in several ways.

1. Like Tricia, stay in tune with your limits. When you "run out of steam," take a break. Ask for help from other relatives or friends, or consider hiring part-time help if you can afford it.

2. Make sure the person with a spinal cord injury is really taking on all the activities he can. Encourage him to maximize his strength by keeping up with physical therapy or an exercise program if appropriate, and to do everything possible to avoid medical problems. Let him lighten your load when possible—for example, by carrying items on his lap when you are shopping together. Women in the study on marriage mentioned earlier found it very helpful, both practically and psychologically, to support their husband's autonomy and independence. "Although participants were willing to assume a heavier domestic role and/or economic role within their relationships . . . they expected their partners to make contributions . . . commensurate with their abilities, and to share in responsibility when it was feasible."

3. Ask your local rehabilitation center about technological aids that can make your job as a caregiver easier, such as an automatic lift to transfer your family member in and out of bed. Let the doctor or thera-

pist know if you are feeling strained, and ask about ideas and resources for assistance.

4. If the person you are caring for requires constant care, for example, because she uses a ventilator or because of a medical problem, you may want to look into short-term respite care, which many nursing homes can provide. While families often hesitate to "put" their loved one in a nursing home, this is sometimes the only way to get a much needed vacation from the physical demands of caregiving. And it may actually provide your disabled loved one with the temporary luxury of being cared for as much or as little as he wants and not having to push himself to meet family expectations.

Having double roles as spouse and caregiver often creates emotional stress that contributes to burnout. If your spouse with a spinal cord injury needs assistance with bowel and bladder care, you may be perfectly willing to provide it. Yet you might find that emptying your wife's urinary drainage bag or giving your husband the suppository for his bowel program makes you feel more like a parent and less like a spouse. This can interfere with your ability to feel romantic or sexual toward your spouse or to see him or her as a competent, equal partner. If this chore makes you uncomfortable or creates relationship stress, you may want to consider hiring an attendant specifically for bowel and bladder care or asking another relative of the same sex as your spouse to help you out.

Finally, caregivers may be stressed by the multitude of issues that arise from their loved one's injury, especially during the early phases of rehabilitation when so many variables must be considered. When Peter's spinal cord was damaged (see Chapter 3), all his energy went into his physical and spiritual recovery. He wasn't even thinking about finances, insurance, or whether his house would be accessible when he went home. His wife, however, was extremely anxious about whether his hospital bills would be covered by Medicare, whether his pension would cover their living expenses, and whom she could hire to adapt their split-level home for Peter's return. Peter feels that his wife lost a lot more than he did. He thinks that more information from the rehabilitation staff early in his hospitalization would have helped alleviate her worries.

Economically, spinal cord injury can have monumental consequences. Medical attention, mobility aids, therapies, making homes accessible, and finding appropriate transportation add up to a huge economic burden and, often, the need for economic assistance. Although economic re-sources are available for the individual with spinal cord injury (see Chapter 7), families frequently need to fill in gaps in insurance coverage or supplement disability payments. Even with maximal use of benefits, the expense associated with spinal cord injury can result in financial hardship for many families. Yet some families worry that questions about medical insurance, unemployment insurance, or financial assistance are inappropriate at a time when their first concern should be the health and recovery of their loved one. Or perhaps they simply don't know whom to ask.

You can help avoid unnecessary stress by asking to meet with the hospital social worker, who can usually assist you in navigating the complex waters of insurance and disability payment applications, act as a liaison with your or your loved one's employer, and provide information on a variety of social service agencies and economic benefits that may be available to you. Hospital staff understand that you must deal with financial and practical matters affecting your family and that you can't devote all your energy to being emotionally on call for your loved one.

Family members have to evaluate for themselves the physical demands, relationship stresses, and social pressures that can stem from the care-giver role. Some families find that caregiving creates greater closeness in the family, avoids the expense of hired attendant care, and is emotionally rewarding for the caregiver. In other families, the strain of caregiving obligations can stress the fabric of family relationships. You can reduce these stresses, using the guidelines given above, or you can choose another option that would be best for your family. Community hospitals and social service agencies frequently offer workshops or support group meetings for caregivers, and several organizations provide support to caregiving families, such as the National Family Care Givers Association (see the Resources section at the end of this book).

Although Tricia has an extra share of physical chores, she and Lee collaborate on many activities. For instance, recently they put up a closet door, with Lee holding it while Tricia put it in place and secured it. Tricia takes out the garbage and does the recycling. She does the yard work, including the mowing, although Lee laughingly says he'd gladly take over if they got a ride-on mower. But Tricia finds yard work a time for solitude while Lee cares for the children. Sometimes, she says, she wishes Lee could do certain things to help her in the garden. But then she sees able-bodied husbands who don't help. Unlike many husbands, Lee does all the holiday cooking. Tricia says he's great in the kitchen!

SPIRITUALITY AND COPING WITH THE SPINAL CORD INJURY OF A LOVED ONE

Spirituality may be enhanced or extinguished when spinal cord injury hits. Depending in part on your individual beliefs and the meaning of spirituality in your daily life, you may find that the crisis of spinal cord injury strengthens your faith or shatters it. Lamar found sustenance in prayer and religious ritual and comfort in believing that God would help her daughter survive. In another family, siblings reacted in opposite ways when a brother was injured in a skiing accident. Janet became very angry with God for allowing this to happen to her vibrant brother. She thought that a good and just God would have prevented this injustice. She dropped out of her congregation and quit praying. But her brother, Vince, in response to the same situation, felt that God had intervened to keep their brother alive and that God would support their family through their brother's rehabilitation. He saw his brother's progress as a sign of God's help and became even more religiously observant.

Spirituality is how some people assign meaning or purpose to the loss their loved one has sustained. Spirituality can take many forms. It may be a belief in a shared consciousness, a higher power, or some other force that connects events and people in "mysterious" ways but ultimately produces personal growth or some other good out of seemingly tragic events (see Chapter 3 for more discussion of spirituality).

Many resources associated with religion and spirituality are available to families. Most hospitals have a chaplain on call for families who want pastoral counseling or support. You can request a clergyman of your own religion, and many hospitals can provide this service. Religiously affiliated hospitals often have their own pastoral counseling department and may offer religious services on site. Many families find contact with clergy helpful, even if of a different religion. Your own house of worship is usually a wonderful source of social, practical, and sometimes economic support, as well as spiritual guidance. And religiously affiliated social service agencies can provide economic and vocational assistance above and beyond that available from government agencies. Don't hesitate to call on these resources even if you are not particularly observant or religious.

FAMILY SUPPORT FROM THE SUPPORT NETWORK

Families experiencing a spinal cord injury usually need information and support, and the best source is usually other families who have a child, parent, or spouse with spinal cord injury.

When Lee was newly injured, he was visited by what would turn out to be his future brother-in-law and sister-in-law. This established a life-long relationship that included both information and support. Lee's family could probably have benefited as much—or more—from contact with these visitors in the early months of Lee's rehabilitation, when they were scared and depressed. Some rehabilitation facilities have established programs for peer support or counseling and may be able to arrange a meeting between your family and a family already living with spinal cord injury. Lamar received visits from parents of people with spinal cord injury and from people with spinal cord injury themselves. They presented different ideas on parenting and on her rights and responsibilities.

Local spinal cord injury associations have a wealth of information to offer families. They often have organized groups of volunteers who visit families or answer their phone calls. You can find them through the National Spinal Cord Injury Association, your local rehabilitation center, or your local government office for people with disabilities (see the Resources section at the end of this book for this and other types of support). Some outpatient rehabilitation programs and spinal cord injury organizations offer support groups specifically for spouses or families of people with spinal cord injury. Others provide fact sheets and other assistance on how to start a support group in your own community if one does not exist.

Other sources of information for families include periodicals and books by and about people with spinal cord injury. The Internet has many sites pertaining to all aspects of spinal cord injury treatment and research and can be used for exchange of information with other families via chat rooms and e-mail service.

Economic, social, and emotional support is often available through houses of worship in the community, many of which have "caring committees" or other organized groups that provide assistance to members during economic or family crises. Social service organizations affiliated with religious groups are excellent resources for a variety of supports. Government and community-sponsored agencies can also provide economic and practical help.

Family members who feel emotionally overwhelmed or unable to function effectively should consider seeking help from a professional psychologist, social worker, or psychiatrist who is experienced in working with families having health crises. Your state psychological, social work, or psychiatric association can usually provide referrals to competent professionals. Many spinal cord injury or rehabilitation centers have mental health professionals on staff. Some rehabilitation programs offer counseling or therapy groups for families of current patients, or may provide family therapy to individual families when needed.

THE WELL-ADJUSTED FAMILY MEMBER

How will you know when you have adjusted to being the relative of someone with a spinal cord injury? When can you say that you've balanced your life in a healthy way? For family members, as for the person with the injury, adjustment is an ongoing process. If you are married to or live with and perhaps care for a person with spinal cord injury, you'll be continually adapting and adjusting as you pass through various stages of life, face new challenges, and cope with additional health problems and limitations that come with aging.

Some family members find it helpful to make contingency plans in anticipation of future needs. When Bailey and his wife built their new home, they included ramps for access to the first and lower levels and a separate bedroom for Bailey's sister, Joan, who uses a power wheelchair. Though Bailey thinks Joan's living with them is "an off-the-wall scenario" given her dogged independence, his wife wanted to be prepared. If Joan needs more help from them in the future, the transition will be much easier for Bailey and his wife because they have anticipated and prepared for the possibility.

On the other hand, you and your adult loved one must resume an adult-to-adult relationship and move beyond the confining roles of "caregiver" and "patient." One clue that your family is getting back to normal is when your perception of your family member with spinal cord injury shifts and you begin to see him as "plain old Joe" rather than "poor Joe, the paraplegic" or "disabled Joe." Although initially you may have treated him as ill or fragile, you'll eventually be willing to argue with him and tease him, or ask him for help, just as you did before his injury. Like Bailey, you'll find that the spinal cord injury becomes "transparent." You will probably start to feel more like yourself, too, as you begin to focus more on your own life again and less on your loved one's needs. Your relationship can once again be freer and more equal, with give and take on both sides.

As you adjust to your new family circumstances, you'll be able to pick up the pieces of your life, turning to things that may have been put on hold while you were attending primarily to the needs of your family member. You should once again be able to function at work, in school, in social relationships, and in other important areas as effectively as you once did. Of course, you may have some modifications in your schedule or level of involvement with certain activities, especially if you've taken on a caregiver role. But, for your mental health, you must have some respite from this role, times when you participate in social and leisure activities that give you a "lift" and restore your energies.

Whatever role or lifestyle you choose, feel free to pursue some of your goals and dreams and attend to your own personal development. If you find your life holds little meaning or interest beyond caring for or worrying about your injured loved one, consider getting some professional counseling. Trying to take control of or "micromanage" the life of your injured family member is not helpful for him. Nor is the person with a spinal cord injury helped by having a family member "in her clutches" at all times. A balancing of each person's needs will avoid prolonged dependence or manipulative behavior and will help promote the development of coping strategies, psychological well-being, and recovery of normal life functions for both the person with the injury and the family members.

Bailey has had to struggle with the conflict between attending to his own life and worrying about his sister's well-being. He has been very involved with Joan from the moment she was injured. Even so, Bailey sometimes feels guilty, wondering if he's doing enough. At times he has even thought of quitting his busi-

ness in order to devote more time to Joan. He has asked himself, should I go over to see her every night? But then he remembers that Joan is an independent adult with her own life and doesn't need his constant companionship. In fact, her schedule is often too crammed to fit in a visit from him! That pleases him immensely.

A well-adjusted family undergoes a constant rebalancing of roles and responsibilities, allowing the needs of each member to be met. Keeping this balance can be tricky when you have a spouse or other family member with special needs. As Tricia discovered, it's important to work together to find ways for the person with a spinal cord injury to contribute so that other family members are not forced to take on a larger share in all aspects of family life.

> *Michaela's life with Scott since his injury is different not only because of Scott's physical limitations and needs but because of their move to the Midwest, which has forced Michaela to make adaptations of her own. Living in a small farming community has been a radical change. She is gradually adapting, taking on new hobbies, such as biking around the nearby lake and berry picking. She and Scott take occasional road trips to major league baseball games. Life is slow paced. They joined a church, but they found getting everyone ready for services on time was a challenge.*
>
> *Michaela has a new friend, and together they have built a business making and selling crafts at craft shows; Michaela says this is perfect for her as she has to be home anyway. Scott and his brother started a business, too.*

By expecting your loved one's competent participation in family life, you'll help him recover his confidence in himself and regain effectiveness in the family and other social relationships. Both family support and the injured person's perceptions of family needs and expectations are important motivators for recovery from spinal cord injury, right from the start.

Christopher Reeve, in his autobiography, *Still Me*, relates his feelings of despair when he first realized the extent of his injury (C1–C2 tetraplegia). He felt that his life was ruined. He wanted to die. But his wife's affirmation of her love and commitment to him and his three-year-old son's eagerness to talk and snuggle with him ended his thoughts of suicide. The interdependence of close relationships gave him the support he needed to recover. And later, his responsibility for his own mental health and productivity allowed him to provide the support his family needed from him. "I know I have to give when sometimes I really want to take. I've realized . . . that it's part of my job as a father now not to cause Will to worry about me. If I were to give in to self pity . . . it would place an unfair burden on this carefree five-year-old." Reeve also spoke about the needs of his older children to get advice from him and his wife's need for companionship and love from him. Family relationships clearly had an important impact on his recovery.

As your relationship with your loved one normalizes, you'll be able to do what all families do: negotiate, delegate tasks, swap roles on occasion, and provide emotional support for each other. You can be a loving wife, husband, companion, parent, sibling, or child without sacrificing your own well-being. And you can help along your loved one's recovery by expecting his or her love and helpfulness, too.

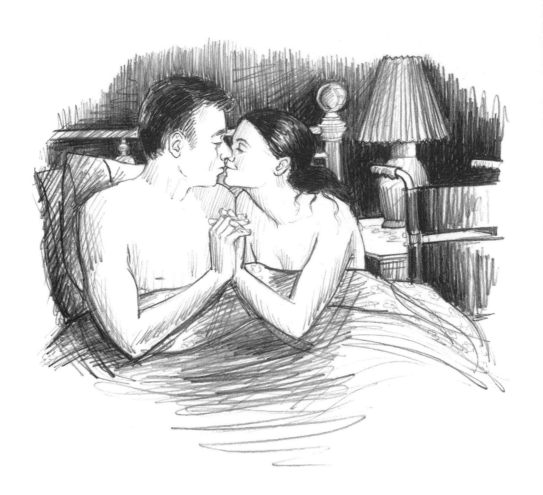

6

Lovers' Lane
Dating, Coupling, and Sexuality

At forty-one, Elliott has been living with tetraplegia for twenty-three years. Following his injury, he married, became a father, got divorced, then dated and remarried. He is employed full-time, drives his own van, and uses a power wheelchair.

Elliott was a precocious teenager, with a steady girlfriend by the age of fifteen. His father had left the family when Elliott was three, cutting off contact with Elliott and his older brother. Elliott's teen years were marked by tension with his stepfather. By sixteen, Elliott had left home and moved to a neighboring state. He easily found jobs in construction and was able to make ends meet. By the age of seventeen he was living like an adult—renting his own place, driving a car, and working full-time. Elliott went home to visit his parents and girlfriend on occasion, but he had no desire to move back home.

During the summer when he was eighteen years old, Elliott was visiting the home of his girlfriend's parents in a bayside town. Eager for a swim, he dived off the dock without stopping to ask about the depth of the water, and his head hit the bottom. He sustained a spinal cord injury at the C5–C6 level, resulting in incomplete tetraplegia.

Elliott recalls his inpatient rehabilitation in a state hospital as "an extremely scary experience." He saw "paras and quads alike that were at home there," unwilling or unable to get on with their lives. "This wasn't for me," he says. His girlfriend was "there" for him from day one: "She never wavered. She did right." She stood by him during the lengthy hospitalization that was typical for tetra-

plegia in the 1970s—almost nine months, plus three months in a residential vocational rehabilitation program.

Elliott had severe motor impairment but much sparing of sensation. "I didn't cut my cord—I've got feeling all over, not perfect feeling, but I know if I'm in pain." He believes that this was partly responsible for his relatively good progress in rehabilitation and helped him avoid many medical complications. Still, the motor impairments made writing, feeding himself, and getting dressed difficult, and he could not use his legs at all.

He had no choice but to move back in with his mother and stepfather after release from the hospital. He didn't yet have independent mobility, didn't drive, and had no means of support. But the relationship with his stepfather was just as strained as ever, and Elliott was eager to find a way out.

Elliott continued to be close to his girlfriend, and a year after he left the hospital they were married. They moved into an apartment, and Elliott went back to school while his wife worked full-time. Elliott enjoyed sex with his wife, though his sexual function was not completely normal. For the first year or so, he could not ejaculate. He had been told that he'd probably be unable to have children. But then "all of a sudden it [ejaculation] just started. So that made it twice as enjoyable. My wife kept saying 'we're gonna have one.' "

Elliott was skeptical about his ability to become a parent, both physically and emotionally. He was having a hard time being so dependent on his wife. He was quite depressed about his job prospects and unsure of what he could do to make a living; he began to feel hopeless. "Suicide had been a contemplation for a while. And then my wife comes home one day and tells me she's pregnant!"

Shortly after that, Elliott heard about a new training opportunity for accounting and decided to give it a try. With the baby on the way, he knew he had to make a living. Motivated by the arrival of his daughter, Elliott got a job as soon as training was complete. He kept the job for twenty years, only recently moving into a new position.

Elliott loved being a parent, but his marriage was floundering. He thinks that his immaturity, injury, and insecurity were the reasons for marital strain. He had gone from a period of premature self-reliance as a teen to complete dependence on the hospital, his parents, and then his wife. He felt that his physical and emotional dependence was a great strain on his wife, yet when he became more self-sufficient, she felt he was withdrawing and they were becoming less close. Elliott and his wife broke up when their daughter was three, but they con-

tinued an amiable relationship. They were both devoted to their daughter, and they worked out flexible childcare and visiting arrangements.

Once Elliott was living alone, he had to confront the obstacles to fuller independence. During this period, he got a power wheelchair and a van with hand controls. He experimented with solutions to problems involving everything from medication side effects to dressing techniques, from wheelchair design to bowel management schedules. The need and the freedom to learn on his own gave Elliott more confidence in himself. Often his ways of solving problems weren't the methods he'd been taught in the rehabilitation program, but they worked better for his particular needs. And he was always vigilant about his skin and bladder management, keeping himself healthy and out of the hospital.

Elliott started to broaden his social life and began dating again, eventually meeting the woman who would become his wife in a new and more successful relationship.

One myth or old wives' tale about people with spinal cord injury or other disability is that they are sexless. Fortunately, this myth has for the most part been dispelled, along with other stigmatizing misconceptions. Most people with spinal cord injury, like Elliott, are as interested in sex as are able-bodied people, and many have active and even adventurous sex lives. Issues of sexuality, sexual function, fertility, and pregnancy are now regularly addressed as part of most rehabilitation programs for teens and adults with spinal cord injury.

In this chapter we first explore sexuality, intimacy, and relationships, then describe the variety of physiological sexual dysfunctions associated with spinal cord injury and their treatment. We address sexual attitudes, communication with a partner or potential partner, romance, and dating. And we discuss fertility and pregnancy for people with spinal cord injuries.

SEXUALITY, SEX DRIVE, AND SEX ACTS

Spinal cord injury often affects one or more *physiological* aspects of sexual function by interrupting nerve pathways necessary for penile erection and ejaculation, vaginal lubrication, genital sensation, orgasm, and muscle control. The *psychological* effects of spinal cord injury on body image, self-esteem, and social relationships can change one's experience of sexuality, perhaps compounding or magnifying any physical dysfunction.

Sex after spinal cord injury can be better understood—and improved—by distinguishing between sexuality, sex drive, and sex acts. Roberta Trieschmann provides clear distinctions between these aspects of sexual experience, which we summarize here.

Sexuality refers to a dynamic process that includes aspects of self-concept and identity, social relationships, and specific sexual behaviors. Sexuality is the sum of the expression of romantic, loving, and sexual feelings, including one's gender identity, sexual orientation, physical attractiveness, communication of sexual interest, sex role behavior, and sexual activities. Sexuality includes the sex drive and sex acts, but it is much more than these. Focusing on sexuality may be helpful in dealing with sexual changes after spinal cord injury and in increasing your ability to maintain a satisfactory sex life with your spouse or partner or to attract and interact with potential new partners.

Sex drive refers to the biologically based urge or need for sexual expression and satisfaction. Sex is a primary drive, just like hunger or thirst. Normally, the sex drive and potential avenues for its expression exist throughout the life span, but they can be impaired by both physical and psychological factors. Spinal cord injury may affect intensity of sex drive but generally does not eliminate it. Sex drive is sometimes referred to as libido, or sexual interest. This can include sexual fantasies, dreams, and interest in erotic books or movies, even in the absence of sex acts. Sex acts are behaviors involving primarily the erogenous zones and genitals, requiring motor activity and producing sensual/sexual pleasure. Despite the cultural emphasis on the importance or primacy of sexual intercourse, the variety of sex acts is almost infinite. When intercourse is made difficult or unsatisfying, perhaps by erectile dysfunction or positioning problems after spinal cord injury, sexual satisfaction can be enhanced by experimenting with a variety of different sex acts.

LOVE AND INTIMACY

The ability to love and experience emotional intimacy is part of normal development. An adolescent, whose capacity for sexual love and intimacy is not yet fully developed, needs to learn or maintain the social skills and opportunities that allow an age-appropriate expression of sexuality, rather than letting a spinal cord injury halt his or her development in this important area. Self-esteem, physical attractiveness, communication, dating, and romance are important issues for teens.

For an adult already involved in a loving sexual relationship at the time of injury, reestablishing a satisfactory relationship is an important part of overall adjustment. Emotional flexibility, experimenting with various sexual activities, and a capacity for playfulness are some factors that can enhance sexual satisfaction. While dating and social skills may not be as important for established couples, some may feel that they are "starting over" after spinal cord injury. Aspects of sexuality that had taken a backseat may again become important in stimulating sexual interest and compatibility—courting, dressing up, going out, creating a romantic atmosphere, and so forth. These are also important to single adults with spinal cord injury who are looking for a new partner.

REESTABLISHING YOUR SEXUAL RELATIONSHIP

For people in a regular intimate relationship, reestablishing a sexual relationship can begin even before leaving the rehabilitation hospital. Many rehabilitation hospitals provide information on sexuality in the form of books, manuals, or videotapes, and they may have sexual education or counseling sessions in which partners are included. Some rehabilitation hospitals have a special suite of rooms, set up like an apartment, where patients can practice daily living skills (cooking, wheelchair transfers, bathing, and so on) along with a spouse or caregiver before going home. An overnight stay here can also afford the opportunity for sexual experimentation with your partner. Ideally, any unexpected sexual problems or concerns can then be talked through with rehabilitation staff before you go home.

Even before you are ready for an independent overnight with your partner, you can begin focusing on sexuality in the context of your overall relationship. This might begin with paying more attention to your grooming, clothing, and overall appearance, making sure you have time alone with your partner during visits, and continuing your usual expressions of affection, such as kissing, hugging, and talking about your sexual or romantic feelings.

If you are a partner of a person with spinal cord injury, keep in mind that your mate isn't "breakable." Don't be afraid to embrace him. If you have any doubts about the safety of any physical activity (such as sitting on his lap while he's in the wheelchair), ask a nurse or doctor. If your partner has significant sensory loss, make sure you ask her what parts feel good to the touch. She may enjoy having her head scratched or stroked, her face and neck caressed, or her back rubbed. Communication and experimentation between partners about pleasurable sensations; physical, verbal, and visual expressions of affection; and openness to asking questions and receiving information on sexuality—all are important aspects of sexuality.

On resuming regular sexual contact outside the hospital, the person with spinal cord injury may need to deal with specific physiological dysfunctions and practical inconveniences—such as difficulty with maintaining an erection or catheter management—as part of the sexual routine. It is most helpful, however, to stay focused on your *sexuality* rather than *the sex act* as you begin to reestablish your sexual relationship. Focusing primarily on intercourse, or any other specific sex act, can produce anxiety about performance or "making it work," with unnecessary experiences of "failure." Try not to turn your sexual experiences into work. Instead, focus on playing around with your partner and having fun! If you focus on mutual pleasure, including emotional, sensual, and sexual elements, some degree of success is guaranteed.

> *David's fiancée was eager to resume their sexual relationship when he came home from rehabilitation (David was introduced in Chapter 3). With a complete spinal cord injury, David has no genital sensation and his sex drive has lessened following his injury. Yet he enjoys the physical intimacy of sex with his fiancée and is willing to experiment with different positions to please her. "I can get into it, but it's more to satisfy her. If I know she's satisfied, then I'm satisfied." At times he misses the intensity of sensation he experienced before his injury, but he feels that the satisfying sexual experiences of the past have helped him adjust to changes in his sexuality since the injury. "By my being older, I've experienced all that. I'm in my forties, I've been there, done that." He accepts that sex will be different, but he still finds satisfaction in relating to his fiancée in a sexual way.*

Your first need is to be comfortable in communicating and experimenting with your partner. Humor and a sense of playfulness can enhance sexual success. Make sure you have plenty of uninterrupted and private time for your initial sexual "sessions." Take the opportunity to express your love verbally as well as physically. Much of sexual arousal is mental, so use your imagination, share your fantasies, and stimulate all your senses. You can create a romantic or sexy atmosphere by using soft lighting and background music, wearing clothes that look or feel exciting, and using perfume, aftershave, or incense to stimulate your sense of smell. A glass of wine, a few chocolates, or a favorite food can add pleasurable taste sensation as a final touch. The keys to this approach are relaxation, stimulation of all your senses, expressions of love, and communication about what feels good.

Some couples whose sex lives have been "conventional," or focused on one specific sex act, may find this open-ended approach to sexual pleasure difficult or even scary. Other couples may have communication or psychological problems that become obstacles to reestablishing a good sex life. And some people with spinal cord injury, or their partners, will be inhibited by embarrassment over altered body appearance, presence of a urinary catheter, or fear of a bowel accident during sex. When these or other factors prevent your reestablishing sexual relations or lead to negative experiences of sexual "failure" or frustration, sexual counseling may be helpful.

Sexual counseling approaches vary. Some are focused on information and education, some on changing one's attitudes about sex and broadening one's acceptance of a variety of sexual behaviors. Others focus on resolving interpersonal conflicts or relationship patterns that affect both emotional and sexual intimacy. Your rehabilitation center or local psychological or psychiatric association can provide referral to a professional marital or sex therapist or can guide you to self-help books and videos on sexuality and spinal cord injury. Some rehabilitation centers sponsor the Sexual Attitude Reassessment (SAR) program, a group seminar for rehabilitation professionals and for patients and their partners that aims to dispel anxieties about discussing sex, to educate people about a wide variety of sex acts, and to stimulate self-awareness and an assessment of sexual values and attitudes.

DATING, ROMANCE, AND FINDING A PARTNER

The "dating game" is stressful even in the best of circumstances. With a spinal cord injury, it may seem truly daunting. Worries about physical appearance, sexual function, and social acceptability may hinder your natural desire to get out and meet potential dates or partners.

Concerns and needs about dating are somewhat different for a teenager with little or no dating or sexual experience than for an experienced adult. Concerns may also vary with stage of life. For example, a teenager or young adult thinking about dating and eventual marriage may be especially worried about birth control, fertility, and pregnancy issues. A middle-aged person may be more concerned about how physical dependency and personal care needs might affect an intimate relationship. And an older adult may be less concerned with appearance or physical prowess than with the burdens a close relationship might place on a partner who is also elderly.

Whatever your age or situation, your success in dating and finding a sexual or romantic partner depends primarily on your personality, your communication skills, and your ability to express your sexuality. Feeling confident in yourself and in your worth as a human being elicits positive responses from others. Social skills such as presenting a positive image, communicating effectively, and being assertive are essential to establishing contact with a potential partner. A willingness to take risks and to expect (and tolerate) some rejection helps broaden your opportunities and encourage perseverance. And avoid stereotyping yourself or others. Don't assume that your injury makes you an undesirable partner or that someone who is interested in you must be a "weirdo."

Elliott started dating shortly after his divorce, before getting his power chair. "I had found places I could go independently, on my own, and there were bars I could go into. And women were picking me up—which was really a surprise. A lot of women at that time seemed to be curious about what a guy in a wheelchair could do or couldn't do [sexually]. I was more than willing to show them!" Elliott found this a big ego boost. As he dated more, his confidence grew. "I was always an outgoing person anyway. If someone doesn't like me because I'm in a wheelchair, then fine. I know who I am . . . I never let it bother me much."

Teenagers

For teenagers, identification with a peer group of teens with similar disabilities may be helpful. If you are a teen with spinal cord injury, you may choose to date another person with a disability. But you are likely to meet many more peers who are able-bodied, and it's best to have the personal and social skills for forming relationships with people in a variety of situations. For presenting an attractive appearance, teenagers recommend cleanliness and smelling good (using perfume or cologne), developing a style of dress that is practical for wheelchair use but still attractive, and looking presentable but not provocative.

All teenagers struggle with issues of fitting in, and the first date is often a badge of acceptance or "making it." Teenagers with disabilities have all the normal concerns about social acceptability and sexuality, but these are compounded by special worries about being different because of wheelchair use, altered appearance, or dependence on others for assistance.

> *Hannah (whom you met in Chapter 5) became paraplegic at age fifteen. She was eager to resume dating. She remembers going on a date to a drive-in movie. At some point, she reached down to move her leg (in which she has no sensation), then realized that "her" leg was really his! Hannah's enthusiasm and sense of fun allowed her to laugh off such potentially embarrassing incidents, and this helped put her dates at ease. In college, she once had a bowel accident while on a date. She matter-of-factly asked her date to take her home and wait in the car while she washed and changed. She then went right back out with him!*

Parents of a teenager with spinal cord injury may have more difficulty than other parents in giving up their protective and caretaking role and in allowing or encouraging their teen to develop the emotional and physical independence necessary for dating. These parents may also find it more difficult to watch their child take risks, get rejected, or experience the pain of first love, even though these are normal teen experiences.

If you are a parent of a teen with spinal cord injury, keep in mind the normal course of adolescent development. Assume that your teen with a spinal cord injury is a sexual being just like any able-bodied teenager.

He or she will want to wear the same attractive or "in" clothing as other teens and have other adolescent privileges such as privacy at home, time alone with peers, and access to social events.

Teenagers with spinal cord injury are more successful socially and sexually if they are given the same sexual information and education as their peers, as well as special information about sexual functions, problems, and solutions unique to their particular disability. They also need to hear the same cautions as all other teens about avoiding sexual exploitation, using birth control methods, and protecting themselves against sexually transmitted diseases.

A sexually inexperienced teenager with a spinal cord injury may feel angry, cheated of the opportunity of a "normal" sex life. Some teens need additional counseling to work through feelings of loss or sort through their confusion. And some need more reinforcement for their positive character traits and other personality or physical attributes in order to build a healthy self-esteem and body image.

Teenagers normally explore their own bodies visually and through masturbation. Autoerotic activities provide sexual pleasure and release tension for teens who are biologically, but not yet socially, ready for sexual relationships with peers. Sensual and sexual self-exploration continues into adulthood, as a form of sexual expression and an important source of information on what "works" sexually. This can enhance sexual experience with a partner. Masturbation and other forms of self-stimulation also provide opportunities for improved body image, self-confidence, and relaxation.

If you are a teenager with no experience of sexual intercourse before your injury, you may get special benefit from this type of "practice" to increase your awareness of your sexual needs and functions before attempting sex with a partner. Masturbation is a normal part of sexuality. It can be a great way to explore your capacity for sexual function and enjoyment, with the same trial-and-error approach you use for other areas of living with spinal cord injury.

For individuals with a high-level cervical injury, with no or very limited hand function, masturbation may not be possible. In this case, you may have to delay sexual exploration of your body until you have a partner, although you will get some idea of how your body responds to touch in the course of your daily care—for example, when you are being dressed, bathed, catheterized, or transferred. Sometimes a very attractive nurse or physical therapist provides personal care that involves touching your body and genitals. Experiencing sexual feelings or developing a "crush" is not unusual in this situation. You may even be tempted to enlist the help of a care provider in your sexual exploration. This is definitely *not* a good idea. Your status as a younger person and a patient makes you vulnerable to emotional damage in any sexual encounter with a health care provider, and providers are ethically and legally prohibited from engaging in sexual contact with patients.

But don't forget the other important avenues for sexual information, aside from touching. Visual exploration and feedback can be extremely helpful. If you have impaired sensation, for example, you may not be able to tell whether you have an erection without looking. Visual examination of your nipples, genitals, and other body parts can also be sexually stimulating and help you feel good about your body. You can ask for help, if necessary, to look in a full-length mirror after bathing or to use smaller mirrors for examining your genitals or other hard-to-see body parts. Asking questions and getting information from your caregivers is important and at times essential in learning about your sexual self. You may want to ask your nurse what is happening during catheterization or bathing. Are you getting "morning erections" or reflex erections? (These can occur in the absence of sensation.) Do your nipples get hard in response to bathing or cold? Are you getting your period? Can you voluntarily control your vaginal muscles even if you don't feel the muscles moving?

These and any other questions about your body can be answered by your nurse or doctor. It's okay to ask about anything you want or need to know. If you sense that your doctor or nurse is uncomfortable with questions about sex or is unable to answer them, ask to be referred to someone else. A urologist or gynecologist may be helpful, or someone on the rehabilitation staff who is designated as the "sexuality expert" and who can talk with you about your concerns.

Finally, especially if physically exploring your own body is impossible, you may benefit from the opportunity to talk with other people who have "been around" after injuries similar to your own. Sometimes this is possible through a peer counseling program. At the very least, watching educational videos about sexuality for people with tetraplegia may be inspiring and will give you some ideas to store away for the future.

Adults

An adult who has been romantically involved and sexually active before spinal cord injury, especially if this was a rewarding and positive part of life, is likely to have the tools and the motivation to find a new partner. But with the added complications of a spinal cord injury, you may need to make some adaptations, sharpen your social skills, and keep your sense of humor handy!

We cannot overemphasize that finding a partner—whether for life or just for a date—depends most of all on your personality and how you connect with others. Your sexuality, which is part of your overall personality or self, often takes center stage when finding a partner is your goal. While "turning on" your sexuality will help you attract a potential partner, the specifics of your sexual functioning need not be a concern when you're meeting a new person or in the early phase of dating. Physiological sexual dysfunctions, or changes necessitated by mobility problems, become important to discuss and "work around" *after* you've established a relationship. During the initial stage of dating and courtship, it's much more helpful to focus on being yourself, as Vanessa did (see Chapter 3), rather than being a "C6" or a "T10." Emphasize your positive attributes, put others at ease by taking the first step in social situations, and be open to new situations and activities that promote social contact.

Of course, some people may react negatively to your physical limitations and your use of a wheelchair or crutches. Limited mobility may also create practical problems for dating, such as finding accessible restaurants and theaters or dealing with the social awkwardness of bringing along your personal care attendant. Some people won't be able to see past your wheelchair or walker. Stigma and social unease can lead others to ignore or actively reject you. But, happily, societal attitudes are changing, as people with disabilities become more active participants in all areas of work and family life. As long as you can make yourself socially available and maintain a positive view of yourself, many people will want to get to know you.

You may even find unexpected social advantages to having an obvious disability. Some men find that being in a wheelchair makes them less physically threatening to women, making it easier to engage a woman in casual conversation in a variety of settings. The wheelchair or disability itself can be a conversation piece, leading to further social interaction. Requesting or accepting offered assistance, such as a ride home or help getting up stairs, can also be an occasion for getting to know someone better.

Keeping a sense of humor is an asset in many potentially embarrassing or frustrating situations, and dating is no exception. One recently divorced man with tetraplegia reports the experience of falling out of his wheelchair and landing on top of his date, who had been riding on his lap. Once it was clear that no one was hurt, they both burst into laughter and ended up taking advantage of literally being thrown together by sharing some hugs and kisses on the ground! Fortunately, the man's attendant was nearby and was able to help him back into his chair.

Another man describes a visit to his date's apartment. Both he and she used wheelchairs, and she was more physically limited. He tried to transfer her from her wheelchair to the couch so they could sit closer together, but this proved very difficult. For a while she was stuck halfway between wheelchair and couch. Instead of panicking or getting frustrated or embarrassed, the woman laughed and enjoyed the absurdity of the moment. The man was eventually able to scoot her slowly onto the couch, where their efforts were rewarded by being "able to smooch the whole afternoon away!"

Aside from its usefulness in potentially embarrassing situations, humor is a great social icebreaker, a tool you can use to put people at ease. Telling jokes, relating funny stories, or making good-natured fun of yourself or your disability are all ways of easing the nervous energy that accompanies most first dates. Being able to laugh at yourself and not taking things too seriously can help others feel more relaxed and comfortable with your disability—and the less anxious they are about that, the more they can focus on you as a person.

People with spinal cord injuries have found some other skills particularly helpful for establishing romantic relationships. In a study of sexuality in women with spinal cord injuries, assertiveness was most often mentioned as a useful social skill. Being outgoing and taking the first step in conversations, smiling, and making good eye contact were recommended. Communication about your feelings is part of being assertive. The physical limitations of your injury might make spontaneous physical contact difficult. You may need to *say* that you have a romantic interest or that you'd like to kiss your partner. Sometimes it's unclear whether you are being included in social activities as a friend or as a potential lover. Don't be afraid to ask "Is this a date?" and to clarify your own intentions.

For many people with spinal cord injuries, presenting a good physical appearance is an important factor in attracting potential partners. Clothes and hairstyles that flatter your best features and are fashionable and appropriate to the social situation make a good first impression. Colorful ties or jewelry that express your individual style can attract positive attention and help counteract the tendency of others to see the wheelchair first.

Getting out to the same social events and situations that you enjoyed before your injury is the best way to meet people. You can still go to parties, restaurants, bars, classes, meetings, and so on, as long as they are accessible. You can participate, perhaps with modifications, in most activities. If you liked ballroom or nightclub dancing, you can dance in your wheelchair. You can participate in wheelchair sports, hiking, or camping activities, attend lectures or college courses, join book clubs or political campaigns—in short, engage in whatever interests you and brings you in contact with other people.

But what if you can't get out as often as you'd like, because of transportation problems, inaccessibility of the places you'd like to go, or periods of physical illness? Many people have found computer chat rooms and virtual cafes a great way to connect with others. Sometimes people meet on the Internet and eventually exchange phone numbers and even arrange meetings that turn into real relationships. (Of course, you should apply the same cautions about first meetings that you would for any blind date: meet in a public place with other people around and don't give out your address until you are comfortable with the new person.) You can also consider using computer dating services and dating services set up specifically for people with disabilities.

Many singles, both able-bodied and disabled, meet through personal ads in local newspapers. These provide initial anonymity and the opportunity to screen a potential date through letters and phone calls before deciding whether to meet. They also give you control over when and how you reveal that you have a spinal cord injury. You can wait until you've established some rapport, or you can disclose your disability immediately and weed out callers for whom this is a reason not to meet you. In either case, placing or answering personal ads can be a good way to make contact when your opportunities are limited. You can decide whether to advertise in publications directed at other physically disabled people or in community or city newspapers with general readership. It's often a good idea to advertise in a publication that represents your interests or peer group, such as age-related, religion-related, or hobby-related magazines.

Gays and Lesbians

To the best of our knowledge, virtually no research exists on sexuality issues specific to gays and lesbians with spinal cord injury. In terms of sexual function, gay men are affected in the same way as heterosexuals; that is, depending on the level and completeness of their spinal cord injury, they may experience dysfunction in sensation, erection, orgasm, and ejaculation. Lesbian women with spinal cord injury may experience difficulty with sensation, lubrication, and orgasm, as do heterosexual women with similar injuries (see Sexual Mechanics, below). In terms of sexuality, autobiographical essays by gay people with spinal cord injury suggest that dating, romance, and reestablishment of a satisfactory intimate relationship after spinal cord injury are affected in much the same ways as for heterosexuals. As Ed Gallagher's account of looking for a relationship after his injury illustrates, concerns about self-image, attractiveness, and altered sexual function are prominent after spinal cord injury, as is the need to explore and redefine one's sexuality.

> He is friendly and attractive and you enjoy talking to him. The inevitable "what happened" question comes soon enough . . . he shyly asks about your sensation levels and what your sexual capabilities are like these days. You tell him that things have changed a bit in that area, but that your mouth still possesses mysterious powers . . . He calls the next night and will be coming Friday evening . . . You are flattered, excited, proud. But your [penis]

does not share your feelings. You know in your heart and mind that problems lie ahead . . . Hey, I'm a confident guy. But somehow, confidence in
my sexuality still eludes me . . . no matter how many times my mind shouts,
"Every bit of sex doesn't have to come through your [penis]" . . . I love kissing and touching able-bodied guys . . . But often I've felt like nothing more
than the available catalyst to get them off . . . So I look now to experiment
with "my own type" of man. I've seen many handsome guys with SCI [spinal
cord injury] . . . Seeing a guy like that as gorgeous and vibrant could reju-
venate my sexual self-esteem. It could help me define sex differently . . . I
want to know that what I can give to another guy and get back from him
is enough to create prolonged (even though compromised) excitement and
satisfaction for both of us . . . We'll discover a more passionate and insight-
ful definition of . . . sex as we are. As we are in these chairs.

If you are a gay man or lesbian who was already in a partnership at
the time of your injury, reestablishing a sexual relationship with your
partner involves similar issues as those discussed for heterosexual couples: good communication, willingness to experiment, patience, and emotional support.

After surgery for a spinal tumor resulting in tetraplegia, John R. Killacky recalls:

While still in the hospital, my husband spent each day loving me back to
existence . . . Caressing my body that could not respond, often he would
lie with me in bed, trying to soothe the blinding pain. One evening, he
closed the curtains and kissed me. As he became visibly excited, I felt desir-
able again and hopeful that our life would return to a semblance of normalcy. As someone who was quite phallocentric, I have been forced to reorient my sexuality. With almost no sensation in my genitals now, my only
indication of an orgasm is violent spasticity in my left arm and leg. Recip-
rocating with my enfeebled fingers and locked-in neck is often very short
lived. Yet the unconditional love of my husband has allowed new patterns
to emerge; light massage and hugging are central to our relating.

For lesbians with spinal cord injury, as for heterosexual women, sexual
"performance" is not as important as it is for many heterosexual and gay
men. The participation of a lesbian woman with spinal cord injury in sex

with her partner is affected primarily by limitations in motor functioning, which may make positioning or active participation in some sexual acts difficult. Experimentation, communication, and mutual affection are the necessary ingredients for redefining your sexual relationship after spinal cord injury.

If you live in an area with an organized gay community, you may be able to get informal support and information on sexuality and disability issues. Many urban areas have health and mental health centers that serve the gay and lesbian community. All of the information on treatment options for sexual dysfunction in the following section apply to people with spinal cord injury regardless of sexual orientation.

SEXUAL "MECHANICS"—FUNCTION AND DYSFUNCTION AFTER SPINAL CORD INJURY

Effects of Spinal Cord Injury on Sexual Function

Spinal cord injury affects sexual function by disrupting the nerve impulses, or messages, between the brain and the rest of the body (see Chapter 1). When the genitals are stimulated, the brain registers excitement. When the brain is stimulated (for example, by sexual fantasies or talking to a partner about sex), the body may respond with physical excitement. If the spinal cord is damaged, these messages are disrupted, the extent of disruption depending on the level and completeness of the injury.

A woman with spinal cord injury can continue to participate in sexual intercourse and other sex acts regardless of her level of motor impairment, though limited mobility may affect positioning and the extent to which she can take a physically active role. Her sexual function is affected primarily by loss of sensation. Vaginal lubrication, sexual excitation, and orgasm may be affected. Complete injuries result in greater disruption. Incomplete injuries have a greater likelihood of leaving a full range of sexual experience. Female fertility is *not* affected by spinal cord injury at any level.

Men with spinal cord injury also have varying degrees of sensory and motor impairment that affect excitement, orgasm, positioning, and mobility during sex. Spinal cord injury also directly affects the ability to have an erection. Normally, men can get an erection in several ways. Psychogenic erections are caused by mental stimulus (sexual thoughts, seeing your partner naked, reading a story about sex): the brain sends messages through the spinal cord to the penis, causing an erection. Erections of this type do not occur after complete spinal cord injury, but can occur after incomplete lesions in some individuals.

Reflexogenic erections are caused by direct stimulation of the penis, such as rubbing or stroking. These erections do not require communication between the penis and the brain. They are caused by a spinal reflex involving communication between sensory and motor nerves within the sacral spinal cord. (A similar mechanism causes limbs to move involuntarily during a spasm, even though your brain cannot make them move voluntarily.) Men with injuries at the cervical or thoracic levels can usually get reflexogenic erections. These can result from direct stimulation that is nonsexual, such as pulling on your catheter or friction from bed sheets or clothing.

Spontaneous erections occur in response to internal physical stimuli, such as a full bladder; "morning erection" is a good example. Spontaneous erections, like reflexogenic erections, are caused by spinal reflexes.

Most men with complete injuries in the lumbar or sacral regions cannot get erections of any type.

Treatment for Erectile Dysfunction

Most men with spinal cord injury experience some type of erectile dysfunction—difficulty getting or sustaining an erection or inability to achieve full erection—that makes sexual intercourse difficult. Sometimes, erectile function improves over time as spontaneous recovery occurs.

In men with injuries at a higher level of the spinal cord, reflexogenic erections can result from sexual or nonsexual stimulation to the genital area or penis. These erections are not necessarily related to sexual arousal, but with practice, couples can sometimes learn stimulation techniques to make these erections last long enough to have satisfactory intercourse. A satisfying sexual relationship may be possible whether you have reflexogenic erections, partial erections, or none at all. But many men and their partners want to have intercourse and may wish to use a treatment technique to create or sustain an erection firm enough for this purpose.

Several options now exist, including vacuum devices, injections, medications, and penile implants.

A vacuum device, or pump, is a simple tube that fits over the penis and creates an erection as air is pumped out of the tube and blood is drawn into the penis. A ring is then inserted over the base of the penis to maintain the erection by keeping the blood in the penis. After intercourse, the ring is removed and the erection dissipates. (Some people use a penis ring alone to maintain erections that occur naturally. Your urologist can tell you if this method is safe for you and can advise you on how long to use it, what size ring to use, and so forth.) The vacuum devices are generally safe, effective, and inexpensive.

Another method for achieving erection is direct injection of papaverine or other vasodilator (a substance that dilates blood vessels and increases blood flow) into the penis. Men with good hand function can inject themselves, or a partner can perform the injection with minimal training by the urologist. This method is generally quite safe. Possible side effects are priapism (an erection lasting over an hour, which can be medically dangerous) or damage to the penis by overuse or improper administration of injections.

Vasodilator drugs (for example, Viagra, Cialis) are now being used for erectile problems caused by a variety of medical conditions including spinal cord injury. The advantage of these drugs is that they can be taken by mouth before intercourse (thirty minutes to thirty-six hours before, depending on the drug), and erection then occurs during the course of normal foreplay. This is more "natural" and esthetically pleasing for many people and allows sexual activity to progress from foreplay to intercourse without interruption. These drugs do not work for all people with spinal cord injury. You may need to experiment with dosages and the time interval between taking the drug and intercourse. Also, vasodilators can have harmful effects in some patients with blood pressure or cardiac abnormalities. Overdosing can be dangerous.

Penile implants are another option for treating erectile problems, but given their invasiveness, permanence, and higher risk of side effects, these should be considered as a last resort, after all other methods have failed. If you had trauma to your penis at the same time as your spinal cord injury or have a vascular disorder, a penile implant may be the only type of successful treatment. An implant is surgically inserted into the space inside the penis that normally fills with blood during erection. There are two types, semi-rigid and inflatable. The semi-rigid implant is very effective for intercourse and can be bent into a variety of positions. However, it may move around in the course of normal activity, creating the embarrassing appearance of an erection in nonsexual situations. The inflatable implant includes a fluid reservoir inserted into the abdomen. When ready for sexual activity, you pump a small bulb in the scrotum and fluid flows into the implant chambers. The erection is deflated by squeezing the bulb again when sexual activity is completed. The advantage of the inflatable implant is that erections do not occur at unwanted times.

Side effects of implants are rare but can include infection, rejection of the implant, and mechanical failure. Should the implant have to be surgically removed because of infection, permanent damage to the penis is possible, making alternative methods less likely to work.

All of these methods for producing erection require a prescription from a urologist. You need to get a urological exam to make the best choice of treatment for your particular situation. Remember, too, that these methods affect *erection only*. They do not improve sensation or affect ejaculation, orgasm, or fertility. However, the psychological arousal of seeing your erection and the ability to have intercourse with your partner may enhance your libido and make possible a variety of sexual behaviors so that, overall, you can have more satisfying sexual activity.

Female Sexual Function after Spinal Cord Injury

As noted above, a woman's spinal cord injury often results in altered genital sensation but has no direct effect on her ability to "perform" sexual intercourse. If vaginal lubrication is affected, an artificial, water-soluble lubricant such as K-Y Jelly makes penetration possible without irritation to the vagina.

The only other specific "dysfunctions" women experience are due to limitations in mobility and positioning, which may make certain sex acts impossible, difficult, or painful. By experimenting with a variety of positioning aids, such as pillows, adjustable beds, and so forth, and different positions for sex (sitting, lying down, side lying, and so on), you can solve most of these problems.

Orgasm and Ejaculation

The ability to have an orgasm (sexual "climax") after spinal cord injury varies widely from person to person. Many women can still experience orgasm with sexual stimulation, though the sensations may be different from those experienced before the injury. You may find orgasm is enhanced by more intense stimulation, such as with a vibrator, by stimulation of other erogenous zones such as nipples and lips, and through fantasy, visual stimulation, or "sex talk" with your partner.

Some men can experience an orgasm after spinal cord injury, even if not until months or even years after the initial trauma. Many men and women have "phantom orgasms," which differ from genital orgasms but have the same feeling of intense excitement and release, involve the whole body, and produce a feeling of elation. This experience, sometimes referred to as psychological or emotional orgasm, usually results from a combination of direct sexual stimulation, fantasy, and memories of past orgasmic experience; visual and auditory stimulation; physical stimulation of areas that retain sensory feeling; and emotional closeness and communication. You are more likely to have this type of orgasm if you have a sexual relationship that includes trust and emotional closeness, and at a time when you can experiment, practice, and relax.

Ejaculation may or may not occur for men with spinal cord injury, depending on the level of injury and other factors. Ejaculation may be absent initially, then spontaneously recovered, as in Elliott's case. The mechanisms of sensation, erection, and ejaculation are neurologically distinct: sometimes ejaculation occurs without erection or the feeling of climax, or orgasm occurs without ejaculation.

Men can sometimes elicit orgasm or ejaculation by using a vibrator, which can be incorporated into sexual activity with a partner or used for masturbation. Other clinical techniques are used to produce ejaculation for the purpose of collecting sperm, as described later in the chapter when we discuss fertility.

Practical Preparations for Sex

Sexual activity after a spinal cord injury is usually more successful if you do some advance planning. You need to consider mobility issues, such as transferring and positioning, and muscle spasms. More important, you probably want to minimize the risk of a bowel or bladder accident during sex. Emptying your bladder before sexual activity will help. If you are on a regular bowel program, the chance of a bowel accident is small. But if your bowels are not regular, you may want to empty them before sex. Protective pads on the bed make quick cleanup easier in the event of an accident. Keeping towels on hand is also useful. Avoiding eating or drinking just before sex, or limiting your fluid intake for several hours before sex, can help minimize bladder and bowel accidents.

If you use intermittent catheterization, you can catheterize just before sex to empty your bladder. Both men and women can have sex with an indwelling catheter in place. A woman should tape the catheter to her abdomen with surgical tape to avoid dislodging it during sex. A man can fold the catheter back along the side of his penis and cover both with a condom before intercourse. Of course, if you prefer, the catheter can be removed before sex and then reinserted.

A woman using a diaphragm for birth control may need help from her partner to insert it. You may want to include this in your sexual encounter or prepare ahead by inserting the diaphragm yourself or getting assistance.

If you have any questions about how to make physical preparations for sex, how to minimize accidents, or how to avoid spasms during sex, ask your doctor. Once you are fully informed, communicate with your partner about the necessary preparations, who will perform them, and the possibility of accidents and how you'll deal with them. The better you prepare your partner, the more relaxed both of you will be and the greater the likelihood of a pleasurable experience.

MAKING LOVE

The first step to a rewarding sex life is establishing a relationship in which intimacy and sexual expressions of love are both desired and possible. You can then explore the many possibilities for sexual pleasure and experience the emotional satisfaction of physical closeness to your lover. If necessary, make use of the options discussed above for inducing and maintaining erection or increasing vaginal lubrication. The proper sexual "mechanics" and a willingness to explore sexual possibilities provide a great starting point. And for some couples, that's all they need for a satisfying sex life.

But making love requires more than the right mechanics, and, as in other areas of life, you'll find it hard to have a good attitude if you're focusing on losses.

> *Don, whose spinal cord injury resulted in loss of all pelvic sensation, was able to get an erection with papaverine injections and to have intercourse with his wife. "I might as well be playing with a piece of wood," he quipped, referring to his lack of genital sensation. Although his wife enjoyed their sexual contact, Don felt he was just going through the motions. Sex began to feel empty and alien, and Don started to pull away emotionally from his wife and to feel deprived and inadequate. Don's wife felt his emotional absence during sex and wanted very much to restore the feeling of making love.*

Don, like many people with spinal cord injury, wanted to find sexual and sensual pleasure but didn't know where or how to look for it. He needed specific suggestions for creating pleasure and involving himself in the emotional and physical give and take that differentiates making love from having sex. The following suggestions may help you get started.

Find Your Erogenous Zones

In most cases of spinal cord injury, some or even a great deal of body sensation is left intact. Sensation is present above the level of the injury, and people with incomplete injuries often have an area or areas of sensation below the injury, too. You and your partner can explore your whole body, taking a sensation "inventory." Being touched in different ways—with a feather, fingertips, or broad hand strokes, for example—may produce different results. This can help you identify what types of stimulation are pleasurable in different body areas. Many people report that areas just above the level where sensation is lost, or areas of partial sensation, become highly sensitive after injury. Stimulation in these areas, possibly chest, belly, or neck, can be sexually exciting. Areas of spared or partially preserved sensation in the pelvic region can also become new erogenous zones, such as the anus, buttocks, or groin.

Of course, all people have non-genital erogenous zones, such as the mouth, lips, and tongue, nipples and breasts, neck and ears, and abdomen and lower back. Stimulation of these areas may have been part of foreplay before your injury. Now this may become part of the "main event."

Focusing attention on erogenous and sensually pleasurable areas can reprogram your experience of sexual excitement. Combined with visual and emotional stimulation and the psychological excitement of giving pleasure to your partner, stimulation of erogenous zones can produce a very satisfying sexual experience and sometimes orgasm. It is a way for your partner to make love to you and for you to be actively involved in the process of discovery and sharing of pleasure.

Try New Techniques

Many individuals and couples are set in their sexual ways. As in other aspects of life, we may discover something that "works" sexually and then stick with it, perhaps not realizing we are excluding other potentially enjoyable activities. But after a spinal cord injury, certain sexual positions and actions may not be possible because of mobility and sensory changes. Innovation and change are now needed for success in making love, just as they are for success in work, parenting, and leisure activities.

Cultural, religious, or personal taboos and fears may hinder your exploration of different sexual activities. And lack of communication with your partner can lead to embarrassment, anger, or disgust. You may need to explore your sexual values with your partner or perhaps seek help from a religious counselor or sex therapist in order to decide which sexual activities are acceptable to you. You'll need to be open with your partner in discussing your sexual needs, desires, and intentions before introducing a new and potentially unwanted sexual practice.

Motor impairments following spinal cord injury often require new positions for sexual intercourse. Finding a position that allows penetration may be fairly easy, but more experimentation may be useful in finding one that is the most pleasurable. In one study of thirty-one women with spinal cord injury, eleven different positions for sexual intercourse were recommended by different individuals!

Some people with spinal cord injury prefer to make love in a wheelchair or other chair, rather than in a bed. Some prefer a waterbed, which provides motion, or an adjustable bed that assists with positioning.

While muscle spasms can be an annoyance during sexual activity, they can usually be controlled by shifting position or putting pressure on the limb in spasm. However, some people find spasms an asset during sex, making it easier to sustain a pleasurable position, enhance stimulation of their partner's body, or elicit an erection. With practice, you may be able to trigger a spasm that enhances sexual pleasure.

Other sexual acts may be more pleasurable than genital intercourse after spinal cord injury. A man who is unable to engage in intercourse because of limited mobility or erectile dysfunction can usually find a position in which he can orally stimulate his partner's genitals. This can be a satisfying alternative to intercourse for his partner, while providing exciting tactile stimulation to the man's lips, mouth, and tongue, where sensation is intact, as well as stimulation of other senses (taste, smell, vision). Similarly, a woman with spinal cord injury who has limited genital sensation may prefer to stimulate her partner orally so she can enjoy these tactile, taste, and olfactory sensations. Men or women with spinal cord injury who have some genital sensation may enjoy receiving oral sex. Combinations of oral sex and manual stimulation can be pleasurable to both partners.

Both men and women may enjoy anal intercourse or stimulation, if this is an area of spared sensation. For men with spinal cord injury, pleasure during intercourse and the ability to maintain an erection may be enhanced by anal stimulation. Of course, for both men and women, anal stimulation increases the chance of a bowel accident and thus requires more careful attention to the mechanics of preparation for sex.

Vibrators can provide intense stimulation, which may be helpful in producing sexual response even when sensation is limited, for both men and women. They can also be used for masturbation by people whose decreased physical dexterity or mobility makes manual masturbation impossible. A vibrator can be adapted with a special handle (similar to one you might use on a fork or pen) for people with limited hand use. Vibrators are generally safe, but sometimes cause autonomic dysreflexia (a sudden, potentially dangerous rise in blood pressure with headache; see Chapter 1). Signs to watch for are reddening of the skin, dizziness or lightheadedness, or your heart pounding in your chest. If any of these signs occur, stop using the vibrator. Ask your doctor about its safety before trying again.

In the section on sexual mechanics earlier in this chapter, we discussed some medical interventions for producing erection. One technique for sexual intercourse that doesn't require medical intervention and is helpful for some men with erectile dysfunction is called the "stuffing technique." Rather than waiting for an erection before attempting penetration, the man stuffs his flaccid or semi-erect penis into his partner's vagina, and the stimulation by her vaginal muscles helps promote erection. Even if full erection is not possible, this technique can allow successful intercourse with enough stimulation of the vagina and clitoris to be satisfying to the female partner.

Imagination, experimentation, and motivation are the keys to successful lovemaking after spinal cord injury. Willingness to try new techniques and methods and to educate yourself and your partner about sexuality are also important. Most people who have a loving partnership, with trust, caring, and affection, are able to find some way to make love and express their sexuality after spinal cord injury.

FERTILITY, PREGNANCY, AND FAMILY PLANNING

Fertility

Female fertility is not affected by spinal cord injury: for a woman of childbearing age, the ability to become pregnant persists unless she has some unrelated fertility problem. Menstruation may stop immediately after the injury, but usually resumes within six months. Keep in mind, however, that even during this early time, ovulation continues and you *can* become pregnant. The length and duration of your menstrual cycle may change after injury, and bleeding may be lighter or heavier.

If you don't want to become pregnant, some form of birth control is just as necessary after spinal cord injury as before. If you do become pregnant, there are special considerations for ensuring the health of you and your child, as discussed shortly.

Male fertility after spinal cord injury is a more complex matter. For most men with spinal cord injury, fertility problems result from inability to ejaculate, from retrograde ejaculation (ejection of semen into the bladder rather than out of the penis), or from lowered sperm counts or decreased motility of sperm.

Several techniques are available for obtaining sperm from men with spinal cord injury, for use in artificial insemination of a partner or for in vitro fertilization (fertilization, in the laboratory, of an egg that has been removed from the woman's body and will be reimplanted as an embryo).

In vibratory stimulation, a vibrator is applied to the penis to produce reflex ejaculation. This technique must be used with medical supervision owing to the risk of autonomic dysreflexia. The technique usually works only for men with lesions above T12, because thoracic and sacral pathways are necessary for the reflex.

Another technique for obtaining sperm is electroejaculation, electrical stimulation of the prostate gland and seminal vesicles that produces muscle contraction and ejaculation. A specially trained clinician places the device in the man's rectum and stimulates the genitals electrically through the intervening tissue, producing ejaculation. The procedure can be scheduled when the man's partner is ovulating, and artificial insemination can be done immediately after. Or the sperm sample can be used for in vitro fertilization.

A new technique for in vitro fertilization is intracytoplasmic sperm injection. This technique improves the chances of fertilization by selecting only the healthiest sperm cells in a given sample and then directly injecting the sperm into the egg cell using microscopic equipment.

Depending on your individual situation, you may be able to father a child without medical intervention or with one of the techniques described above. A urologist who specializes in fertility can provide a thorough assessment of your individual situation and help you explore your options. The American Society of Reproductive Medicine can supply you with a list of medical centers that provide infertility treatments of all types.

Birth Control

Both men and women with spinal cord injury who are sexually active and do not want a pregnancy must use a birth control method, even if you think ejaculation is unlikely. Keep in mind that *erection and ejaculation are separate functions*. Some men with paraplegia can ejaculate despite the lack of erection or sensation of orgasm. Therefore, if you are having sex and wish to avoid pregnancy, birth control is essential.

All birth control options available to able-bodied people are possible for people with spinal cord injury. Birth control pills and intrauterine devices have the advantage of greater effectiveness in preventing pregnancy but may have higher medical risks for women with spinal cord injury. Barrier methods such as the diaphragm and condoms have the advantage of also protecting against sexually transmitted diseases, but they may be difficult to use because of mobility impairments. Permanent contraceptive methods such as tubal ligation or vasectomy are an option for individuals or couples who are sure they do not want children. The best way to decide on the method that is right for you is to consult your doctor. Together you can explore the options and weigh the risks and benefits of each type of contraception.

Pregnancy and Childbirth

Childbirth is possible for a woman with spinal cord injury at any level. Healthy babies have even been born to women who were injured during their pregnancy. If you are emotionally ready to have a child and have considered the physical aspects of parenting, being pregnant and becoming a mother should be an exciting and fulfilling experience.

You need to consider several potential complications of pregnancy, however, if you have a spinal cord injury. Pressure sores may occur more often during pregnancy because of increased body weight or anemia, and you need to do more frequent weight shifting or pressure releases. Urinary tract infection is more likely during pregnancy but can generally be managed with antibiotic treatment. An increased risk of autonomic dysreflexia occurs as the pregnancy progresses. This can be caused by sexual activity, and it may be advisable to avoid sexual intercourse after the seventh month to reduce the risk of complications.

The risk of autonomic dysreflexia increases during labor and requires close medical supervision. Other complications include the possibility of early delivery or the inability to feel contractions that indicate the start of labor. These problems can be managed by frequent medical checkups after the thirty-second week of pregnancy. Once dilation has begun, hospitalization and bed rest are usually advisable so the course of the labor can be closely monitored. Delivery may be vaginal or by cesarean section, depending on the individual needs of mother and baby. Episiotomy (surgical incision of the perineum to assist with delivery) may or may not be necessary. Finding an obstetrician who has some experience with spinal cord injury, or coordinating care between your obstetrician and physiatrist, is the best way to ensure a healthy pregnancy and delivery.

Breast-feeding your newborn may be possible, perhaps with some help in positioning. Consult with your doctor or a nurse lactation specialist if you want to breast-feed your baby. Keep in mind, too, that breast-feeding is not essential for the well-being of your child, and you and your infant can form a strong emotional bond through bottle-feeding, snuggling, and other forms of nurturing and closeness.

Parenting Options for Infertile Couples

Some men with spinal cord injury are not able to impregnate their partners because they are unable to produce viable sperm. But there are other options for having a family that you and your partner might want to explore.

One possibility is artificial insemination with donor sperm. Sperm banks collect sperm samples from healthy anonymous donors. Use of donated sperm allows a couple to go through the experience of pregnancy together and to begin parenting the child from the moment it is born. For some couples, however, the "imbalance" of having a child genetically related to the mother but not the father is unacceptable and a reason not to pursue this option.

A second possibility is adoption. The adoption procedure may involve extensive evaluation of you, your partner, and your home by the adoption agency, long waiting lists for an available child, and a series of evaluations and court proceedings before the adoption is legally finalized. Adoption agencies may have discriminatory attitudes toward parents with a disability, but your application to adopt a child cannot be refused solely on the basis of your disability. A private (non-agency) adoption is an alternative, but this can be extremely expensive and result in much disappointment if the birth mother decides not to relinquish the child.

If you wish to adopt a child, consult with other adoptive parents who have disabilities and inquire at several adoption agencies to find one that is best suited to your needs. If you are willing to persevere, adoption can be a rewarding way to become a parent.

Elliott looks back on the day his first wife announced her pregnancy as a turning point in his recovery. He recalls the surprise and happiness in finding out he could father a child, his wife's enthusiasm, and a dawning sense of responsibility. For more than two years Elliott had been dependent on others. Now he would have to take care of someone else. At the age of twenty-two, he wasn't "real hot" about having a child—until he found out he was going to have one! "The real point at which I knew I was trapped and there was no way out, and I didn't want any way out, was when I saw her born. I was there in the delivery room. She had me wrapped around her little pinky from the day she was born!"

After his divorce, Elliott lived alone for three years, rebuilding his self-confidence and independence, working, dating, getting his power wheelchair and van. Then he met the woman who would become his second wife, and they lived together for a few years before marrying.

In this marriage, Elliott feels he is an equal partner. He sometimes asks his wife for assistance with particularly difficult or time-consuming tasks, but he functions independently for the most part. He has been steadily employed during their marriage, recently switching to a better job. His daughter, always a frequent visitor, moved in with them during high school and is now starting college. Elliott's second wife has never had children. Now in her mid-thirties she and Elliott are thinking about having a child together.

Elliott was fortunate in having substantial recovery of his sexual function and being able to father a child without medical intervention. But his story also illustrates the interaction between physical and psychological factors in dating, developing romantic and sexual relationships, and being a responsible and loving parent. Elliott found that the road to becoming an attractive sexual partner and succeeding in a long-term relationship required self-confidence, some social risk-taking, a sense of humor, a relish for relationships, and responsibility for his own life.

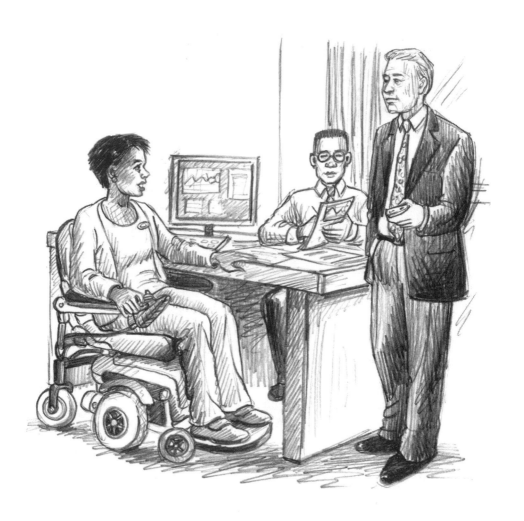

Life Goes On
Independent Living

Nora was a twenty-four-year-old expectant mother with two toddlers. She and her husband, John, were busy and worked hard, running a small manufacturing business, raising a young family, and involved in a large extended family.

For about seven months Nora had been experiencing unusual sensations: backaches, fatigue, legs that wouldn't support her going up and down steps, and spasms. Her gait had changed, and sometimes she would fall. One night she had finished her sewing, removed the needle, and stuck it into her slacks. Immediately she realized that she'd pushed the needle into her leg, yet with no sensation of pain. She felt nothing.

Over the next few weeks, she "rested" while relatives came to her home to help her. The symptoms persisted. Her doctor referred her to two neurosurgeons, who soon whisked her into surgery.

Attempting to do a myelogram, the surgeons found they couldn't penetrate the area where they usually draw a sample of spinal fluid. A delicate operation revealed that the arachnoid, a thin membrane surrounding the spinal cord, had become inflamed so that spinal fluid was unable to flow. Nora's spinal fluid protein count was a hundred times higher than normal. The two operating surgeons made different prognoses: one predicted imminent death; the other thought Nora had a good chance to live. They operated, but her spinal cord was already seriously damaged. Although this procedure ensured her survival, it resulted in paraplegia.

Nora and her family lived on the second floor of the two-story duplex home that they owned. Her husband notified the tenants on the first level that they would need to move so that he and Nora could live on the lower floor. John made a ramp over the steps to the front door, and family members helped move furniture to make more room for Nora to maneuver her wheelchair. Her father installed grab bars in the bathroom.

On her return home, Nora found that Tim and Dan, the toddlers, were confused about who was "the boss" because of the coming and going of the various family members and friends who'd been taking care of them. Nora soon began reasserting her role as mother. The family, including her mother and her mother-in-law, continued to give frequent help so that, at first, Nora was not alone.

Shortly after Nora's return home, John wanted to go to the store when none of their "helpers" were around. Nora told John about her fear of being alone and responsible for the two little boys. John replied, "You have to do this sometime. I'm just going around the corner." They survived.

After that, the "disability moved in but it didn't dominate" life, says Nora. The focus was on the activity of the family. "It helped having kids, wanting to get home to them. The family wanted me to know that I had a place and they depended on me." Nora used the wheelchair to transport her boys around the house.

Nora vividly recalls how, on the first anniversary of her spinal surgery, she really grasped the finality of her disability. She was feeding Joey, the baby born after her spinal surgery. She remembers thinking, "Forget the thought that I'll ever walk again." She mourned the fact that she couldn't push the new baby in the buggy, taking the other children along for a walk.

Clearly, children were Nora and John's focus. They planned to have a large family. She soon became pregnant with Kathleen, and the year after Kathleen's arrival, Maureen was born. After the fifth child, Nora's doctor advised her that a further pregnancy was unwise, that there always had to be a youngest child in the family and it might as well be Maureen.

Because they wouldn't have more children of their own, John approached a local adoption agency. The agency was very receptive until the staff learned that Nora had a disability. A mother with a disability would create an "unfit home," they said. (At that time, none of the current protections against this type of blatant discrimination were in place. For more information on parenting and adoption, see Chapter 6.)

Soon after Nora's return home, she and John had become involved in an organization for people with paraplegia. They both held offices locally, doing whatever was needed, and even housed the association in their home for a time. Answering the telephone for the organization was the beginning of her advocacy career, Nora says.

When the local organization found "real" office space, it offered Nora the job of executive director. She was instrumental in improving building code legislation to increase accessibility and was a driving force in the campaign for her state's legislation to require curb-cuts, enabling people using wheelchairs to cross streets independently (the first such legislation in the country). She also campaigned to have all new county-owned buses made accessible to the disabled.

Shortly after Nora became executive director, her husband died. Nora was now a single mother with five teenagers. Each member of the family was given responsibilities in managing the household. Sunday was family day, with the teenagers planning dinner. After dinner they held family meetings, "some of which were down and out battles between two kids." But they all got their feelings out, Nora remembers.

In 1982 Nora was selected to head her state's Governor's Committee for Employment of the Handicapped. She moved to the state capital, where she remained for the following seven years, renting an apartment. When her children arrived to attend college in the city, she bartered good home-cooked meals for vacuuming and taking out the garbage.

Seven years later Nora accepted a government job in another large city, where she still lives and works. Although living in a major urban center with public transportation, Nora prefers to drive her own two-door car with hand controls, putting her wheelchair in the back seat. She flies frequently, attending conferences and meetings as part of her job assignment.

Nora has chosen several aids to make the practical aspects of life more manageable. For example, when in her wheelchair she uses bungee cords (elastic cords with hooks at each end, available in a variety of lengths at hardware stores) to keep items such as grocery bags in place on her lap or on the footrest. She also keeps lightweight, foldable, cloth shopping bags in her purse to use when shopping so that individual items don't fall off her lap. Another ingenious idea is her use of "lap anchors," small pieces of rubberized material normally used to anchor throw rugs. She has stashed them throughout her apartment to use when she needs to secure something on her lap.

Nora has had some difficulties with the medical community. Two years ago she broke her leg for the third time. The ER doctor refused to believe it was bro-

ken because she was not in pain. She told him she had broken a leg twice before and knew what to look for. After convincing the doctor that the leg was indeed broken, she directed him in how to set it.

Nora emphasizes the importance of getting complete information about any medications. At one time a doctor suggested that Nora take Valium for her spasms. When she took the medication during the daytime, she became oblivious to everything around her. She decided to take it at night so she could get the benefits of the medication without feeling so groggy in the daytime.

In her midlife, Nora finds that her job allows less time for hobbies than she would like. But she sews and fits her own clothing (using a hand to operate the foot pedal on her sewing machine). She is putting photograph albums together for each of her children. And she loves to read about the Irish and listen to Irish music.

Nora says that her disability opened doors for her, creating the possibility for her career. Before her spinal cord injury she was a homemaker and had no particular plans apart from having a very large family. She now enjoys both a very busy career and a rewarding family life.

In Chapter 4 we described the transition from rehabilitation hospital to home, with all of its accompanying physical logistics and emotional significance. In this chapter we focus on the next crucial step after adjustment to the return home: reentry into the wider world, reengagement with life so as to become, once again, a contributing member of society. Nora's story illustrates how one person negotiated these transitions. Nora has created a satisfying, independent life for herself, while addressing a series of challenges.

The "how to" of independent living, especially when you have a disability, depends on many well-oiled gears meshing in life's machine. To be as independent as possible in making decisions and taking action, you need a well-greased support mechanism that moves smoothly and easily. And you need to set these gears in motion—and constantly maintain them—for all aspects of your life: housing, transportation, vocational and economic support, and educational and social support. You need to be an advocate for yourself. Your ability to speak for yourself when the mechanisms don't mesh is vitally important.

HOUSING

The major part of our lives is spent at home, whether in a duplex with five children or a bachelor apartment in a big-city high rise. We carry on the essential activities of living—eating, sleeping, relaxing, dressing, being with friends and family, having intimate relationships, disciplining the children, paying the bills—in this space that is uniquely ours. Selecting and arranging our home has a major effect on our lives.

As Nora's story illustrates, different types of housing meet our needs during the different seasons of our lives. Homes come in a variety of sizes, styles, locations, and prices: single-family homes, apartments, condominiums, multiple-family dwellings, rented rooms. Sometimes home is a room in a nursing home (see Chapter 9).

If you have a disability, "home" takes on new dimensions. It may feel like prison or like liberation: imprisoning when it limits or constricts your movement or ability to come and go; liberating when it allows you free range of movement and the opportunity to get out into the world. Where once steps went unnoticed, they now become major obstacles. Doors that are too heavy or too narrow to let you pass become entrapments. You begin to look at your needs in an entirely new light.

In addition to accessibility, your choice of living site will be based on your financial resources, the amount and type of physical assistance and accessibility you need, geographic location, and personal preferences.

Single-Family Homes

Most people whose stories we have told in this book returned to their family homes after rehabilitation. In most instances, these homes were single-family dwellings where modifications were made to allow the newly disabled person to move about with the greatest possible freedom. Joan's family relocated her bedroom, built a ramp, and made other modifications. Lee's parents, already planning a new house, scrapped their old blueprints and chose a completely accessible one-story home. Yet in another locale and economy, Lee and his wife could not afford the square-footage costs of a home on one level. Instead, they built a two-story home with an elevator. Bella and her family purchased a lovely one-level home for her in the suburbs, installing ramps over the one-step or two-step entryways. (Joan's story is told in Chapter 4; Lee's in Chapter 10; Bella's in Chapter 9.)

Some modifications are inexpensive and can be made by family or friends—a ramp over a couple of steps, for example. However, when undertaking a building project with accessibility in mind, some standards—such as door widths or ramps with "do-able" inclines—are very helpful. In response to the growing numbers of senior citizens in the United States, a trend has arisen among enlightened architects to emphasize accessibility. The two types of homes designed are visitable and universal. As described in *En-able Magazine,* a visitable home is one "that provides the essentials of barrier-free access such as zero-step or sloped entrances, doorways at least 32 inches wide, electrical outlets at reachable heights and reinforced bathroom walls for grab bars."

A universal home, on the other hand, "offers a wide range of accessibility and convenience features to accommodate a broad range of human ability and age groups." Universal design goes beyond the barrier-free design concept. It eliminates the need for special features that can be stigmatizing, different looking, and usually more expensive. Ron Mace (the "father of universal design") notes, "The features of a Universal Design Home make it appealing and marketable to persons of all ages and abilities." Sources of information on universal design are included in the Resources section at the end of this book.

The importance of visitability is highlighted when relatives and friends of a person with spinal cord injury find that he or she cannot attend social events at their houses because of inaccessibility. Lee and Tricia have found the lack of access to friends' homes to be difficult; Tricia usually checks out the homes of new friends to see if it's possible to visit.

If you are searching for an older house or even a newly constructed house, you'll benefit from working with a realtor who is knowledgeable about what is required for accessibility. Uninformed realtors can be a source of frustration, as Lee and Tricia found when they decided to move closer to their son's school. They found that most realtors "don't understand disability issues and don't listen to the family's needs." Check advertisements in the newspaper, call the real estate board to inquire about realtors with accessibility specialties, or get information from friends who have used realtors to find accessible homes. Of course, budget is always a consideration in buying a home, and often requires compromise. If possible, it's helpful to anticipate changes in your abilities that may come with age so that you can make accommodations that will be sufficient for the future. Moving when you are older is more economically difficult and can be more physically stressful. Lee, for example, found that even though his house had an elevator, he sometimes had to drag himself upstairs during a power outage. As he began to get arthritis in his shoulders, this was more difficult, and he looked for a house with a master bedroom on the first floor. Such homes tend to be more expensive, and Tricia notes that it may not be feasible at their income level. Since they just invested in a wonderfully accessible van, she teases Lee, "you'll just have to live in the car and the office!"

Apartments

After Joan completed her education, she chose to live in an apartment community (see Chapter 4). This decision was based on her desire to be as independent as possible. Located in a bustling urban area, the apartment complex houses many essentials for living, such as a grocery store, cleaners, restaurant, small shops, and a bar for socializing. The complex has a personal care attendant on site, hired by the people with disabilities who live in the high rise.

Discrimination based on disability in renting, purchasing housing, or obtaining financing is illegal. Under the Fair Housing Amendments Act, a landlord cannot have two different rental agreements, one for people with disabilities and one for those without.

Most people with disabilities require some environmental changes so that they can carry out the activities of daily living. What are "reasonable accommodations" (a term used in the Americans with Disabilities Act, discussed later in the chapter) to achieve this independent living? Someone who uses a wheelchair needs room under the kitchen sink to fit the chair. Someone who uses crutches needs a parking space close to his apartment entry. Another person needs a curb-cut to move from the parking lot to the sidewalk in her wheelchair. Other modifications might be needed in various rooms. Some common needs are raised toilet seats, bathroom grab bars, roll-in showers, widened doorways, door levers or automatic door openers, lowered kitchen cabinets, appliances with reachable controls, and lowered call-buttons in elevators.

All such alterations are charged to the renter, unless the landlord receives funding from the federal government. According to the pamphlet *Fair Housing: How to Make the Law Work for You,* available from the Paralyzed Veterans of America, the renter has to agree to restore the unit to its original condition (allowing for normal wear) on leaving; to give a fair description of the changes to be made; and to assure that the work is done well and that necessary permits are obtained.

Buildings with four or more living units must have basic accessibility for people with disabilities. Entryways, public areas, and common-use areas must be accessible. Doorways must be wide enough for wheelchairs. If you encounter problems that you feel are discriminatory, contact the U.S. Department of Housing and Urban Development, Office of Fair Housing and Equal Opportunity.

Condominiums

A condominium is an apartment or townhouse that is privately owned, usually by the occupant. All the rules that govern the purchase of a single-family house apply here. The difference is that condominiums normally have a governing body of owners that determines policies affecting each unit and the common areas. In some cases condominium boards have discriminated against individuals based on their disabilities.

If your condominium is a townhouse with several different levels, ensuring mobility will be challenging. One option might be to center your primary activities on one level. Another choice is to install either an elevator or a stair-climber. A stair-climber is a device attached to a railing on the wall; it may be a chair in which you sit or a platform on which you ride in your wheelchair. Some power wheelchairs are specifically designed to climb steps.

Some people with paraplegia choose to stay in their multilevel homes and bump up and down the steps on their buttocks. For this exertion, however, you need good arm strength and balance, and you must frequently assess the wear and tear on your backside to guard against skin breakdown.

Condominiums have the advantage over free-standing houses of monthly fees that cover the maintenance of lawns and parking lots and snow removal. And they have an advantage over rental homes in the usual tax advantages of home ownership. On the down side, you need to anticipate escalating condominium fees, which may eventually become unaffordable.

Multiple-Family Dwellings

Although rare in our society, several families or generations sometimes live together, whether by economic necessity or by choice. In this arrangement, accommodations and modifications for the person with spinal cord injury must be agreed to by all involved, and you'll have to educate family members about your needs. On the other hand, you'll have more thinking power and perhaps more willing hands to get things done.

As reported in the *Baltimore Sun* in 1997 and 1998, the story of siblings Naomi Shoemaker and Jason Fleckenstein provides an inspiring example of intergenerational living. Naomi and Jason were young adults with children of their own when they were injured in separate, unrelated car accidents, about two-and-a-half years apart. Both injuries resulted in tetraplegia. Naomi, separated from her husband at the time of the accident, moved with her three children into her parents' home. Jason, separated from his wife, was already living there. His six-year-old son visited the family after school, returning to his mother's house at night.

Naomi and Jason's parents, Victor and Patsy, provide a home for their adult children and their grandchildren, and Patsy acts as personal care attendant. Victor works full-time and helps out at home in the evenings. Living under one roof saves money on resources that would have to be duplicated if Naomi and Jason lived alone. The family borrowed money to install a basement exit and indoor wheelchair lift for Jason's basement quarters, as well as an outside backup lift.

After the first newspaper article about their unusual situation, the family was flooded with donations from strangers and from acquaintances in the community. Victor's union organized a four-state fund drive and set up a trust fund to provide for Naomi's and Jason's care when their parents are no longer able to do so. The union local also secured donations from an anonymous benefactor, including a small bus to transport the multigenerational family and a voice-activated computer to help Jason and Naomi explore home-based business opportunities.

This ordinary working-class family has met unusual adversity with a "can-do" attitude. With the help of their community, they've turned a potentially tragic situation into an opportunity for mutual support and growth. Though Naomi and Jason depend on their own parents for physical assistance, they are able to be full parents for their own children, providing love, guidance, teaching, discipline, help with homework, and setting of limits. All family members, including the children, help out as much as they can. With the physical and emotional contributions of each generation, and the economic and practical assistance of their community, this family has made multigenerational living work.

Economic Assistance for Housing

Several sources of economic housing assistance are available for low-income people with disabilities. Under Section 8 of the U.S. Housing Act, three program areas could be helpful: Section 8: Existing Housing Program; Section 8: Rental Vouchers Program; and Section 8: Home-ownership Vouchers Program.

Under the Section 8: Existing Housing Program, designated units have reduced rent—rent is 30 percent of a person's adjusted income. The units may be scattered throughout the community or clustered in one building. Renters are responsible for modifications in these units.

The Section 8: Rental Vouchers Program can be used in a different way. An individual can go anywhere in the community to find a unit. If the owner agrees to accept subsidized housing, the Housing and Urban Development agency (HUD) pays the difference between the individual's 30 percent contribution and the fair market value. If the owner wants more than fair market value as determined by HUD, the individual can pay more than the 30 percent.

Section 8: Homeownership Vouchers Program allows vouchers to be used for partial mortgage payments. Not all local government public housing agencies participate in this program, and there are often long waiting lists.

Another program exclusively for people with disabilities who live on fixed incomes is Fannie Mae's Home Choice program, featuring a low down payment and a different debt-to-loan ratio (Fannie Mae is the Federal National Mortgage Association). The HOPE 6 Project, intended to replace distressed public housing with home ownership and rental units, is available to people with a wider range of incomes and is covered by Section 504. Modifications are made by the owner. Information about economic assistance for housing can be found through your local Office for Persons with Disabilities, your local public housing agency, or your local HUD office. These agencies can also help you if you feel your civil rights have been violated in the housing arena.

When Kelsie Collins, who had sustained a spinal cord injury in a car accident, was looking for an already-accessible rental unit, she had a real estate agent who believed that "anything was possible," according to the *Baltimore Sun,* in a 1997 article. The agent was convinced that Kelsie could buy her own home, and set out to make this happen. Kelsie was living on a fixed disability income and didn't think she could get financing for her own home. Like many people with spinal cord injury, she had spent a lot of "down time" in the hospital and both her credit and income history had suffered.

The real estate agent thought that a steady income was the bottom line for obtaining a mortgage and that Kelsie's disability income was likely to be her permanent source of income because her disability was so severe (tetraplegia). With the help of an independent living center and a mortgage company that was willing to at least consider Kelsie's application, the agent was able to get the Social Security Administration to confirm that her disability income was projected to be lifelong. With this virtual guarantee, Kelsie's disability check became an asset rather than a liability. She was able to buy a condominium, with mortgage payments only slightly more than her previous rent. The condo was already accessible inside. Only the addition of a ramp was needed to give accessibility to the parking lot.

Kelsie's story illustrates the power of persistence and creative problem-solving in dealing with housing needs. It also provides several insights into home-buying:

1. Seek financial counseling if you need to clear up your credit record.

2. Make a budget or get advice on how to build up savings.
3. Write a letter of explanation if your credit rating has suffered because of lengthy hospitalization or job loss following your injury.
4. Look into FHA (Federal Housing Administration, a division of HUD) mortgages and other federal assistance programs.
5. Shop around for a loan officer and get approved for a loan before you shop for a home.
6. Try to persuade banks to waive some fees.
7. When negotiating the sale, ask the seller to finance home modification costs.

Once you've picked out your home, look to community organizations, church groups, or private firms to help with home modifications. These sources can supplement any federal or state assistance you receive. Above all, don't give up!

TRANSPORTATION

Essential to being a part of society at large is "getting there." Transportation is vital for independent living and participation in the community. You need to travel to the grocery store, your workplace, the bank, your church or synagogue, the theater, the laundry, the dime store, your friend's home, the park. How do you get to your many destinations?

Public Transportation

Buses

If you live in a city with good public transport, you may rely on this system to get from place to place. Buses that "kneel" or have wheelchair lifts open up the world for people with disabilities. Under the Americans with Disabilities Act (discussed more fully later in this chapter), all new fixed-route, public transit buses have to be accessible, and additional para-transit systems must be provided for people unable to use the buses. Although bus system accessibility is mandated, call your transportation authority to confirm you'll be able to get an accessible bus on the route you need and at the right time.

Public para-transit systems provide accessible minibuses or taxis for people with disabilities. Various payment systems are used, so call ahead for information. You may also be eligible for economic assistance. Note that many of these transit systems require advance notice of a day or two for pick-up time, so be sure to plan ahead.

Some counties and cities have special van services available for people with disabilities, at no cost. These services also require advance notice for pick up. Some take people anywhere in the area; others may be available only for transportation to medical appointments.

The use of taxicabs can be fraught with problems if you use a wheelchair. John Hockenberry relates several instances when taxis cruised by him as he hailed them from his wheelchair. He describes the anger and frustration he felt in these situations. Many taxi drivers assume that a wheelchair user needs to be lifted into the cab, or they simply don't want to bother with stowing the wheelchair in the trunk of the taxi. When possible, call a cab company ahead of time if you must rely on a taxi. Some cities have private cab companies that have wheelchair vans. Transportation from airports may often be arranged (in advance of arrival) with these companies.

Rail Systems

Under the Americans with Disabilities Act, rail systems must have at least one accessible car on each train. Railway depots must also be accessible. This means that if you are traveling cross-country with sleeping accommodations, you will have one small compartment, barely large enough to turn a wheelchair around in. There will be a pull-down berth in addition to benches that create a bed, a small table, a commode, and a sink. This car will be your "home" for the duration of your trip as no other cars are accessible. Meals will be brought to you and socialization will be limited to people on their way to the commode on some trains or simply going car to car on others, depending on the location of the accessible compartment. If you need assistance, attendants must take you off at stops if you so desire. Because of lack of maintenance on the rails, trains may rock back and forth, or side to side. Make sure to brake your chair while the train is in motion. Try to do transfers (for example, bathroom use) while the train is at a stop.

If you are traveling between cities on the Eastern seaboard, you can sit on a regular car with wheelchair carve-out and an accessible bath-room. But as on other trains, you cannot move to other cars, including the club car, so you must ask for food to be brought to you if you intend to eat. If you do request accessible seating, ask about discounts off the price of your ticket.

City dwellers depend on subway systems for much of their commut-ing. People with disabilities who want to use the subway should check whether elevators are available and if they are in working order. Not all subway stops have elevators, so you may need to plan to embark or dis-embark at specific stations. A note to new subway users: if you use a wheelchair, check the distance from platform to the subway car as small front wheels sometimes get stuck in the void between them. For this reason, some people like to back onto a car, or if they're wheelchair "jocks," they may prefer to "pop a wheelie" to access the subway.

Air Travel

If you fly, you know the challenges to getting airborne. Informing reser-vation agents of your special needs is the first step to ensuring a safe and comfortable flight. Be specific about your needs, such as requiring assis-tance to your seat, help when transferring between airlines, or a seat assignment in the bulkhead. Be sure to make these requests again at the time of departure so they are not overlooked.

Both the Air Carrier Access Act of 1986 and the Americans with Dis-abilities Act specify that the needs of persons with disabilities must be met both on the ground and in the air. This covers accessible parking near the terminal; signs indicating accessible parking and access to the terminal; accessible medical aid facilities and travelers aid stations; ac-cessible restrooms; accessible drinking fountains; accessible ticketing systems at primary fare-collection areas; amplified telephones; accessible baggage check-in and retrieval areas; accessible jetways and mobile lounges; flat boarding ramps, lifts, and so forth; information systems with both visual and oral components; and signs indicating the location of specific facilities. For more information, contact the U.S. Department of Transportation for its handy little pamphlet, *New Horizons: Informa-tion for the Air Traveler with a Disability.* Another useful booklet is the

Paralyzed Veterans of America's *The Air Carrier Access Act: Make it Work for You.*

You may want to get advice from people with disabilities similar to yours who fly frequently. Some advise not consuming liquids before flights so that you don't have a "call of nature" on the flight. Others advise waiting on the plane after landing until your chair or scooter comes up from the hold. If you leave the plane in a wheelchair provided by the airline, you could be stranded in the airport without your own means of getting about. If you use crutches, expect different rules for their storage, even within the same airline. Some stewards say crutches go in the overhead bins, while others allow you to stow them on the floor beside you. If you are flying coach class, try to get seating in the bulkhead row, the first row in the coach section. This offers more space and thus greater ease in getting in and out of your seat.

Rules about what medical equipment may be taken aboard an airplane vary from airline to airline. Using that equipment aboard the airliner is an even thornier problem to resolve. Many users of battery-powered wheelchairs or scooters have experienced problems with mishandling, damage, and loss of parts when this equipment is put in the hold. So when you decide on the equipment you'll take, label it well and have a back-up plan at your destination if there are any problems. One iBOT (a motorized wheelchair that climbs stairs) user will not take his on an airliner because he fears damage to this very expensive equipment. Other users of electric wheelchairs or scooters make sure batteries are disengaged and stored separately. Because of worry about the handling of their wheelchair cushions, most people keep them in the cabin, sitting on them or stowing them in overhead bins.

Transporting portable respirators and ventilators may require documentation and a letter from your physician so that you can take them aboard an airliner. This equipment, usually operated by sensitive computers, has to be handled carefully; explain to the flight personnel the need to keep it in the cabin near you in a secure place. There are also those who need to use their equipment in flight; this requires advance communication with the airline. Some people carry prescriptions or letters of medical necessity to show when necessary.

Ships and Ferries

As the American population ages, the call for accessible ships, including cruise ships, is increasing—an advantage for persons with disabilities. When new ships are introduced into ship lines, they are required to be physically accessible. This includes accessible bathrooms in the cabins. Problems for those with physical disabilities arise when excursions on land are planned. Although some ports have docks where passengers can leave the ship via stairs or ramps, many ports have to be "tendered," which means that passengers are taken ashore on smaller boats (tenders). Transferring to a tender in a wheelchair is usually impossible. If you are planning a cruise, ask in advance about tendered and non-tendered ports and whether each port has accessible transportation and general accessibility. If you need a wheelchair-accessible cabin, make sure you book well in advance because those cabins are requested early. Sources of information abound (see the Resources section at the end of this book).

Ferries are an essential mode of transportation in some parts of the world. One example is the state system of ferries plying the inland waterway in southeast Alaska, which is a basic way to travel for many Alaskans as well as for visitors who want to "get the feel" of real Alaska. These huge ferries are wheelchair accessible with the exception of some entries onto the decks, which have one step.

Private Transportation

The first issue to settle is whether you can still drive your vehicle after spinal cord injury, with or without some type of adaptation. This may require a driving evaluation and assessment for adaptive equipment. Most states require drivers to report a physical disability that might significantly affect their driving status and require that these drivers be re-examined. If you do not report your disability, your automobile insurance carrier may not be obliged to cover you in the event of an accident. Check with your insurance company and state Motor Vehicles Department before driving your adapted vehicle. Driver education for persons with disabilities is usually available through rehabilitation centers. You can get more information from your state Department of Rehabilitation. Of course, private driver training programs are also available.

After the proper driving training, you'll need to make decisions about types of vehicles and special accommodations. Basic decisions will center on:

1. Will you be the driver or the passenger?
2. If you are the driver, what needs do you have?
   – Can you drive without any accommodation?
   – Do you need hand controls?
   – If so, do you have the necessary strength to lift your wheelchair into the back seat?
   – If not, do you want to drive a sedan, a van, or a minivan?

If you decide on an accessible minivan, it will probably have a lowered floor and a "kneeling" (lowering) capability so that the incline of the ramp to run your chair up will not be too steep. Ramps, by the way, may be in-dwelling under the floor and slide out with remote control or may simply fold up or down, also automatically, by the side door. There are also rear door ramp and lift systems available. And the cost? New vans almost double in cost when equipped with manufacturer built-in ramps. Some large automobile companies have programs that give a rebate toward the cost of modification.

There are various ways for a driver to get a wheelchair in and out of the car. Vans can be fitted with a wheelchair lift or a ramp that folds down so that you can wheel inside, as described above. Some people with power wheelchairs prefer to remove the driver's seat and adapt the vehicle so they can drive while seated in the wheelchair. Others stow the power chair behind the front seat, transferring into the car seat to drive. Some people with manual chairs drive two-door cars with wide doors and more access to the back seat, which allows them to fold the chair and put it in the back. If you have some walking ability, you can put a chair or scooter on a lift on the back of the car and walk to the driver's seat. Also available are lifts that put a wheelchair into the back seat of the car.

If you prefer to drive a sedan, containers called chair toppers can be purchased to install on top of your vehicle. These ingenious contraptions automatically lower a hook from an overhead compartment, which resembles a car-top luggage carrier. The hook slips under the seat of the wheelchair (which is easily collapsed by pulling up on the seat) and carries it vertically upward until it flips on its side and slips into the open container. The container then closes, to store and protect the chair. An advantage of this device is that you can transfer from the chair to the car seat, hook the chair, and push the button in the car to raise it. This is helpful for those unable to walk or without sufficient strength to lift the wheelchair into the back seat of the car. One caution: the height of the vehicle plus the container will dictate which parking garages you can patronize; a sign over the entrance usually states the height limit allowed. When you are buying a new vehicle, check with the manufacturer about cash allowances for modifications. Ford, General Motors, and Chrysler all give some rebate toward hand controls, pedal adaptations, van conversions, or lifts. Dealers usually have brochures available on the dollar amounts their manufacturers grant. This allowance can be a major economic boost in these expensive purchases.

If you do not drive, perhaps a personal care attendant or family member can drive your vehicle. Your personal safety is important, so make sure you have proper tie-downs for the wheelchair. Other issues to consider include an attendant's valid driver's license and good driving record, and insurance to cover the driver and passengers in the car.

A note on technological aids in driving: before investing in the latest technology to aid in your driving, talk with others who have used the device about pros and cons. Some items require sensitive care and frequent fine-tuning. If you know in advance that a technological device needs tender loving care, you may be less stressed about the time you spend taking your car or van to the shop.

When considering hand controls, think about what type of driving you are likely to do. Some hand controls are permanently mounted in the vehicle. If you travel and rent cars often, or own more than one vehicle, you may want to buy portable hand controls. These can be switched from one car to another and are easily installed and removed without permanently altering the car. They are also useful if another family member will sometimes be driving the same car using the foot pedals.

MEETING THE CHALLENGE OF WORK

Robert was injured in a car accident on a winter night in 1983, when he was twenty-four. He was on his way home from his job in a nuclear power plant when he fell asleep at the wheel. Robert was a Midwest grain farmer, who, like other farmers, had to take a second job to sustain his farm. He remembers getting up at 5:00 a.m. to do chores in order to get to work at the power plant by 7:00 a.m. After an exhausting day, he had an hour's drive home and then more chores after his 6:30 p.m. arrival home. The grain farm also had chickens, a small cattle herd, and other animals for the family's meat.

On the night of his accident, he had set the cruise control he'd rigged up on his old pickup truck. When he fell asleep, the truck crossed the center line, rolled, and ejected him into a ditch. Normally he wore coveralls at work, removing them prior to his drive home. That evening he had not taken them off. The warmth had caused him to fall asleep at the wheel but also saved him from freezing as he waited to be discovered. He remembers hearing the truck's radio play on and on. Sometime later, he was found by a neighbor, who got some lumber from his truck and jury-rigged a litter that he used to drag Robert up the embankment to the truck. "My right side was broken. Head to toe." Robert had dislocation of his T4, T5, and T6 vertebrae, and sustained a T4 spinal cord injury.

Ever the hard worker, Robert applied himself strenuously to his rehabilitation, and began to think about work immediately upon returning home. During the year following his inpatient rehab, Robert tried to return to farming. But he found no adaptive farm equipment and his home community was largely inaccessible.

Although he had not been successful going to college after high school, he decided to give it another try. With the support of the State Department of Vocational Rehabilitation, he started off at a small college, and eventually transferred to a large university in a big city. He moved to the city, went to school, worked out at a rehabilitation center, and got involved in athletics, which built his confidence. During the summer he worked at a camp for kids with disabilities. During his second year of college, he met and moved in with his girlfriend, a manufacturers sales representative. After he graduated from college with a degree in exercise physiology, his girlfriend was transferred by her company to the West Coast, and he followed her.

Robert began to pursue a graduate degree in urban design, but left the pro-

gram before getting his degree, when his girlfriend was transferred again, this time to the East Coast, where they got married. Robert had trouble finding a job. He finally went to a series of résumé-building seminars for persons with disabilities. He saw an announcement for director of accessibility seating at a sports arena. He called that Monday and went for the interview that afternoon; impressed with his knowledge and his own accomplishments in sports, they offered him the job the same day. He worked for several years directly under the owner, orienting staff and helping people with disabilities enjoy events in the arena. As the arena expanded services to people with disabilities, Robert was put in charge of the education of staff on sensitivity to issues of disability, and worked on signing, seating, and restroom accessibility. In his position he met a number of national celebrities and enjoyed his job tremendously.

Robert's third career began when he met a member of the city's accessibility board on the subway, and they talked. This man suggested that Robert apply for an opening on the board, that of accessibility specialist working on outdoor accessibility guidelines. The three areas of guidelines he works on include play areas/playgrounds, recreation facilities/amusement parks, and outdoor developed areas like beaches, camping, and picnic areas. He also does training all over the county in these areas. Robert's work, which is part of his active lifestyle, has been a highly satisfying part of his life.

Work is the backbone of many people's lives. It provides some definition of who we are. Work will probably be a key issue as you reenter the "real world."

You may have no difficulty reentering your old profession. If you are an accountant, an English teacher, an editor, or a computer specialist, job modifications may be minor. If you are a dancer, a window installer, or a professional soccer player, you'll have to think about switching careers. However, before deciding on a change, stop and consider: if you love your line of work, look for a creative way to continue. If you were a professional baseball player, what about coaching or managing a team? And dance companies need choreographers and managers, whose work can be done primarily on computer. You may need additional training to stay in your chosen career in a new, creative way.

Jerome Lee's story, as told in *Newsweek* magazine, is an interesting example of creativity in combining an old career with new limitations and new skills. Jerome worked in construction for twenty-two years before a random shooting injury caused his paraplegia. During rehabilitation, his positive attitude helped motivate and encourage many younger patients. When he left the rehabilitation hospital for a vocational training program, it seemed logical to work in human services. Jerome earned certification as a human services assistant, but although he liked helping people, he hated to throw away all those years of experience and all that he knew and loved about construction work.

After many consultations with the business opportunities division of his vocational training program, Jerome worked out a way to combine his old skills in construction and site management with his new skills in human services and motivation. He became the manager of the painting crew for the large outpatient center that housed the vocational training program, recruiting many workers with disabilities. "I bid on jobs, organize the workload, order supplies, assemble the work teams, supervise the jobs, and do a lot of the plastering and painting myself . . . I teach my crew members a trade they can really use . . . We sometimes surprise people who don't expect to see individuals with disabilities doing this kind of work. To me, we are proof that no one should be denied the chance to work because he or she has a disability."

Keith Thompson, a police officer in Omaha, Nebraska, was injured in a car accident while pursuing a stolen vehicle. The initial accident resulted in a head trauma and a twenty-day coma. When he awoke from the coma, he underwent surgery to repair a damaged aorta. During the surgery the doctors had to cut off the blood supply to his spine; this resulted in paraplegia. After his hospitalization and rehabilitation, Keith was enrolled in Goodwill's Head Injury Rehabilitation and Employment Program. Here he honed his skills and received job-coaching. Coaches worked with him by calling in mock police reports, which Keith had to record following a specific protocol. With this training, he returned to the police department, where he now works with the Telephone Response Unit, taking calls about auto theft, destruction of property, hit-and-run accidents, and other problems.

Chelsea had been a flight attendant then a homemaker and mother for fifteen years before her spinal cord injury. Unlike Keith and Jerome, who returned to familiar job arenas, Chelsea struck out on a new venture. After she returned from rehabilitation and had some time to reorganize her home and family life, she decided to run her own business. With financial backing from the Small Business Administration, she opened her own culinary shop, specializing in spices.

If you are young and just starting to think about what careers are interesting to you, or if you need to change to another line of work, you can take advantage of a number of resources. While in the hospital, you'll probably be linked up with your state's Department of Rehabilitation Services or Department of Vocational Rehabilitation. A counselor will help you make career decisions, based on an assessment of your physical and mental abilities and your interest in various vocations as measured by interviews, tests, and questionnaires. Vocational rehabilitation services also include job training, job placement, and sometimes follow-up support services once you are in a new job. Sometimes, vocational rehabilitation services also include other supports you need to make employment possible. Noah (introduced in Chapter 8), for example, got assistance from his state's vocational program to prepare him for success in college and the workplace. The agency provided him with certain medical supports, such as a personal care attendant for sixteen hours a day and a case manager to make phone calls and advocate for his needs when necessary. In addition, the program funded some of the technical and mechanical aids that increase his independence for work-related activities, such as computer access.

Some federal programs provide tax incentives for employers who hire people with disabilities. Keep this in mind when looking for a job. Some larger companies also have affirmative action programs in place to hire individuals with disabilities. Your counselor should be able to provide further information.

Some excellent private vocational rehabilitation services are also available. Be sure to get two references before paying for these services. Similar services may also be provided by local religious organizations or community colleges. Using a variety of services almost always provides the best chance to find employment.

A cruel irony of our system is that sometimes individuals are caught in a bind in which disability payments are more than they can earn in a job. Sometimes receiving a government payment, such as Social Security Disability, precludes accepting employment. Because the costs surrounding disability needs (personal care attendant, supplies, equipment, transportation, housing) may exceed what you can earn, you may have to refuse paid work. In this case, finding a job that falls within the income guidelines of the law may be the solution. The Social Security Disability program allows you to supplement your disability payment with part-time work, up to a set dollar amount. You are also entitled to a trial period of full-time work, during which your disability payment continues. If you continue to work past the trial period, your payments are discontinued. If you find that full-time work is not possible, or if you have medical complications that force you to stop working before the end of the trial period, you don't lose your disability benefits. For more specific information, contact your local Social Security office.

Paid employment may be impossible, or you may choose not to work. If you are primarily a homemaker and parent, your rehabilitation center can provide training and adaptive devices to make your work at home easier. Some people opt for volunteer work as an alternative to paid employment. (For more information on volunteering, community service, and other non-vocational lifestyles, see Chapter 9.)

ACCESS TO EDUCATION

If you need a college education or technical training to prepare for work, explore public or private vocational services. Check whether you meet the eligibility requirements (they change periodically). Private career counselors provide testing and direction. You can find them through local or state professional organizations, such as psychological, social work, and rehabilitation counseling associations.

You'll find many ways to get into further education. Access to colleges, universities, and vocational training facilities is easier than it used to be, thanks to legislation, such as the Americans with Disabilities Act, Section 504 of the Rehabilitation Act of 1973, and other laws. And the legislation guaranteeing the rights of persons with disabilities to equal educational opportunity means that colleges, universities, and technical training schools are better prepared to accept students with disabilities and meet their needs than in years past. Most institutions now have an Office for Students with Disabilities, which assists students in obtaining appropriate education. For example, if you need a note-taker or audiotaping assistance, this can be set up. Or if you write very slowly, you may be allowed more time or given access to a computer for taking tests. These programs help the faculty and administrators maximize educational opportunities for students with disabilities.

Most schools have been made more accessible to wheelchairs over the past few years. If some classrooms are inaccessible, however, you can request that classes be relocated. If elevators require the use of keys in particular buildings, the Office for Students with Disabilities can arrange for you to have a key so you can use the elevator when you need it. Some schools are technically accessible because there are no steps, but large, hilly college campuses may be hard to navigate. Joey, who developed incomplete tetraplegia after his second year of college, could use a manual chair for flat surfaces, but was not strong enough to wheel efficiently from one class to another. Since there were no shuttle buses on campus, arrangements were made for Joey to have a student aide push his chair between classes. Ultimately, he was able to get a motorized chair, which gave him independent access to all parts of the campus.

Economic access may be the crucial factor for your schooling. If you qualify, your state vocational rehabilitation department may be helpful in financing your education. Of course, you can apply for the usual student scholarships and loans, and sometimes for local, private scholarship funds specifically for people with disabilities. Some state colleges and public community colleges may waive tuition for people with disabilities. Your local community college, the public library, or the Internet are good sources of information on scholarship funds.

If you are a teenager and still in high school, your local public school is legally obligated to accommodate you with accessible classes and whatever adaptations you need to get your education. If medical complications preclude attendance at school temporarily, the public school system provides in-home tutoring. Some teenagers choose to complete a high school equivalency degree rather than return to school. Much of the studying for this degree can be done at home, but you still need access to some classrooms and to the building and room where the equivalency examination is given. Some teenagers who acquire a spinal cord injury during their high school years may choose to return to inaccessible private schools rather than switch to an unfamiliar public school.

When Andrew returned home from a rehabilitation center after a shooting injury left him with paraplegia, he wanted to take his place in the small private school he had attended before he was wounded. The only hang-up was the total inaccessibility of the school. But Andrew was determined to return and the school was equally committed to it. Although the school did not make structural accommodations for Andrew, he arranged for other students to carry him up and down the steps between classes. While not an ideal situation, this solution was satisfactory from Andrew's viewpoint.

BECOMING AN ADVOCATE FOR YOURSELF

Although we sometimes wish that other people could read our minds and go to bat for us, in reality no one knows our needs and desires better than we do. While you are in the rehabilitation center, the professionals who work there serve as your advocates. When you leave, you have to become your own advocate.

What does "advocating" mean? Basically it means standing up for yourself and communicating the importance of your needs to those who can meet them or who can help you achieve your goals. To advocate effectively, you must believe yourself worthy of having your needs met.

Bella (whose story is in Chapter 9) says, "When I was told I would be living as a handicapped person, my reaction was 'I don't think so.' What is a handicap/disability? It is a state of mind, an attitude that is not political but personal, and it is a barrier. We have choices: how we go forward. The best way is to acknowledge the existence of the condition, find out all that's possible to find out about it, then make a plan, elicit support, find role models, and get to work."

Different people have different levels of comfort in speaking for themselves, and we're generally more comfortable doing so in some situations than in others. An extrovert may find communicating easy, while an introvert might find it intimidating. Comfort levels are also affected by the amount of stress in our lives.

Gwen, an attorney, was usually quite competent in dealing with situations that involved gaining entry using her wheelchair. One Saturday night she went to the movies with a couple of friends. Arriving at the theater, they waited in line in the freezing cold to buy tickets. They eventually got their tickets and entered the theater, only to be met by the manager, who told them that Gwen wouldn't be able to see the movie because it was on the second level and the theater had no elevator. Gwen, who'd had a stressful week litigating a case and caring for her aging mother, burst into tears. This was the proverbial "straw that broke the camel's back," she thought.

In another time and place, Gwen would have handled the situation with her usual professional demeanor, imparting information with a sense of humor. Her experience at the movie theater illustrates how emotions change, depending on what is happening in our lives. When advocating for yourself, give yourself some slack. Don't expect to be "perfect" in being educational and understanding in every situation.

When you have the emotional resources, what sorts of skills do you need to be your own advocate? Most people agree that advocacy involves the following steps:

1. Identify the problem.
2. Identify the desired solution.
3. Identify various ways to reach the solution.

Each step requires clear thinking, the ability to articulate, and the willingness to hear other people's ideas, appreciate them, and incorporate compromises if necessary.

How do you learn to advocate for yourself? First, be informed; know what you are talking about. What are your rights? Read further in this chapter about the basic rights set forth in the Americans with Disabilities Act and know the fundamentals of Section 504 of the Rehabilitation Act for a good legal grounding.

Second, learn assertiveness and advocacy skills. Programs that teach advocacy skills are most likely sponsored by your local Office for Persons with Disabilities or Commission for Women. You can also learn these skills through mainstream organizations that teach public speaking.

Some rehabilitation programs provide social skills training, and many community colleges and mental health facilities offer assertiveness training classes for the general public. On a very practical level, you can learn from watching how other people with spinal cord injury or members of their families gain the attention they need to achieve their goals. For example, Jane's work, initially on behalf of her son, has benefited many others over the years. Her story illustrates that family members can play an important role in advocating for their loved ones with spinal cord injury, especially their children and teenagers.

> *About 7:30 on a snowy winter evening, Jane, her husband, and her two sons, ages twelve and two years old, were returning home from a party for the two-year-old's nursery school class. Jane and twelve-year-old Andrew were in one car, while her husband and the two-year-old were in a second. As they parked near their home, a third car without headlights drew up. The boyfriend of their former nanny jumped from his car, aiming a gun at Jane's husband, and fired several shots in his direction. Andrew shouted to his stepfather, "Get out of the way!" The shooter heard the call, faced the boy, and shot him as Andrew raced to duck into the car. Andrew fell to the ground in the softly falling snow. The ex-boyfriend, once a trusted friend of the family, sped away in his car.*
>
> *Thinking that the man had been firing blanks because he had not been hit, Jane's husband went to Andrew, thinking he was just scared by the gunfire. "I can't feel my legs," Andrew said. Jane recalls trying to reassure him, "Honey, those were blanks; you're just traumatized." Then they "stupidly" carried Andrew into the house, where they soon discovered that he had been shot and was paralyzed.*
>
> *The rescue squad arrived soon, along with hordes of neighbors and friends and TV trucks. Andrew was transported to a pediatric hospital where Jane was told that he was paralyzed with a complete T10 injury; one bullet was embedded in his spine and one was in his shoulder (it had just missed the aorta). Andrew was placed in the ICU. "They kept assigning words to him, like 'paraplegic.' I had to run out of the room because I was going to throw up. It was too big for my mind."*
>
> *Jane was also terrified that the shooter would come back to the house to hurt them, especially her two-year-old. They learned later that the gunman had driven to a bar in a nearby city where he shot and killed himself. This brought some relief to Jane, who "couldn't have lived knowing he was around; he had known and played with my children."*
>
> *During the first hours of Andrew's treatment, Jane and her family had tremendous support; seventy people filled the hospital waiting room after hearing of Andrew's injury, and a friend of the family, a doctor, translated medical jargon into understandable terms. Jane recalls that "I didn't lose it but I was terrified."*

She remembers telling her friend, "I always felt something would happen to Andrew. It was a dread. But now I know why I'm here: to take care of Andrew."

Andrew had a variety of complications during his first month after injury, including blood in his chest, infections, fevers, and hallucinations. Jane continued to hope for a cure for Andrew, and when his legs moved involuntarily in a spasm, Jane imagined that motor control was returning.

Jane was confronted with the multiple demands of raising a now frightened two-year-old and caring for Andrew. Her marriage had been strained before the shooting; it now became more so, as she had little energy to extend beyond her two boys. Her concerns for her younger son led her to seek professional counseling to help him cope with his brother's injury and the trauma of the shooting. Her finances were stressed, and she was not able to afford all the home modifications that would have been ideal for Andrew. So when Andrew came home, between his acute hospital stay and his admission to a rehabilitation center, Jane carried him up and down the steps to his bedroom. Real estate agents encouraged them to move to the outer suburbs to find a home on one level, but Jane did not want to "punish Andrew more by taking him away from his friends." Finally, they found a house with an elevator and a bank gave her a mortgage; she wound up $20,000 in debt.

Jane found a newly opened state-of-the-art rehabilitation center for Andrew. It was cheerful and lively, and served many young people like Andrew. Parents could visit on weekends. While there, Andrew began to study for his bar mitzvah, scheduled for June. Although friends urged her to postpone the event, Jane was firm in her belief that Andrew could prepare for and participate in the ceremony on schedule. Coordinating with the center's staff, study sessions via phone were slated for specific times ("they called it the Tele-Torah!"). Often Andrew couldn't be found when the calls came. He spent much of his free time in the room of Katie, a five-year-old girl he had met at the pediatric hospital; she had a brain injury incurred in an automobile accident.

Andrew was discharged from the rehabilitation center one week before his bar mitzvah, when he was twelve-and-a-half years old. He wrote his bar mitzvah speech about Katie and delivered his speech standing in his leg braces. This was his welcome back to his community. He stayed in touch with Katie's family for years.

Jane became an advocate for her son and others with disabilities. "When Andrew came home I took my anger and fear and turned it into advocacy. I did what I do best: I knew how to be angry and how to get information. I got twenty-

seven curb-cuts in my neighborhood so that Andrew could go where he wanted to go."

Finding resources is important and county governments have many free resources available, Jane says. She has found money just sitting there, waiting to be used; people just don't know to call. "If I'm after something, I'll find it. I used whoever was around, for instance, the staff in the hospital. Find the people with the skills who want to help."

She feels it equally important for parents to advocate for themselves, to deal with their own issues. "Get counseling with someone who knows about spinal cord injury. Have your own private time and dump everything on your therapist. Then go back to advocate!"

While a tireless advocate for Andrew, Jane also "was tough on him . . . He did chores, what everyone else did, dishes, cleaning his room." She worked hard at supporting Andrew's independence, and not babying him because of his injury. She allowed him to take an accessible subway to school, and to get his driver's license at sixteen, like his peers. She supported his involvement in wheelchair athletics, though this took Andrew on trips away from home at a young age. She expected Andrew to be responsible for his own choices and accomplishments.

Jane says proudly that when Andrew (now an accomplished professional) speaks in public, he often says, "My mother opened the doors and I chose whether to go through them."

THE AMERICANS WITH DISABILITIES ACT

In 1990, in Washington, D.C., President George H. W. Bush signed into law the Americans with Disabilities Act (ADA), which ensures the rights of Americans with physical or mental disabilities in the areas of employment, public services, public accommodations, transportation, and telecommunications. It was a landmark day in the lives of those who had fought for this legislation and for all those who would benefit from it. As the years have passed and the law has been implemented, it has been the subject of much heated debate and interpreted in many different contexts.

Title I of the Americans with Disabilities Act bans discrimination in employment against qualified persons with disabilities. Employers must make "reasonable accommodations" to the needs of the qualified applicant. Accommodations might include making the work area accessible, providing or changing equipment to make it usable, changing work schedules or restructuring jobs, and providing readers or interpreters. The use of selection tests that screen out persons with disabilities, as well as pre-employment medical examinations, is banned. Title I permits the use of medical exams after a job has been offered, if all persons in the same job category have to submit to such an exam and the results are treated as a confidential medical record. Questions about the ability of a job applicant to perform job-related skills are appropriate. If your disability makes job performance impossible or dangerous, even with accommodations, you can be screened out. But you cannot be questioned about medical or physical problems that are unrelated to specific task performance. These rules apply to businesses with fifteen or more employees; smaller businesses may be exempt.

In order to be protected from job discrimination under the ADA, you must be able to perform the essential elements of a job, with or without reasonable accommodation. According to the U.S. Equal Employment Opportunity Commission, "First, you must satisfy the employer's requirements for the job, such as education, employment experience, skills or licenses. Second, you must be able to perform the essential functions of the job with or without reasonable accommodation. Essential functions are the fundamental job duties that you must be able to perform on your own or with the help of reasonable accommodation."

Title II of the act mandates that services and programs of local and state governments be made accessible and that all new buses be accessible. Para-transit or other special transportation must be provided for those who cannot use regular routes. All new rail vehicles and stations must be accessible, and all rail systems must have one accessible car per train. Title II also states that local and state governments cannot discriminate or exclude people from public programs or activities based on disability.

Title III relates to public accommodations, such as sales, rental, and service businesses. It requires auxiliary aids to ensure full participation of persons with visual, hearing, or sensory disabilities, as long as this will not be an "undue burden" on the business. The law gives business owners flexibility to choose various alternatives for providing clear communication. In existing public accommodations, Title III requires barriers to be removed when "readily achievable," meaning when it can be done easily and with little expense. Accessibility is required in new constructions and in alterations of older buildings, except that elevators are not required in structures less than three stories high or less than three thousand square feet per story.

Title IV amended the Communications Act of 1934 to require telephone companies to provide telecommunication relay systems. Speech-impaired or hearing-impaired persons who use a Telecommunication Device for the Deaf (an electronic device for text communication via a telephone line) or other non-voice systems must have the same opportunities for communication provided to other customers.

Title V bans any coercion or retaliation against persons pursuing their rights under the ADA, along with other miscellaneous issues such as a special federal wilderness provision and technical assistance guidelines. Specific avenues to address grievances go through the Attorney General's Office, the Equal Employment Opportunity Commission, and the Department of Justice.

ATTAINING YOUR LIFE GOALS

This century will no doubt bring both new demands and new means of meeting them. Many of those "I dare you" challenges for people with spinal cord injuries will move from fantasy to reality. Already, you can come closer than ever before to structuring the kind of life you had before your injury, or the kind of life you dreamed of having. Your disability exists; it is real. But you can find technological, legal, social, and educational solutions to obstacles (both physical and psychological) that will help you reach your goals.

As a person with spinal cord injury, your work is threefold. First, identify what you want; second, believe that you deserve to achieve your goals; and third, fully tap your internal sources of energy and motivation, as well as the wealth of external supports.

PART III

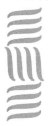

SUCCESSFUL LIVING
WITH SPINAL CORD INJURY

Having survived the early trauma, rehabilitation, and reentry into the bustling workaday world, you now enter the challenging and most fulfilling part of your journey. Your focus now is deciding what a "successful life" with spinal cord injury consists of and how you can achieve that goal.

Chapter 8 provides information on procedures, devices, and scientific advances that can help you do what you want to do. It also provides some ideas on how to maintain your health, maximize the physical integrity of your body, and prevent physical complications as you age. A discussion of the current work on spinal cord regeneration and other research innovations is included.

In Chapter 9 the theme is reconnecting all those puzzle pieces that make up your life. It concentrates on activities that can help you adjust, adapt, and reconcile your pre-injury life with the challenges posed by injury—healing old wounds, checking out coping patterns, reframing self-image, owning your spinal cord injury, and working on relations with others. And it illustrates some successful lifestyle options after injury.

Chapter 10 summarizes some ways in which you can build a more enjoyable and satisfying life and address the aging process. We also give you some ideas about how you can share your wisdom with others who are just beginning the journey. This final chapter finds you in a place far removed from the wilderness you entered when you first had your spinal cord injury. From that initial feeling of free falling, you at last find yourself grounded, in control, balancing what is doable. This chapter gives you a true appreciation of the breadth and depth of your victory—the balance in your life—that you have achieved.

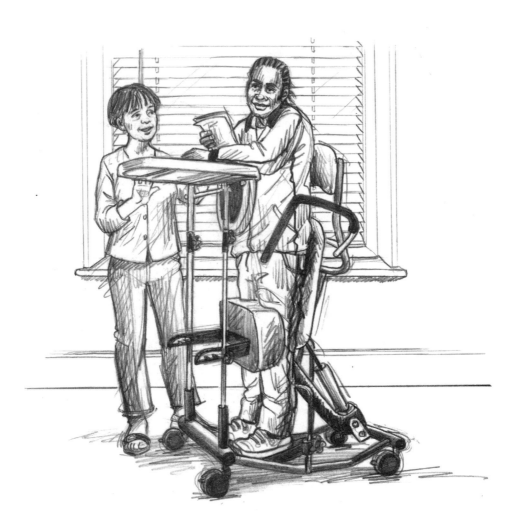

8

The Next Frontier
Spinal Cord Injury Research

with contributions by John W. McDonald, M.D., Ph.D.,
and Cristina L. Sadowsky, M.D.

Newly separated from her husband, Lark was in her first year of business school, concentrating on marketing and strategy in preparation for starting her own business. One weekend, while at a party with friends, she was pushed into the pool and injured her neck. She had an incomplete C5–C6 spinal cord injury.

Lark was the oldest child in a large family, and she was thankful that the accident hadn't happened to one of her brothers or sisters. Being so committed to her family, Lark felt she needed to be "up" for her family members, to make it easier for them. Lark's mother was an actress and often worked at night, and Lark had become a second mother to her siblings. She did the cooking, bathed the younger children, and drove them about while their mother was working at the theater.

Lark's passion was golf, and her first questions following the accident were "Can I have children? Can I play golf again?" She thought she'd be miserable if she couldn't play golf. Life wouldn't be worth living. At first, she says, "It was all I could do not to think about golf."

After her rehabilitation, Lark tried to play golf in her wheelchair, but found it frustrating because she had very limited strength in her arms and upper body. "I couldn't even play it as well as others with disabilities. It was a heart breaker." To keep up with her interest in golf, she helped out at tournaments, bet on tournaments, and watched golf on television.

Looking back, she sees how her interests gradually changed. She has replaced her passion for golf with other activities and no longer feels the keen sense of loss. Lark tells other people who have spinal cord injuries, "Your interests will change. You will find activities to fill the needs of your old ones."

Lark is aware, however, that you can't convince anyone still in rehabilitation that life will get better. Each individual has to figure that out for herself or himself, says Lark. Some people with spinal cord injury refuse therapy because they think that everything they have lost will come back, that they will be cured. Others resist rehabilitation efforts because of despair over what they have lost. They feel their efforts will be useless.

Rehabilitation doctors and therapists have a difficult message to deliver, says Lark. They must explain how to hold two ideas in your head at the same time: understanding the worst, that you may always be disabled, and hoping for the best, a cure for spinal cord injury. These seemingly opposing ideas can motivate the same behavior: making the most of your physical functioning. If you're going to be permanently disabled, maximizing your strength and function will mean fewer problems and a better life. If a cure comes along, such as regeneration of the spinal cord, you'll be better prepared if your body is in the best possible condition.

At the time of her injury, Lark had been helping a national organization that focuses on disability issues to organize a fundraising event. After her injury, the director of the organization, who also has C5–C6 tetraplegia, called her to say, "Boy, are we lucky to have you! We'll get you working on things to do with disability!" Indeed, soon after the accident, Lark did a TV spot on pool safety. She remembers that her head was shaved on both sides, she wore "goofy-looking" glasses because she couldn't wear her contact lenses, and her neck was supported by a collar. That was her initiation into her informal public relations role: filming TV spots, making speeches for the hospital, and lobbying for its interests.

Lark feels that all this activity delayed her acknowledgment of her loss. She was held up as an example and felt she couldn't let people down by "crashing." Organizations "piled" awards on her, though she wasn't actually doing anything. "People can't imagine going through this, so they give you an award for living with it. All I am doing is getting back into life—sailing, skiing, and taking up flying. I don't feel it's extraordinary."

Like many people with spinal cord injury, Lark had some misconceptions about the physiology of the spinal cord. Soon after her injury, she read that myelin, the substance making up the layer that surrounds the spinal cord, is largely cholesterol. Deducing that she needed to "replace the cholesterol," Lark went on a high-cholesterol diet that included shrimp, eggs, and butter. Her favorite was lobster with drawn butter! She abandoned this "restorative diet" after further study, as she learned that it could not help; myelin cannot be replaced by a high-cholesterol diet once it is lost. In the long run, she realized, this diet could even damage her health.

Lark emphasizes the importance of physical conditioning in her life. She has a personal fitness instructor who plans her exercise program, and she works out five times a week. Using an FES machine (functional electrical stimulation machine, discussed in this chapter), Lark rides an electric stationary bicycle. She wears special shorts with implanted electrodes through which the FES machine stimulates her quadriceps, producing sufficient muscle contraction for her to pedal the bike. Lark considers this activity critical for improving circulation, maintaining muscle mass, and strengthening bones. She also finds it exciting and thoroughly enjoyable. "It's wild, kind of a high!" This is her only aerobic exercise, the only activity in which she gets out of breath, and that's an exhilarating feeling.

Lark also lifts weights, using a specialized upper-body exercise system that doesn't require hand mobility. She says, "I do everything to stay healthy, concentrating on heart, circulation, and saving muscle tone." In addition to its overall health benefits, the exercise boosts her self-esteem and mental well-being. Lark says it's fun to talk at parties about weight systems, body-building, and your personal fitness trainer. "People identify you by what you do," she says. Though she can no longer play golf, Lark's continuing interest in fitness is shared by her peers and is a social asset.

Lark's story illustrates the importance of adapting to a spinal cord injury by maintaining hope for future recovery while making the most of all remaining abilities. By rechanneling her athletic abilities after her failed attempt to play wheelchair golf, and by setting aside her high-fat diet when she learned it would not restore her nerve tissue, Lark was sorting out what works from what doesn't and evaluating information about treatments and technologies. This type of evaluation of advances in rehabilitation is essential for people with spinal cord injury.

As you probably know from newspaper stories and accounts in the television news, numerous research laboratories worldwide are working on problems related to spinal cord injury. Some are developing ways to reduce or repair the damage to an injured spinal cord. Others are working to reduce the effects of spinal cord injury on other body systems (such as the bowel and bladder). Still others are developing innovative approaches to rehabilitation.

In this chapter we discuss some of the important work being done in these laboratories, to help you understand the state of the art in spinal cord research. We also discuss how research gets funded and reported, how to decide whether to participate in a research project, and how to interpret stories that appear in the news media, in order to distinguish between what is worth serious consideration and what is not truly a viable option for you in the near future. The political aspects of research into a cure for spinal cord injury, and of the use of animals in research, are also discussed.

HEALING THE SPINAL CORD

The primary area of research on spinal cord injury looks at ways to reduce the damage caused by the injury and to repair the spinal cord. To explain this work, we first need to review some mechanisms of spinal cord injury.

As we noted in Chapter 1, the spinal cord can be damaged by traumatic injury or by disease. Traumatic injuries usually cause damage by direct mechanical injury (crushing, stretching, or cutting the cord) or by destroying the blood supply to the spinal cord, which can kill the cord's nerve cells. In the first few minutes or hours after a traumatic spinal cord injury, a variety of toxic chemicals released from damaged cells and tissues may cause further damage to nerve cells in the cord.

Diseases can damage the spinal cord by the same mechanisms. For instance, a tumor or bone spur can compress the spinal cord, causing direct mechanical injury or compressing essential blood vessels that supply the cord. Other diseases affect the spinal cord by producing inflammation, by causing degeneration of spinal nerve cells, or by impairing the ability of the spinal cord to carry nerve impulses.

Regardless of how the spinal cord is injured, some recovery occurs without any medical intervention—but generally this is a limited amount. The spinal cord is very delicate. Once its nerve cells are killed, they have little ability to grow back. However, many nerve cells that are damaged in a spinal cord injury are not actually killed.

As we explained in Chapter 1, the spinal cord is, in large part, a bundle of nerve fibers (white matter) that carry nerve impulses up and down the neck and back between the brain and the rest of the body. Each nerve fiber is an extension of a single nerve cell that has its main portion, or cell body (gray matter), in the spinal cord or brain. If the cell body is killed, the entire nerve cell dies. If a nerve fiber is damaged, the cell body can survive and the fiber may be able to regrow. Once a nerve fiber is damaged at a particular point along its length, however, it cannot simply grow back to fill in the damaged portion. It must regrow all the way from the damaged area to its far end—the end farthest from the cell body—where it connects with other nerve cells. Unfortunately, this regrowth does not work very well, and the greater the damage, the less the chance that nerve fibers will regrow.

As Lark discovered in her reading, long nerve fibers in the spinal cord are coated with a protein and lipid substance called myelin, which helps the fibers to conduct impulses. All forms of injuries or diseases of the spinal cord cause a loss of this coating, a process called demyelination, which interferes with nerve impulse conduction. In mild cases conduction is slowed, but in severe cases it can be completely blocked in the area of demyelination. Even if the nerve fiber itself is completely intact, it cannot conduct impulses properly if its myelin coating is damaged. Even the loss of two segments of myelin (of the thousands that cover each nerve fiber) in a row eliminates function in the entire nerve fiber.

The Body's Response to Spinal Cord Injury: Three Phases of Injury

Before discussing research efforts to heal the spinal cord, it is helpful to review in more detail what happens when the spinal cord is injured.

Acute Injury

Acute injury begins when a mechanical force strikes the spine. This force dislocates the vertebrae that normally protect the spinal cord and tears the ligaments that hold each section together. As a result, the spinal column becomes unstable. Fragments of shattered bone press on the soft spinal cord, which has the consistency of Jell-O. Although the cord is normally as thick as your index finger, sudden impact makes it swell rapidly. The spinal cord is contained within a hollow tubular structure called the spinal canal, which is one-and-a-half to two times wider than the cord and rigid. When the spinal cord swells, it pushes against the walls of the canal, creating pressure. Ultimately, this pressure causes blood flow to stop, which means that critical nutrients and oxygen can no longer be delivered to the swollen segment, especially to the center of the spinal cord. Thus, the center of the cord suffers a "stroke," which causes the core of the spinal cord to die; tissue toward the outside of the spinal cord usually survives because it receives some blood. Typically, the spinal cord swells several segments above and below the initial injury site, but most of the damage occurs within two levels.

This swelling creates a state of shock, which prevents the affected portion of the spinal cord from functioning. As a result, a person who has just suffered spinal cord trauma becomes completely paralyzed below the injury level. Spinal shock usually lasts for less than a week, though it may persist for longer, especially in children. It is not possible to accurately predict the extent of injury or permanent loss of function until spinal shock subsides. After spinal shock resolves, reflexes return, but some or all motor and sensory function is lost because motor and sensory circuits are interrupted.

Secondary Injury

A secondary wave of damage follows the death of cells in the spinal cord. The dying cells release chemicals that kill neighboring, previously intact cells. This secondary injury, which begins within minutes, extends over hours to days. More recent work suggests that a further wave of cells' deaths occurs primarily in the spinal cord's white matter in the days to weeks after injury. This progressive cell death further compounds the dysfunction of the spinal cord.

Most of current knowledge about secondary injury is based on studies of head trauma and stroke in the brain. The progressive loss of blood supply following the acute injury kills additional nervous tissue. Impairment of the microcirculation (blood circulation in tiny vessels within the spinal cord), ruptured blood vessels, and damaged nerve cells increase the concentration of chemicals that kill nerve fibers not initially damaged by trauma. These chemicals also kill oligodendrocytes, specialized cells that make the insulating covering—myelin—that allows nerve cells (neurons) to function. In turn, the loss of myelin (demyelination) causes the release of additional harmful chemicals.

A substance called glutamate is one of the chemicals released by damaged neurons and their nerve fibers (axons). At normal concentrations, glutamate is an essential part of the nervous system because it carries messages between nerve cells. When its concentration rises to abnormal levels, however, it overexcites neighboring neurons, causing them to produce chemicals that kill previously healthy neurons. This process is known as excitotoxicity.

Excitotoxicity is very harmful to the oligodendrocytes. Because one oligodendrocyte myelinates ten to sixty different axons, loss of even a single oligodendrocyte can contribute to the demyelination of several axons that remain intact following the primary injury. Oligodendrocytes may also "commit suicide" after spinal cord injury, even when they are as far as four segments away from the initial trauma site, thus magnifying the original injury. Collectively, the events that occur during secondary injury result in greater cell death and demyelination in the previously normal tissue immediately adjacent to the spinal cord injury epicenter, which leads to a larger area of damage and the start of scar formation (see Figure 8.1).

Research on the process of oligodendrocyte death in humans, which might proceed for several months, is an important step toward developing therapies to protect the spinal cord. For example, it was once thought that the immune system exacerbated nervous system injury, but recent findings have challenged this view. In animals, chemicals that cause inflammation help prevent spinal cord injury. New evidence suggests that some immune cells, called T cells, might participate in nerve cell repair, and help limit secondary injury. Indeed, T cell–based vaccines are being studied as potential therapies for the early stages of spinal cord injury.

Many secondary mechanisms of injury are common to traumatic and non-traumatic spinal cord injury. Chronic loss of myelin seen in secondary spinal cord injury is similar to the demyelination that occurs in chronic degenerative nerve disorders, such as multiple sclerosis. Thus, treatments developed to limit the effects of secondary spinal cord injury may potentially be effective for people with multiple sclerosis and related disorders.

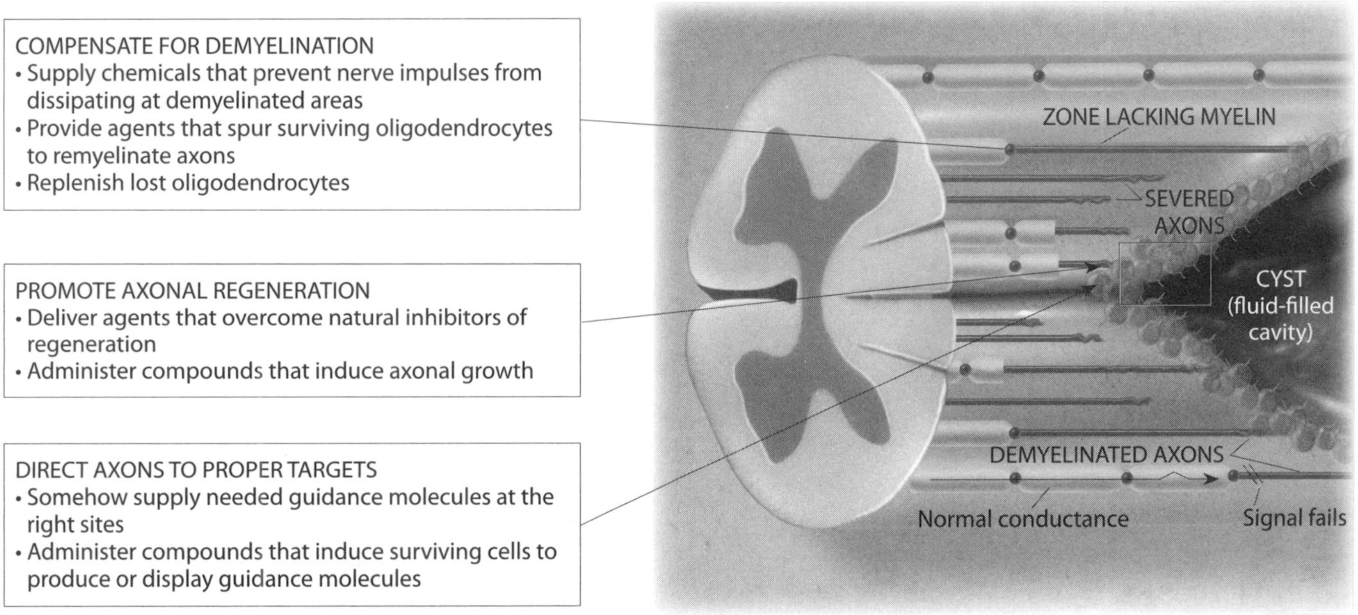

COMPENSATE FOR DEMYELINATION
- Supply chemicals that prevent nerve impulses from dissipating at demyelinated areas
- Provide agents that spur surviving oligodendrocytes to remyelinate axons
- Replenish lost oligodendrocytes

PROMOTE AXONAL REGENERATION
- Deliver agents that overcome natural inhibitors of regeneration
- Administer compounds that induce axonal growth

DIRECT AXONS TO PROPER TARGETS
- Somehow supply needed guidance molecules at the right sites
- Administer compounds that induce surviving cells to produce or display guidance molecules

ZONE LACKING MYELIN
SEVERED AXONS
CYST (fluid-filled cavity)
DEMYELINATED AXONS
Normal conductance
Signal fails

Figure 8.1 The zone of injury. A spinal cord injury often affects a small area at first, but it triggers secondary processes that expand the area of damage. Many axons (nerve fibers) die because they are directly damaged (crushed or cut) or lose their blood supply. Other axons lose their coating of myelin, necessary for conducting nerve signals. These demyelinated axons cannot carry nerve signals up or down the spinal cord across the area of injury. Axons in the spinal cord normally do not regrow. But even if they did, they would still meet barriers. One is a fluid-filled cavity—a cyst—that forms where nerve cells and fibers have died. This cyst is often surrounded by a scar composed of specialized cells. These cells release substances that prevent regrowth of nerve fibers. In many cases, only a thin layer of intact axons remains at the rim of the area of injury.

© Edmond Alexander

Chronic Injury

The subchronic stage of spinal cord injury, which follows primary and secondary injury, is characterized by further death of oligodendrocytes in the spinal cord. In humans, this stage may last for months. Consequently, a large number of nerve cells and their circuitry stop functioning, even though they remain physically intact. Another prominent feature of subchronic spinal cord injury is the growth of a scar around the lesion. This scar tissue forms a barrier to nerve regeneration (see Figure 8.1).

In the chronic phase of spinal cord injury, the scar is well formed and contains much debris. As well as acting as a physical barrier, the scar tissue produces molecules that inhibit the growth of nerves. These inhibitor molecules normally guide growing nerve connections to their correct locations during nervous system development. After spinal cord injury, these roadmap signs become rearranged in a nonsensical manner, leading to nerve regeneration that is nonfunctional.

The end result of spinal cord injury is evident by the chronic phase of injury. Typically, the central cavity (cyst) spans one to one-and-a-half segments of the spinal cord and is filled with fluid. The remaining donut-like rim of white matter (nerve fibers) surrounds this cyst (see Figure 8.1). In complete spinal cord injury, signals from the brain cannot reach below the level of the injury, resulting in loss of normal movement below the injury level. Normally, the brain sends inhibiting signals to the spinal cord that suppress reflex activity. These signals are also disrupted in spinal cord injury, resulting in increased reflex activity after injury. This leads to abnormal function, including spasticity of the limbs, bladder and bowel dysfunction, sexual dysfunction, pain, and autonomic dysreflexia. Such chronic neurological dysfunctions contribute to the progressive worsening of overall health. The aging process also affects spinal cord injury, but the underlying mechanisms are not understood. It is theorized that the injured nervous system is vulnerable to accelerated aging. Further research is needed to develop treatments tailored to offset this process.

Medications to Reduce Secondary Injury

Clinical Trials and Development of New Drugs

Many potential drugs for treating spinal cord injury are being studied in the laboratory, but drug development typically takes twenty to thirty years. The initial laboratory work is most time consuming. Imagine that scientists are trying to find a new drug to prevent the loss of oligodendrocytes after traumatic spinal cord injury. The first step would be to identify the mechanisms that contribute most significantly to the delayed death of oligodendrocytes. Often, this involves screening a large number of compounds to see how they affect oligodendrocytes' survival or death. More modern approaches assess compounds' effects on the genes, proteins, and biology of spinal cord cells. The thousands of compounds that give positive results are then tested in laboratory cultures that model the major features of spinal cord injury. For example, promising compounds could be tested for their ability to limit the death of cultured oligodendrocytes exposed to high concentrations of glutamate. This second phase of research might reduce the original thousand candidates to perhaps fifty. More extensive testing could then be used to identify a few drugs to be tested on animals with spinal cord injury. Once the most promising candidate is chosen, extensive studies must be performed, usually in rodents, to determine safety and side effects of the drug; further studies with larger animals are often required before approval for testing in humans will be granted by the U.S. Food and Drug Administration (FDA).

Generally, the FDA requires data from three phases of testing in humans before it will consider approving a drug for human use. Phase I evaluates safety by administering the compound to a small number of subjects—usually fewer than fifty. Once the drug's safety is determined, a phase II study, which typically involves between twenty and two hundred subjects, determines which dosages to use and which clinical measurements will best test whether the potential drug is having the desired therapeutic effect. Phase III is a much larger study, called a randomized clinical trial, or prospective trial, conducted at multiple research centers. Subjects are randomly assigned to groups; one group receives a placebo (an inert substance, such as a "sugar pill") and one group receives the drug. This phase determines the effectiveness of the drug when compared to other drugs or to no treatment. The average cost of a phase III trial is on the order of $50 million.

The three phases of a clinical trial typically take ten to fifteen years to complete, and the treatment becomes available to humans only if it is shown to be both safe and effective. These trials involve collaboration among the federal government, which funds much of the basic research, scientists in universities and other institutions who perform the laboratory studies, and pharmaceutical companies, which help fund clinical trials and then produce and market the drug. Even when these collaborators are ready to move forward, however, politics can hinder their progress. For example, many scientists, the American public, and many congressional representatives and senators are excited about the potential of human embryonic stem cells to repair damaged nerve tissue. However, research with embryonic stem cells in the United States has lagged behind that in other countries, because of opposition from some religious groups and government figures.

Several prospective clinical trials of potential drugs for treating the initial stages of spinal cord injury have been completed. They have assessed the safety and efficacy of a number of drugs, including methylprednisolone, which is now readily available for use in treating spinal cord injury.

Methylprednisolone

Methylprednisolone, a steroid, was the first drug to be approved by the FDA for inhibiting the events leading to secondary injury. Most medical centers administer this drug within twenty-four hours of injury. However, research indicates that methylprednisolone works best when delivered within the first eight hours, and animal studies suggest that within three hours is the most beneficial time. Therefore, it is important for emergency medical workers to give an injured person the first dose of methylprednisolone as quickly as possible after the injury. Although this drug cannot reverse the damage already done, it can minimize the ongoing damage and result in better spinal cord function. How methylprednisolone works is not known, but it may interfere with the action of the toxic chemicals released by damaged cells.

Methylprednisolone treatment is now in widespread use around the world. It results in a small but significant improvement in recovery from spinal cord injury. For example, a patient who might have had a completely paralyzed hand without methylprednisolone treatment may instead have a weak but functional hand. Thousands of patients have benefited from this drug, and its use has been an important breakthrough in the treatment of spinal cord injury. A number of other drugs with a similar function are currently under development.

High-dose steroids can have significant side effects. They can suppress the immune system, weaken the body's response to infection, and delay healing. However, early mobilization (physical therapy) of people with spinal cord injury soon after admission to the hospital has greatly reduced the risks associated with methylprednisolone treatment.

GM-1 Ganglioside

In the early 1990s a large clinical trial with monosialo-tetrahexosyl-ganglioside (GM-1 ganglioside) was conducted in the United States. Within seventy-two hours of injury, an initial dose of GM-1 ganglioside was given intravenously, after methylpredinose had been administered; then a daily dose was given for the following fifty-six days. Although the study did not prove that GM-1 produced greater recovery, those study subjects with incomplete spinal cord injury made a faster neurological recovery. Improvements were observed in motor and sensory function, bowel and bladder function, sacral sensation, and anal contraction. While GM-1 was approved by the FDA, it was produced only in Europe, and it is no longer readily available in the United States.

Another area of research is the development of medications to reduce demyelination after a spinal cord injury. As noted above, demyelination impairs nerve impulse conduction, even in nerve fibers that are otherwise intact. Reducing the extent of demyelination by medical treatment should result in better function of the nerve fibers.

The difficulty of clinical trials, described above, combined with the complexity of spinal cord injury, has led to slow progress in developing medications for treating spinal cord injury.

SPINAL CORD REGENERATION

The great unsolved problem in spinal cord injury research is how to make the spinal cord repair and regenerate itself. Just a few years ago, spinal cord regeneration was thought to be completely impossible. Scientists thought that damaged nerve cells in the brain and spinal cord could not regrow. However, recent studies have shown that both the spinal cord and the brain are capable of some regeneration after damage. Indeed, partial regeneration is more the rule than the exception. But the amount of spinal cord regeneration is small. Medications called nerve growth factors are now being developed that can promote the growth of nerve cells.

Once injured nerve cells begin to regrow, the next problem is to direct that growth so that the nerve fibers extend to reach their original targets (the nerve cells with which they originally connected). Nerve cells may have to regrow over a long distance—up to several feet. Investigators don't yet know how to ensure that a growing fiber will find its way over such a distance or to a specific target. For optimal recovery, the regrown nerve fiber would have to reattach precisely to the same target cell to which the original fiber was attached.

A vast amount of research is going on; scientists are working on repairing the damaged spinal cord by replacing damaged tissue or making the cord repair itself. Some research groups are studying the signals that tell nerve cells when and where to grow during their normal development. Others are developing surgical techniques to assist damaged spinal nerve cells to begin growing back in the right direction, toward the correct targets. Still others are searching for newer and better nerve growth factors to promote cell growth.

It is important to point out that partial repair of the cord can lead to significant improvement in function and could greatly improve an individual's quality of life. Fortunately, some of the functions important to people with spinal cord injury are frequently recoverable. These include bowel, bladder, and sexual functions, which are controlled by the lowest portion of the spinal cord. Improvements in hand function or enhancing trunk balance can also greatly improve quality of life. Restoration of walking is a top priority for many people with spinal cord injury. This will take much longer to achieve in individuals with ASIA A spinal cord injury (see Chapter 1), because it would require extensive repair of the spinal cord. However, progress in research on spinal cord recovery and nerve regeneration is encouraging, and there is hope that this research may lead to restoration of walking in the future (see section on Promoting Recovery of Function, below).

Stem Cell Research

An important area of study is the role of stem cells in spinal cord regeneration. Not long ago, it was believed that the nervous system contained all of its cells at birth and could not replace those cells. One remarkable discovery of the last decade is that the mature central nervous system contains stem cells. These so-called endogenous stem cells are found in the spinal cord of infants and children as well as adults. Stem cells are precursors to functional nerve cells and continually give rise to the three major types of nerve cells. We now know that neurons are born constantly in at least two areas of the brain and that stem cells reside around the central canal of the spinal cord. Related progenitor cells, cells that are capable of further differentiation, are located throughout the gray and white matter of the spinal cord. Astonishingly, an estimated 500,000 to 2 million new cells are born every day in the spinal cord of an adult rat one month after spinal cord injury, but only a fraction of these cells become functional in the nervous system. Critical goals of future research include understanding how to stimulate endogenous stem cells to grow, how to specify what types of nerve cells they become, and how to control the direction of their growth to the correct location in the nervous system, so that they can communicate normally with other cells.

Embryonic stem cells come from blastocysts. The blastocyst is the earliest stage of growth of a new organism from a fertilized egg. Embryonic stem cells are especially important to medical research on spinal cord regeneration because they have the potential to become many different kinds of cells, and scientists know how to make embryonic stem cells develop into nerve cells. But because embryonic stem cells come from fertilized eggs, there are political, religious, and ethical objections to their use, and lack of suitable cells for transplantation is one of the largest barriers to stem cell transplantation. However, techniques exist to make unfertilized egg cells duplicate their DNA and create embryonic stem cells without being fertilized; this process is called parthenogenesis.

Within a week of growth in a laboratory culture, embryonic stem cells spontaneously differentiate into the specific types of nerve cells. The neurons form electrical circuits, and the oligodendrocytes myelinate the nerve fibers. These nerve cell cultures display normal physiological responses. Likewise, research has shown that some embryonic stem cells can develop and function normally after being transplanted into the injured spinal cord of rats. Embryonic stem cell transplantation may someday lead to recovery of spinal cord function in people with spinal cord injury.

Transplanted neural stem cells can aid regeneration in several ways. They do not merely replace lost cells; they also produce regenerative growth factors (chemicals that encourage cell growth) and release enzymes that break down scar tissue in the spinal cord. Recent studies suggest that descendants of embryonic stem cells can produce minute tunnels through the scar tissue in the spinal cord, through which nerve fibers can grow.

Various techniques are being used by scientists to make stem cells suitable for transplantation to humans, such as transferring the DNA from a person's skin cells into these stem cells to create a genetic match to the person; this process is called somatic cell nuclear transfer (SCNT). The genetic makeup of the transplanted cells should match that of the recipient to avoid the problem of transplant rejection. People with spinal cord injury cannot be treated for long periods with anti-rejection drugs, because these drugs are immunosuppressants and cause increased vulnerability to infection. Donor cells should be nervous system cells, not blood cells or umbilical cord stem cells.

The recent discovery of "transdifferentiation" of stem cells, where stem cells from one organ system can become cells from another organ system, has generated excitement in the research community and may eventually lead to additional sources of stem cells for transplantation, but this technology is a long way from being applicable to spinal cord injury in humans.

Replacement of neurons lost at the injury site is a long-term goal of research on spinal cord regeneration. It is important to understand that it is not currently possible to re-create the complex neuronal circuitry in the injured spinal cord. However, even partial restoration of nerve function in the spinal cord can result in recovery of important functions. As stated earlier, there is evidence that some regeneration of the nerves occurs spontaneously; there is a growing consensus that spontaneous regeneration might not be limited to a short period after injury, but rather could continue throughout life.

The Role of Imaging in Spinal Cord Regeneration Research

The lack of noninvasive methods for determining the severity of injury has hampered spinal cord injury research and the development of therapies. Conventional magnetic resonance imaging, or MRI, is not very useful for predicting how much movement or sensation someone will have after injury, in part because it does not distinguish between functional tissue and scar tissue. Development of new MRI-based methods that can differentiate between functional tissue and scar tissue will be important for determining injury severity and prognosis for recovery after spinal cord injury. Development of new MRI tools will contribute to better design of clinical trials and potentially to individualized regenerative treatment plans.

Recent development of advanced imaging techniques, such as diffusion tensor imaging (DTI) and magnetization transfer (MT), is promising for evaluating the extent of spinal cord injury. Development and application of functional MRI (fMRI; currently used in research on brain function) to the spinal cord will greatly advance research on regeneration. These advances in imaging allow tracking of the distribution and movements of transplanted cells after they are placed in a living animal. In the future, it should also be possible to learn more about these processes by combining advanced imaging techniques with advances in molecular biology.

Research on stem cell transplantation and regeneration in the spinal cord is exciting, but its clinical application in humans still lies in the future. Research on spinal cord regeneration will continue, as will efforts to overcome the political and social barriers to use of stem cells and other techniques for regeneration. Research on methods for improving rehabilitation of function and quality of life for individuals now living with functional impairments due to spinal cord injury is equally important. To this end, research laboratories are developing ways to improve bodily functions, prevent medical complications, and develop innovative approaches to the rehabilitation of individuals with spinal cord injury.

PROMOTING RECOVERY OF FUNCTION

Neural activity—communication between nerve cells—provides instructions for the birth, survival, differentiation, and maturation of new nerve cells, for myelination, and for many other tasks necessary to promote the normal development of the central nervous system before and after birth. Because the same tasks are necessary to nervous system regeneration, it is hypothesized that regeneration may be related to increasing neural activity.

Both before and after birth, limb movement is a major stimulant of nerve cell communication. If fetal limb movements become restricted during pregnancy, central nervous system development is profoundly hampered, resulting in abnormal nervous system structure and functional disabilities. Similarly, lack of limb movements after spinal cord injury could shut down neural activity below the injury level, preventing the spinal cord from healing itself.

This concept has begun to influence strategies for rehabilitation. Certain types of physical therapy administered during the acute phase of rehabilitation, or even years later, may prove to promote spontaneous regeneration of spinal cord tissue and functional recovery. These physical therapy programs include partial body weight-supported walking, functional electrical stimulation (FES), and activity-based restoration therapy (ABRT), discussed below.

Restoration of walking is the ultimate goal for many people with spinal cord injury. Two of the questions being asked by scientists are: (1) How much of the spinal cord has to be restored to achieve significant recovery of walking (and other functions)? (2) What is the mechanism for recovery of walking in people who have significant spinal cord damage?

In cats with experimental spinal cord injury, roughly 10 percent of spinal nerve fibers appear sufficient for recovery of spontaneous walking without external support. In monkeys with spinal cord injury, about 25 percent of spinal nerve tissue allows the animals to regain functional use of their hind limbs. Clinical observations in humans support the concept that only a portion of the spinal cord tissue is required to retain function. For example, the spinal cords of cancer patients who had surgical destruction of part of the cord for pain relief of intractable pain, but whose ability to walk had been only mildly or temporarily affected by the procedure, were examined postmortem. Over 50 percent transection of the spinal cord had occurred in many of these patients, indicating that less than half the cord is required for walking. Sometimes, in spite of significant loss of nerve fibers and cell bodies in the spinal cord, humans are able to walk again after injury.

Central Pattern Generators and Recovery of Walking

One mechanism related to recovery of walking and other motor functions after spinal cord injury is that of central pattern generators (CPGs), which control complex patterns of neural activity in both lower animals and humans and can be activated by sensory and electrophysiological stimuli.

According to the traditional understanding of human movement, all neural centers that control movement are in the brain, and the spinal cord is a conduit for information, with little or no ability to process information and control functional movement.

This view is slowly changing. We have known for some time that lower vertebrate animals have movement control centers outside the brain; some animals, for example, can learn to walk again after complete spinal cord injuries.

Recently, scientists have described a CPG for functional control of walking (gait) in the lumbar portion of the spinal cord. Similar pattern generators exist for the arm/hand motion with walking, located in the lower cervical or upper thoracic spinal cord, and for breathing, located in the cervical spinal cord. Because the majority of spinal cord injuries occur in the cervical and thoracic areas of the cord, they leave the lumbar gait CPG intact. Multiple researchers are studying how to use the potential of the gait CPG for retraining walking in those recovering from spinal cord injury or other disorders causing gait difficulties.

There is some communication between the lumbar gait CPG and the arm/hand CPG. In some individuals with C1–C5 spinal cord injuries, upper arm movements that are similar to normal movements coordinated with gait are elicited when their legs are actively cycled using a FES bicycle (see below). The key point is that this link of the arm/hand and gait CPGs occurs with active FES-induced cycling but not with passive leg motion. This suggests that feedback from muscle use in the legs activates the CPG for the arms through nervous system "cross talk." Partial weight-supported walking and functional electrical stimulation (FES) are two mechanisms thought to stimulate the CPG for walking and thus encourage recovery of function.

Partial Weight-Supported Walking

Partial weight-supported walking may improve gait in individuals with incomplete spinal cord injury. With this technique, the person is positioned on a treadmill while supported by a harness and a pneumatic suspension device, and the legs are passively moved with a reciprocal walking-like pattern. After weeks of such exercise, some individuals find that their legs seem to "learn" to move in a repetitive cycle—something previously thought to be impossible. This potential treatment can be used by people with spinal cord injury who have enough control of their legs to begin walking (ASIA C-D grade injuries; see Chapter 1). The Christopher and Dana Reeve Foundation has created a NeuroRecovery Network designed to employ and test the usefulness of partial body weight-supported walking. Functional gait in rodents is improved with partial body weight-supported walking and further enhanced when locomotor training is combined with FES.

Functional Electrical Stimulation (FES)

People with spinal cord injury, despite their impaired mobility, benefit just as much from exercise as able-bodied people. Although it has been challenging to devise exercises for people who are completely or partly paralyzed, advances in rehabilitation technology are providing some solutions. Connections between the spinal cord and muscles below the injury level remain intact. Although they can no longer receive nerve signals from the brain, these muscles can respond to electrical stimulation. Functional electrical stimulation (FES) is an important therapeutic technique for exercise in patients with spinal cord injury.

In FES, electrodes placed on the skin over a muscle deliver electrical stimulation to make the muscle contract and move the limb. Modern electronic control systems can deliver complex patterns of electrical stimulation to different muscles, producing patterns of muscle activity that mimic functional limb movement. In fact, a six-channel controller the size of a pager and electrodes placed on the thigh, buttock, and hamstring muscles of the upper leg can generate leg movements that are sufficiently coordinated for riding a stationary bike. The addition of a mechanical motorized pedal system can provide resistance training during FES, which can slow or reverse bone loss and improve muscle mass and blood flow.

Some FES systems reproduce walking, but engineering complexities and high human energy requirements preclude their routine use. However, using FES to facilitate standing can improve blood flow to paralyzed legs and potentially enhance quality of life. FES is also used for strength training and cardiovascular retraining.

New research suggests that delayed recovery of function may be stimulated when therapies such as FES are delivered with sufficient frequency and intensity. Christopher Reeve, for example, began to recover five to eight years after having a severe spinal cord injury at level C1–C2. For the first five years after injury, he showed no recovery. But over the next three years, after participating in an intensive physical therapy and FES regimen, he regained sensation in much of his body and began to move his joints. This movement was limited and did not result in improved function, but it demonstrated that late recovery was beginning to occur. Additionally, the significant improvement in his sensation improved his quality of life.

Scientists are working on solving several technical problems with FES; these include electrode design, tissue tolerance, and detection and processing of the relevant sensory information.

The problems with electrode design are due, in part, to the difficulty in controlling each muscle individually. When a muscle is stimulated through the skin, all nearby muscles are stimulated indiscriminately. And deep muscles cannot be stimulated through the skin at all. To address this problem, several laboratories are working on tiny stimulating electrodes that can be implanted surgically, so that electrical stimulation can be delivered more directly to the target nerve or muscle. Because the electrode wires tend to weaken and may break over time, new materials are being developed to do the job better. FES with implanted electrodes has also been used to improve breathing and enhance bladder function (see Reducing Long-Term Medical Complications, later in this chapter).

The tissue tolerance problem relates to scarring at the site of stimulation. (This is not a problem for FES delivered through electrodes on the skin.) In the past, scar formation sometimes resulted in a lack of response after repeated FES with implanted electrodes. However, recent advances in biomaterials have largely overcome the problem of scarring.

The requirement for continuous detection and recording of information about the position of the body in space and the motions of the many joints and muscles creates another problem. Proper control of even a single joint requires constant monitoring of that joint's position, with continuous feedback to the FES computer controlling the motion. The activity of multiple muscles must be properly coordinated to control motion at that joint.

Functional movement involves some interaction with the environment, such as transporting the body through space (as in walking, climbing, lifting, or carrying) or changing the body's orientation in specific ways (as in moving the body from a lying to a sitting position, or turning the dials on a radio); this is even more complex. Control of functional movement requires measuring changes not only in body position but in the body's interaction with the environment. For example, planning foot placement for walking requires a way of measuring the shape of the surface of the ground. Lifting heavy objects requires an assessment of the physical stresses applied to the bones and joints, so as to prevent stress fractures and other damage. And the lifting of fragile, lightweight objects (such as a glass of water) requires measurement of the force applied to the object in order to prevent accidental breakage. Further research on miniaturization of parts and materials will be needed to develop an FES system that is powerful enough to produce complex functional human movement, yet small enough to be practical for use outside the laboratory.

FES is limited in that it does not work for everyone. Injuries of the cauda equina, a bundle of nerve fibers carrying impulses to and from the spinal cord, often results from damage to the lumbar spine (see Chapter 1). When the motor nerves in the cauda equina are damaged, the muscles associated with these nerves do not respond to FES. (It is technically possible to stimulate these muscles electrically to produce contraction, but this requires an enormous and potentially harmful shock.) The same phenomenon may occur with injuries of the spinal cord itself, if there is also damage to the nerve roots at their junction with the spinal cord. In other words, FES will only work on a muscle when the nerves to that muscle are intact.

FES holds great promise for restoring movement to paralyzed muscles and limbs. The greatest success thus far has been with highly specialized systems for performing specific, narrowly defined tasks, such as Joan's use of FES for improved hand function (see Chapter 4) and Lark's use of FES to increase muscle mass by riding a stationary bike. With technological advances in designing electrodes, measuring positions and forces, rapidly processing huge amounts of information, and precisely controlling the electrical output to each individual muscle, FES will steadily become more useful for improving the lives of many people with spinal cord injury.

> It was the summer after Noah's freshman year at college. He was excited about his major in business with an art minor and his selection for the school's highly regarded competitive tennis team. When he had extra time he welded sculptures.
>
> Near the end of the summer he went to the beach on vacation with his family. The first afternoon, he played a round of golf, unpacked, and called his buddies. They decided to meet at the beach. Noah remembers they were boogieboard surfing when he turned, with his back to a wave. "It picked me up and slammed me down," Noah says. He hit the ground with such force that his eyes were rolled back in his head and his swim trunks were torn off. He was injured at the C5 level.
>
> A doctor on the beach observed what was happening and immediately used his PalmPilot to call 911. Noah's father, also a physician, saw what had occurred, ran to his son, and assisted with the rescue process. Noah was airlifted to a regional trauma unit. He spent five weeks there on a mechanical ventilator with

no movement except for a slight one in his left shoulder. His weight plummeted from 185 to 135 pounds as his muscles began to atrophy.

"I was best friends with the wall above me," he says of that time. The Olympics and the U.S. Open on TV helped him get through the day; his family was allowed to see him for limited periods of time. While he was there, two other boys came in with spinal cord injuries that were also caused by beach accidents.

Two frustrating months at a rehabilitation hospital followed. Problems with nursing care left Noah with a bed sore. But he learned to work hard with what he had and when he left he could move his right wrist.

Coming home felt good, but it also emphasized the stark reality of his dependence on technology to live his life. It was hard to fathom. Noah says that he was able to deal with the situation through the support of family and friends. He realized that he needed to work on his "persona," understanding that his mind controlled and directed his being, while reinforcement he received from others was also vital. "A percentage is just you," he says, but help is needed to push, guide, and allow you to "get over the hump." With this mindset, he began his own personal rehabilitation program.

Noah, his physicians, and his father researched promising new technologies and therapies. This research led them to believe that a combination of therapies was needed to make stem cells grow in the spinal cord and to keep the body fit. Noah discovered a new program of intensive physical therapy and exercise (see below), and says he has made some physical progress through his participation. He is now able to wiggle the toes on his right foot and his left arm is "coming back." He has transitioned from a complete to an incomplete injury, according to the ASIA criteria (see Chapter 1).

Noah's comprehensive conditioning and exercise program includes the following elements: physical therapy exercises "on the mat," using various positions, grades, and gravity; FES—on legs, hands, and feet; standing in an elliptical glider frame; using an arm cycle; electromyogram (EMG) biofeedback; and water therapy when available.

Much of this exercise occurs at home, where he has special equipment ordered by his outpatient rehabilitation program or bought on his own after intensive personal research. Much of this equipment was paid for by the vocational rehabilitation program in his state. His parents have installed an elevator in the house, which takes him down to the basement, where he spends five *hours per day working out. He has an electronic lift system to transfer from his wheelchair to the exercise equipment.*

Noah firmly believes that there will be a cure for "chronics who keep their bodies prepared." Because of this conviction, he keeps current on the latest medical research on spinal cord injury, and is especially impressed with work in some foreign countries on combinations of therapies. "You have to be ready to fight," he says, "ready to meet your doctors halfway," by staying fit.

Noah finds that much more planning is needed for post-injury activities. But he still spends weekends "hanging out" with his same old friends. The difference is that someone else drives (at least for now!) and someone helps him get into bed. Because of the physical advances he is making, Noah is hopeful that he will drive his own van in the future.

Noah's hobbies include working and playing on the computer and chess, "my new favorite sport." A poet, Noah especially likes to sit by the pond in the backyard to write. He enjoys "everything" on TV and video games. Walking with his mother and sister is relaxing, especially if the dog is along. Always an athlete, Noah is now gearing up to play "murderball" (wheelchair rugby). As for the future, Noah wants to finish college, start his own health care consulting business, and get married when he's "between twenty-eight and thirty-two."

Activity-Based Restoration Therapy (ABRT)

The dramatic reduction in neuronal activity below the level of a spinal cord injury causes physiological deficiencies leading to increased risk for long-term complications, such as decreased cardiovascular conditioning, reduction in high-density lipoproteins (HDLs—the "good" cholesterol), accelerated osteoporosis and loss of bone density, and muscle wasting. As a result of these problems, individuals may develop glucose intolerance and diabetes or pathological bone fractures, and they may be at increased risk for stroke, heart attack, or skin breakdown. Physical rehabilitation and exercise can ameliorate these problems to some extent. But the difficulty for individuals with complete paralysis to perform effective exercise is significant. The benefits of passive movements or weight bearing are very limited in people with complete paralysis, since passive movements do not strengthen muscle. Training with FES-induced movements against resistance shows promise for rebuilding muscle and improving fitness.

For those with disabilities, time is the greatest obstacle to participation in a clinic-based rehabilitation program. A potentially more efficient approach, allowing physical reconditioning to take place in the home, has recently been developed. This novel activity-based restoration therapy (ABRT) can be accomplished in about six hours per week. The main goals of the program are to encourage spontaneous regeneration and to maximize the physical integrity of the body through exercise. This is accomplished through a physical activity regimen that tries to approach the amount of physical activity normally achieved by an able-bodied person. Preliminary studies suggest that participants in an ABRT home-based program have fewer medical complications and reversal of physical deterioration. The program includes: (1) an intensive day-treatment ABRT program designed to rapidly advance physical conditioning (typically four hours per day, three to five days per week, one to six weeks in length), (2) training in ABRT methods, and (3) development and implementation of an individualized, lifelong, home-based ABRT program.

This program is built on a theoretical model, based primarily on research with animals, that links neural activity produced by physical activity (for example, cyclical movements of the legs) with spontaneous regeneration of the spinal cord and increased functional recovery. The idea that inducing patterned neural activity in the spinal cord might harness the restorative potential of endogenous stem cells was recently examined in rats that were injured in the mid-thoracic region of the spinal cord. Gait-like activity in the hind limbs was produced by linking an FES device to nerves in the legs. One-hour periods of gait-like activity, three times a day for two weeks, enhanced the birth of new nerve cells below the level of the injury by 60 to 70 percent. Similar studies have shown that activity also optimized axonal regeneration, cell survival, and myelination in rats with embryonic stem cell transplants. The molecular mechanisms through which FES induces neuronal recovery are not known and are an active area of investigation.

While the use of ABRT to improve neurological recovery in humans is supported only by preliminary clinical trials, studies with animals support the potential effectiveness of this approach. Like Noah (and Lark, who developed her own workout program) participants enjoy the physical and psychological benefits of regular exercise and the opportunity to keep their bodies "ready for a cure." Many scientists are hopeful that this work will eventually result in methods for restoring motor and sensory functions, and ultimately walking, in people with complete spinal cord injuries.

Surgery to Restore Function

Tendon Transfer

The loss of hand function, perceived by most individuals with tetraplegia as their greatest disability, can be partially regained by tendon transfer surgery. Tendons of "redundant" muscles that are unaffected by the spinal cord injury (that is, one of two functioning muscles that can perform the same movement) can be surgically rerouted to muscles that are no longer receiving nerve signals from the brain. These muscles can be trained to take over lost motor functions. The most frequently performed tendon transfers restore voluntary thumb pinch, improve grip strength, and restore active elbow and wrist extension. Exciting recent work in humans indicates that transfer of partial nerves can accomplish the same goal as functional tendon transfers.

Correcting Scoliosis

Recently, advances are being made in the surgical approach to scoliosis, or curvature of the spine, which is a common complication of spinal cord injury, especially in children (see Chapter 1). Traditional approaches to scoliosis focused on bracing, which limited the child's mobility, contributing to further weakening of trunk muscles already impaired by the injury. Recent work suggests that promotion of activity and strengthening the trunk muscles can help prevent the development of scoliosis. An innovative approach to treating scoliosis, currently under development, maintains mobility of the spinal column despite surgical correction. This allows the trunk muscles more freedom of movement. The new procedure involves placement of pie-shaped titanium wedges between vertebrae in the space normally occupied by the intervertebral disk; the large side of the pie piece functionally reverses the curved segments of the spinal column. Instead of fusing the spinal column, which prevents movement, this procedure stabilizes the vertebrae but allows for more normal movement and does not interfere with further growth and development of the spinal column in young children. FDA approval for this type of surgery is currently being sought; if approved, this could be a major advance in pediatric spinal cord injury care.

REDUCING LONG-TERM MEDICAL COMPLICATIONS

The indirect effects of spinal cord injury on body systems, including the urinary tract, the skin, and the respiratory system, can produce major changes in body function, lifestyle, and health. In fact, when individuals with spinal cord injury become ill and require hospitalization, it is almost always because of complications involving other body systems (that is, not the spinal cord itself). The complications (see Chapter 1) can be serious and may be fatal.

Progressively shorter periods of inpatient rehabilitation for spinal cord injury have created the need for more outpatient treatment of medical conditions associated with injury. In addition to participation in exercise programs, people with spinal cord injury should have annual medical and functional evaluations by a physiatrist or other expert in spinal cord injury medicine. Such experts can help combat loss of function by tailoring physical fitness programs and other treatment regimens to each individual, taking into consideration the most current scientific and clinical advances. The goal is to minimize the long-term medical consequences of spinal cord injury, improve function, and maintain overall health and quality of life. A major focus of current research is analyzing the precise mechanisms by which spinal cord injury affects other body systems and developing ways to prevent medical complications and improve health.

Urinary Tract

The kidneys usually function well after spinal cord injury. However, voluntary control of the bladder is usually lost. The bladder can become overfilled, resulting in high bladder pressures, and backing up of urine into the upper urinary tract can lead to serious complications, including kidney failure. At one time, kidney failure was a common cause of death in people with spinal cord injury, but it is now a rare complication. Modern techniques for bladder management, especially intermittent catheterization, have revolutionized the care of individuals with spinal cord injury. But some major problems with bladder care persist.

Some individuals with spinal cord injury cannot retain urine in their bladder and urinate involuntarily, even when taking medications designed to suppress bladder contraction. Scientists are working to develop better methods of preventing this involuntary bladder contraction. Some people have an incompetent, or "leaky," urethral sphincter, which allows urine to leak from the bladder at inconvenient times. Urologists can sometimes inject artificial material directly into the sphincter to tighten it. Urologists and biomedical engineers are working to develop an implantable artificial urethral sphincter, but we don't yet know whether these efforts will be successful.

For people who retain urine in the bladder and are unable to urinate, scientists are now developing methods for computerized electrical control of the bladder. In one system, FES produces contraction of the bladder's muscles, causing it to empty. This research is still at an early stage but may someday lead to an implantable, artificial system for overall bladder control. The device would keep track of the volume of urine in the bladder, signal when the bladder is full, then stimulate the bladder to empty when so instructed. For some people, electrical stimulation of the bladder may need to be combined with an artificial sphincter system to achieve complete bladder control.

Skin

The skin is the body's largest organ. It has several essential roles in maintaining health, of which the most obvious is preventing infectious organisms (such as bacteria and viruses) from entering the body and causing serious infections.

Many individuals with spinal cord injury develop decubitus ulcers (pressure sores or bed sores), open sores caused by prolonged pressure on the skin (see Chapter 1). Unlike able-bodied people, individuals with spinal cord injury often have impaired sensation and cannot feel the pain or pressure that would normally cause them to change positions. Because of impaired mobility, many people with spinal cord injury cannot shift their weight or change positions easily when sitting or lying down for long periods, even if they are able to sense pressure. Thus, both sensory and motor impairments contribute to the development of decubitus ulcers.

Researchers have taken several approaches to preventing and treating decubitus ulcers. The best "treatment" is to prevent them. This is done only by preventing persistent pressure on the skin, which is best accomplished by changing body position frequently to take the pressure off vulnerable areas. Specialized mattresses, beds, chairs, and cushions have been developed to distribute the pressure over a larger area, so the person can stay in one position longer before needing to move. A routine method of prevention is pressure releases, if necessary with the use of a power wheelchair (described later in this chapter).

Scientists and engineers have developed devices to measure the pressure on the skin that results from lying or sitting in any given position, and these devices are being used to test the effectiveness of new methods for reducing pressure. No method is available for strengthening the skin to prevent decubitus ulcers.

Some research is looking at better ways of treating decubitus ulcers once they have developed. The basic approach is always the same: remove the pressure and keep the skin clean. Once the pressure is removed, a decubitus ulcer usually heals naturally. Sometimes special dressings are necessary to protect the healing skin, to remove unhealthy tissue, and to prevent infectious organisms from entering the wound. Researchers are actively working on new dressing materials that will provide better protection for the healing tissue. Others are experimenting with physical agents such as therapeutic electrical stimulation to enhance wound healing. A recent development, currently in use, is a vacuum suction device to help close the wound and keep it clean.

A final area of active research is the development of better surgical techniques for treating decubitus ulcers that are too large to heal on their own. Surgeons can sometimes remove an ulcer by cutting out the dead tissue, closing the resulting defect with an adjoining area of healthy tissue (sometimes referred to as a "surgical flap"). This is usually done as a last resort for treating non-healing ulcers.

Breathing

People with spinal cord injury at C4 or higher typically need mechanical ventilation to assist with breathing, due to weakness or paralysis of the diaphragm muscles. The need for a ventilator twenty-four hours a day can be a tremendous burden, because the ventilator must be kept available and in working order at all times.

Some people have sufficient strength in their breathing muscles to manage without the ventilator for short periods of time, and other devices can sometimes be used to extend this period off the ventilator. If one or both phrenic nerves to the diaphragm are still intact, an implantable phrenic nerve stimulator can be used to promote breathing. Stimulating the phrenic nerve electrically causes the diaphragm to contract. (Recall from Chapter 1 that the diaphragm receives nerve impulses primarily via the phrenic nerves.) By careful control of the stimulation, the diaphragm can contract with enough strength to fill the lungs with air, as in normal breathing.

An electrical stimulator can sometimes be implanted in the body surgically. Its stimulation of the phrenic nerves then produces artificial breathing. This technique has several problems, however. First, it can be used only with certain types of spinal cord injury. Second, it rarely works full-time; rather, it provides part-time relief from the mechanical ventilator. Third, the device may fail unexpectedly, so a mechanical ventilator must be available in case of emergency. This greatly reduces the benefit of the phrenic nerve stimulator: a primary reason for developing this device was to avoid the inconvenience of keeping a mechanical ventilator available at all times. Still, the potential benefits of artificial breathing are great, and several laboratories are working on methods to increase the effectiveness and reliability of the electrical stimulator. One method currently being studied involves controlling the movement of the diaphragm with electrodes that are implanted in the diaphragm muscle laparoscopically (through tiny holes in the abdomen) in a simple outpatient procedure. By placing the stimulating electrodes directly on the diaphragm (where the phrenic nerve endings are located), this approach overcomes some limitations of directly stimulating the phrenic nerves; it requires less invasive surgery and has less potential for nerve scarring.

An additional problem with breathing after spinal cord injury is weakness of the muscles of expiration (breathing out). The key muscles of expiration are the abdominal and chest muscles, which get their nerve supply from the thoracic levels of the spinal cord. Anyone with a spinal cord lesion above T6 is likely to have some weakness of expiration, even if the diaphragm is working well. Breathing is certainly possible without expiratory muscles, but we need these muscles to exhale forcefully, to shout, and, most important, to cough. As we described in Chapter 1, coughing is essential for keeping the lungs clear and preventing infection, especially pneumonia. Patients with cervical spinal cord injury are highly vulnerable to respiratory tract infections because they cannot cough.

"Quad coughing" (see Chapter 1) is a very effective method of clearing the lungs, but it requires another individual's assistance. Although no method is yet available for a person with tetraplegia to cough effectively without assistance, researchers are working on several methods for independent artificial coughing. The first is a mechanical method, such as a specially made body jacket that squeezes the abdomen and chest to help generate a cough. The second method is electrical stimulation of the expiratory muscles, causing muscle contraction and forcing air out of the chest. These methods for independent artificial coughing are not yet available for clinical use outside of clinical research trials.

Another method for artificial coughing uses a mechanical device that has air pumps. The device first blows air into the lungs (exsufflation), then forcefully sucks it out of the lungs (insufflation) at high velocity. This device is commercially available, and some patients can learn to use it for independent artificial coughing. Further research is needed to determine whether this device is more effective at clearing the lungs than routine quad coughing.

Spasticity

Often the result of spinal cord injury, spasticity can affect function, comfort, self-image, and even the delivery of care. Spasticity can contribute to secondary complications, such as fractures, pressure sores, and pain. Treatment options for spasticity include physical therapy, splinting, nerve blocks, Botox injections, general and regional pharmacologic interventions (dantrolene, oral or intrathecal Baclofen, tizanidine, clonidine, benzodiazepines, gabapentine), and surgery (posterior rhizotomy). In rats with experimental spinal cord injury, Baclofen, a commonly used anti-spasticity drug, was associated with a dramatic reduction in the number of spinal cord stem cells. The drug also reduced the differentiation of neural cells and impaired recovery of gait in these rats. Results of this research mean that clinicians may need to rethink the use of Baclofen (and related drugs) for spasticity in spinal cord injury, because it may impair regeneration and functional recovery in humans, too. On the other hand, patients who regain the ability to walk may need to take Baclofen, because severe spasticity can interfere with functional walking. The development of implantable pumps, such as a Baclofen pump, provides an important treatment option for spasticity. The pump allows direct delivery of Baclofen to the spinal fluid, provides more effective treatment, and avoids the side effects associated with oral Baclofen, such as sedation.

Chronic Pain

Many people with spinal cord injury have chronic pain, and about one-third rate their pain as severe. Current treatments involve a variety of pharmacologic (oral or intrathecal opioids, alpha-adrenergic agonists, antidepressants, anticonvulsants, local anesthetics, N-methyl-D-aspartate [NMDA] receptor antagonists, Baclofen), surgical, physical, and psychological approaches. However, there is limited scientific evidence for the efficacy of many of these treatments. Pain can occur above, at, or below the injury level. It is classified as nociceptive (from muscle, skin, tendon, bones, or organs) or neuropathic (from nerves).

Above the level of injury, nociceptive pain is felt in the same way as before the injury, but it occurs more frequently because of excessive wear and tear on muscles and tendons. Neuropathic pain above the injury level also develops more frequently in individuals with spinal cord injury than in the normal population because of excessive wear and tear on nerves or spinal cord in that region. If vertebrae in the neck were fused together after the original injury, the spinal segments above and below the fusion are more likely to be stressed when motion occurs, just as a chain might bend a bit more above and below two rusty links. This can produce pressure on spinal nerve roots, causing pain. This type of pain can be achy, sharp, or burning, and usually travels up and down the arm.

Pain at the injury level is more likely to be neuropathic than nociceptive. It feels like a tight band that squeezes, burns, and tingles because of sensory nerve damage. This pain is hard to control but is usually managed with medications, such as antidepressants and anti-seizure drugs that affect the levels of chemical substances that travel through nerves.

Below the injury level, some people experience a dull aching or vague pain sensation that is hard to localize or describe, and is sometimes associated with autonomic dysreflexia (see Chapter 1). This type of neuropathic pain is sometimes called central pain, and it can be managed but not generally eliminated.

Sexuality and Fertility

Most of the recent developments in sexuality and fertility after spinal cord injury focus on male sexual function. Several medical and surgical techniques have been developed for treating erectile dysfunction resulting from spinal cord injury. (Erectile dysfunction and other aspects of sexual function and sexuality following spinal cord injury are discussed in detail in Chapter 6.)

On the medical front, medications to treat impotence—especially Viagra, Levitra, and Cialis, which have received a great deal of attention in the press—may be very effective for some men with spinal cord injury, making genital intercourse possible. Caverject, a naturally occurring prostaglandin (hormone-like substance), injected directly into the penis or delivered through a urethral suppository can help achieve erection. Another recent development is the use of a suction pump that can be applied to the penis to help create an erection. Surgical techniques include two types of penile implant, one that keeps the penis in a semi-erect condition and another that uses a miniature internal pump to create a full artificial erection. Unfortunately, the pumps have not been very successful because they are susceptible to mechanical failure.

Treatment of infertility in men with spinal cord injury has improved greatly. In Chapter 6 we discussed various methods of inducing ejaculation in men with spinal cord injury to obtain sperm for artificial insemination or in vitro fertilization. A testicular biopsy, in which a small piece of testicular tissue is removed, can also be used to collect sperm cells directly from the testes.

Perhaps the most disturbing aspect of sexual dysfunction after spinal cord injury, for both men and women, is the loss of genital sensation. This sensory loss is a direct result of damage to nerve fibers carrying sensory information between the genitals and the brain through the spinal cord. Unfortunately, there is currently no way to repair these nerve fibers. However, research is underway in many laboratories (see Healing the Spinal Cord earlier in this chapter).

PREVENTIVE CARE

"An ounce of prevention is worth a pound of cure" applies to most health conditions. It is especially important for people with spinal cord injury, because of their increased risk for medical problems. As discussed earlier, regular medical care and checkups are recommended to prevent complications and maintain health. Your periodic medical examination should include assessment and treatment of medical conditions associated with your spinal cord injury, as well as common medical conditions that can occur in any person. The following list offers some suggestions for examinations, tests, and vaccines that can protect you from becoming sick or detect problems at an early, treatable stage:

1. *Pulmonary (lungs).* Pneumonia vaccine every six years and flu vaccine yearly.
2. *Cardiovascular (heart and blood vessels).* Fasting lipid profile (a blood test) yearly; cardiovascular endurance exercise program three times per week.
3. *Gastrointestinal (esophagus, stomach, and bowels).* Daily fiber intake of 24 grams or more; test for blood in the stool annually after age forty; sigmoidoscopy or colonoscopy every three to five years after age fifty.
4. *Genitourinary (bladder, kidneys, reproductive organs).* Kidney scan, ultrasound, and BUN/creatinine (blood tests for kidney function) yearly for the first ten years after injury, then every three years thereafter; urodynamic (bladder function) testing to determine whether additional treatment is needed for bladder management

and health; PSA (prostate specific antigen) measurement yearly in men over forty to test for prostate cancer; Pap smear yearly in sexually active women (every three years otherwise) to test for cervical cancer; yearly breast exam performed by a physician, and yearly mammogram starting at age forty for women, to test for breast cancer (monthly self-examination of breasts is also recommended for women who are physically able to do so); urine cytology (a test for cancer or inflammation) yearly for individuals who use indwelling catheters for long periods.

5. *Metabolic/endocrine (nutrients and hormones)*. Yearly bone health (DEXA bone densitometry) exam; yearly free and total testosterone measurements in men; yearly blood levels of calcium; daily intake of calcium of 1,200 milligrams (pregnant or lactating women require 1,500 milligrams), daily Vitamin D intake of 600 to 800 units.

6. *Skin*. Appropriate sitting surface; tetanus vaccine booster every ten years.

7. *Musculoskeletal*. Periodic evaluation for appropriate mobility device (power versus manual wheelchair); home exercise equipment; periodic reevaluation of splinting and bracing needs (for function and exercise).

INNOVATIONS IN REHABILITATION TECHNOLOGY

Orthotics and Prosthetics

Another area of importance to spinal cord injury is orthotics, the design and making of devices to assist with function (such as braces and splints), and prosthetics, the design of devices to substitute for functions the person cannot perform (such as pacemakers and artificial limbs). Many people with spinal cord injury can benefit from appropriate bracing and splinting of the limbs and trunk. Bracing is very important for preserving stability of the spine after it is injured, keeping it in the proper alignment. For individuals with paraplegia, lower extremity bracing often allows walking with crutches. Upper extremity splinting can greatly enhance hand function in people with tetraplegia. Of particular note is the wrist-driven flexor hinge splint (also called a tenodesis splint), which uses wrist extensor muscles to give power for gripping objects between the thumb and fingers (with a pinch-type grip). (Extensor muscles contract to straighten a limb; flexor muscles contract to bend it.) New materials for braces and splints are under development. As these materials improve, braces become lighter and sturdier, making them more durable and more efficient.

Powered orthotics—motorized braces and splints—are also being developed, which are particularly important in combination with FES. As we noted above, FES is sometimes impractical because of the great number of muscles involved in controlling the movement of a particular joint. Some laboratories are working on systems that combine FES and powered braces. For example, one approach to restoring the ability to walk in people with paraplegia is the use of FES to provide control of the knees and ankles, a rigid spinal brace to control the trunk, and a powered joint to control the hip. Another FES-powered brace (WalkAid, Ness) prevents paralysis-induced foot drop. And yet another hand FES-powered brace (Ness H200) enhances hand function in individuals with spinal cord injury or stroke.

Bracing of the hip is a major challenge in orthotics. The human hip has enormous flexibility, with freedom of motion in many directions. It also undergoes a great deal of physical stress during normal daily activities. The design of an external, mechanical joint that can support the hip of individuals with paraplegia is therefore a challenge. The standard approach has been to use a metal joint on the side of each hip (the lateral sides), with motion in at least one axis of rotation. However, this device takes up too much space and makes sitting in a normal chair or in a typical wheelchair difficult. The use of this brace is therefore impractical. Most individuals with paraplegia need to be able to switch easily and quickly between walking (with crutches and braces) and using a wheelchair. An approach to this problem is the development of a joint that sits medially (between the thighs) instead of laterally (at the outside of the hip). A single midline metal joint positioned below the groin can substitute for both hip joints, providing a tremendous advantage for stability in the upright position and making walking much easier.

FES technology can also be used to help restore hand grasp and release to individuals who have lost hand function due to spinal cord injury; this is a type of neuro-prosthesis. Several multi-channel implanted FES systems are currently undergoing clinical trials for use as neuroprostheses in humans. Other researchers are developing implantable, computerized devices that interface with parts of the brain to bypass damaged motor pathways; these could one day be used to restore sensory and motor functions lost through injury or disease. Current efforts to develop smaller hardware should eventually make such systems less expensive and easier to implant.

Assistive Devices Technology

The term *assistive devices technology* refers to the range of tools used by people with disabilities to interact more effectively with the environment. In the broadest sense, assistive devices include braces, splints, canes, crutches, walkers, wheelchairs, reachers, grab bars, powered hospital beds, communication systems, and even personal computers. Advances in assistive devices technology have a huge impact on the lives of individuals with spinal cord injuries.

One critical area is wheelchair design. For an individual who spends much of the day in a wheelchair, the characteristics of that chair are critically important. The chair must be comfortable, lightweight, sturdy, and maneuverable. For individuals with tetraplegia, a power wheelchair is often necessary. Sophisticated control devices have been developed for individuals with injuries of the upper cervical spinal cord, who may have difficulty controlling a power wheelchair. These devices include modified joystick controls, "sip and puff" controls, tongue switches, head controls, chin controls, and even eye controls.

A particular problem for people with tetraplegia is performing the pressure releases necessary to prevent decubitus ulcers—many find these difficult or even impossible to perform independently. Sophisticated power wheelchairs often can perform automated pressure releases. The entire positioning system of the chair can tilt backward, under the control of a small accessible switch: the seat, backrest, and headrest all tip backward, and the leg rests tip upward, taking the weight of the body off the sitting surface. This restores blood flow to the skin under the buttocks and prevents skin breakdown. Some wheelchairs are able to change from sitting to standing position. This provides a method for pressure relief and also enhances function, allowing individuals to reach high kitchen cupboards, book shelves, and so forth. And even more sophisticated wheel-chairs can negotiate harsh terrains and even climb stairs (iBOT Mobility System).

Another important area of assistive devices technology is the environmental control unit. This device enables a person with severe physical disability to control electronic devices in the environment, such as lighting, telephones, radios, televisions, air conditioners, and computers. A key element of an environmental control unit is the interface with the user, which may be a simple on/off switch or a complex, sophisticated, personal computer with specialized software. The environmental control unit interfaces with the appliances or devices in the environment by direct wiring or by remote control using radio waves or infrared light.

> In addition to his participating in therapies designed to restore function, Noah utilizes a variety of assistive devices technologies to help him function better with his current limitations. His bedroom, "command central," is on the second floor of the family home, which he reaches by an elevator. In his bedroom, Noah uses an ECU (environmental control unit) to monitor bed movement, the telephone, and a chime system to summon help. He has a computer station above his bed that includes a wireless earpiece for house telephone and computer, and a wireless mouse and keyboard. An extra LCD computer screen rolls over his bed, along with a Kurzweil on which he puts his books to read. Bluetooth wireless signals operate the phone with voice signal. Noah also has an electronic lift system for transfers. Noah comments, "As technology evolves, opportunity expands and my freedom expands."

> After some research, Bella, who has incomplete C4 tetraplegia (see Chapter 9), has acquired a variety of technological innovations that let her manage her life more independently. In her bedroom she has a portable heater with a timer that turns the heat on and off during the night and a fan with the same features. Her speakerphone picks up automatically on the third ring and hangs up automatically when the other person hangs up. An X-10 internal board on her computer links to addressable electrical boxes that control lights, stereo, TV, VCR, electrical doors, bells and buzzers, and appliances throughout the house.

A final important area of assistive devices technology is augmentative communications, electronic and mechanical devices that enable individuals with speech and language impairments to have spoken or written communication. Augmentative communication has limited applicability for people with spinal cord injury, because most individuals with paraplegia or tetraplegia have no difficulty speaking and understanding speech. However, some individuals who require long-term use of a mechanical ventilator are unable to speak independently and can benefit from augmentative communications systems.

A related communication technology is the voice-activated computer, which can be useful for people with limited hand function. Pauline, whose job involves writing long reports, used to rely on hired stenographers to transcribe her dictations after her C4–C5 injury. She now uses a voice-activated computer. This evolving technology is becoming less costly and more effective. Pauline also uses a voice-activated switch for the call-light in her nursing home room. This allows her to communicate easily with nursing staff when she needs assistance. Previously, she had to shout down the hall because she couldn't turn on the light switch. This has changed everything, from her sleeping habits to her personality, says Pauline. (Pauline's use of a nursing home for her living quarters is described in Chapter 10.)

ISSUES AND CONTROVERSIES IN SCIENTIFIC RESEARCH

Medical research has clearly produced marked improvements in the lives of people with spinal cord injury, and further research will undoubtedly present new opportunities to improve neurological recovery, reduce the incidence and severity of medical complications, and enhance rehabilitation techniques, thus ensuring even more active and productive lives. However, dealing with the flood of medical information in the media can be difficult. With so many sources of information—often conflicting—it is difficult to know which reports are truly important, and it is also hard to understand the technical language used in scientific publications.

How can you understand what you read and hear about the latest research? How do advances in spinal cord research affect your choice of treatments? Is it safe to be a volunteer for medical research? Should we focus all our resources on research for a cure? Is animal research really necessary? We address these difficult questions in the remainder of this chapter.

How to Interpret What You Read

How can you protect yourself from exaggerated claims? How can you tell which medical reports are legitimate, realistic, and relevant to your situation? There is no easy answer. Obviously, not every person with spinal cord injury can become an expert in basic medical science, reading and interpreting all the relevant research publications. On the contrary, the job of physicians, nurses, and therapists who care for people with spinal cord injuries is to keep abreast of new developments in medical and scientific research and to know when these developments have direct relevance to the care of their patients. Many sources of reliable information on spinal cord injury exist. But the best way to get accurate information is to have a trusting relationship with a personal physician who is familiar with the field of spinal cord injury treatment and research, and to use that physician as a resource for assessing the validity of stories in the media or any claim of a startling new medical breakthrough. Discuss what you read with your doctor. If you want further advice, you can consult with a spinal cord specialist at a major university medical center.

How to Make Decisions about New Treatments

Be aware that many treatments and therapies, including some discussed in this chapter, can contribute to overall fitness or well-being or help prevent medical complications. You may choose to use a variety of treatments for these benefits. You may also elect to try out therapies that are based on a theoretical or animal research model of spinal cord recovery, even though they are not proven to work in humans. Before embarking on any experimental treatment for spinal cord injury (especially one that promises a cure), get another opinion from an accredited, hospital-based or university-based rehabilitation program or a board certified physiatrist. This will help you to ensure that the treatment in question is not harmful, and to evaluate the potential benefits. But you should be aware that, at the present time, there is no complete cure for spinal cord injury.

Becoming a Research Subject

One way to help advance research on spinal cord injury is by participating in research. During the course of your rehabilitation, or at a routine follow-up visit with your doctor, you may be asked to participate in a research study on some aspect of rehabilitation. How can you decide whether or not to volunteer to be a research subject? This is a highly personal decision.

One consideration is whether the research has scientific merit. Any study that is performed in a reputable research institution must be reviewed and approved by the Institutional Review Board (IRB) for human subjects research. This board consists of a group of physicians and other clinicians from the institution and representatives of the lay public. The IRB is charged with determining whether the proposed study has scientific credibility (in other words, is relevant and well-designed) and whether the ratio of potential risks to potential benefits is acceptable (relatively small risk to individual subjects and a relatively good chance that the drug or technology will prove beneficial for a particular condition).

All studies involving medication, surgery, or any significant risk require a written document that explains the rationale, the risks, and the expected benefits of the study to potential subjects. For an approved study, you will be asked to review and sign this document, called an Informed Consent. If you are not offered such a document, be wary about participating in the study. You may not be adequately informed or protected against potential harm. If a study has not been approved in writing by the applicable IRB, you would be unwise to participate.

Another consideration in deciding whether to participate in a study is whether it could have direct benefit for you. Some research studies might involve teaching you a new skill (for example, relaxation training) or providing a medication with the potential to alleviate pain or spasticity. Other studies may have the potential for helping others in the future, but no possibility of an immediate benefit to you as a subject. You should clearly understand whether a study has the potential for direct benefit or not, and this may be an important factor in your decision to participate. In some cases, participation in one study may prevent you from becoming a subject in other studies. This is the case, for example, with embryonic stem cell transplantation. Experimental embryonic stem cell transplant surgery carries the risks of further paralysis, infection, and blood loss, as well as the risk of malfunctioning of the transplanted cells. Because of these risks, and the likelihood of being excluded from later, potentially beneficial clinical trials, you may want to wait until the technology is more advanced before becoming a subject in an embryonic stem cell trial. Even with an IRB-approved study, it is wise to check with your own physician before volunteering.

Cure versus Care

Some people in the spinal cord injury community are fundamentally opposed to spending research dollars on rehabilitation research. This position is based on the notion that the cure for spinal cord injury is really close, if we'd just commit sufficient resources to cure-oriented research. In this view, supporting rehabilitation research is counterproductive, because it takes away money that could be more productively used in finding the cure.

As we have discussed above, healing the injured spinal cord is an active and necessary area of research, but the complexity of the problems to be solved will take time. Working toward a cure for spinal cord injury remains important, but not to the exclusion of research on innovative approaches to rehabilitation, including FES, assistive devices, and maximizing the functions of the respiratory system, bowel, bladder, and skin. It is critical to have support for efforts toward both a cure *and* improvement of current care, because the two are interdependent; there will be no cure without improvements in medical care and rehabilitative methods for maintaining and optimizing the physical health of the body.

Is it reasonable to hope for a cure of your own spinal cord injury? Of course. Hope is an essential aspect of human psychological function. Without it, we'd have little ability to tolerate adverse events. There is every reason to hope that a cure for spinal cord injury will be found someday, perhaps within your lifetime. Hope for a cure is motivating and energizing for people with spinal cord injury and for scientists. Hope for a better quality of life *with* spinal cord injury is also important to well-being and motivates participation in medical treatment, therapy, and self-care activities that are necessary for effective rehabilitation and for participating in the world of family, social life, and involvement in the community. It would be detrimental for anyone with a spinal cord injury to reject existing treatments and therapies because he or she is "waiting" for a cure. In fact, keeping your body as healthy and fit as possible will maximize your potential to benefit from medical or surgical cures that may be developed in the future. Thus, research must continue on cure *and* care in order to fully meet the needs of people with spinal cord injury.

The Importance of Animal Research

Much of the research on spinal cord injury involves the design and implementation of sophisticated mechanical and electrical engineering systems for FES and assistive devices. These studies often rely on the participation of volunteers with spinal cord injury. But studies on the basic neuroscience of spinal cord injury cannot be done with human subjects. These studies require invasive methods, which include producing specific types of spinal cord injuries in order to study aspects of recovery. These studies, in which a spinal cord lesion is produced artificially, can be done only with experimental animals, as discussed earlier in this chapter. Such studies allow the investigation of what happens in the damaged spinal cord during the first few minutes, hours, and days after injury. Only by detailed study of these processes will we be able to understand the changes at the cellular and molecular levels. This sort of detailed information is absolutely essential for any attempt to develop new medications and surgical approaches for reducing the long-term effects of spinal cord injury.

Some individuals and organizations have raised objections to this research, claiming that it is immoral, unethical, and even cruel to use experimental animals in this way. But, as yet, we have no other way of studying these processes. Given the enormous burden of human suffering associated with spinal cord injury, it seems not only reasonable but absolutely necessary that we continue to study experimental animals. Of course, the treatment of experimental animals should be humane and compassionate. Scientists and ethicists have developed comprehensive regulations to ensure that experimental animals are protected from excessive pain and are not misused.

IN THIS CHAPTER, WE'VE DISCUSSED SEVERAL AREAS of research and technology that hold promise for improving the health and functional abilities of people with spinal cord injury and, ultimately, for the repair of nerve damage in the spinal cord. Many new developments are likely over the next several decades. As a person living with a spinal cord injury, you'll find it helpful to keep abreast of these developments. You can rely on your doctor, your local rehabilitation hospital, spinal cord injury associations, popular and scholarly science journals, and medical school Internet sites for gathering information on new findings that may be relevant to your own rehabilitation, recovery, or health. You may also want to get directly involved by becoming a research subject, by volunteering as a research assistant, or by contributing money to research associations or university departments.

Being an informed consumer helps you communicate better with your health care providers, participate more fully in decisions about your care, and maintain a positive outlook on the future. And, as we've emphasized throughout this book, taking an active role in learning about and discussing all issues relevant to spinal cord injury will help you make the most of your potential for a fulfilling life.

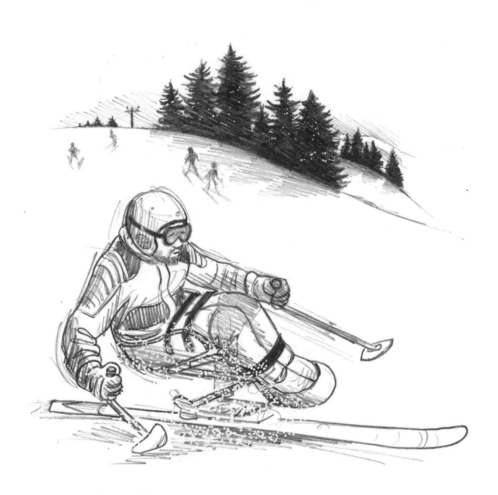

9

The Journey Continues
Finding Yourself

On a glorious spring day, twenty-two-year-old Bella and her young husband—just starting their life together in his home in Europe—borrowed a friend's powerful motorcycle to drive into the countryside. As they were driving along a small, winding road, the car three vehicles ahead of them suddenly stopped short to turn off into a field. The next car jammed on its brakes and turned off to the side of the road; the third car did the same.

As Bella and her husband were just in the process of passing the third car, their motorcycle was forced into the oncoming traffic lane and fell off the road. Bella was carried with the bike off the road.

"Then a car comes around the bend at high speed and, in order to avoid hitting my husband, who's lying in the road, pulls off to the side of the road and hits me as I am getting up. That's accident number two. Then they put me onto an ambulance stretcher and forget to tie the stretcher directly to the ambulance. That is accident number three. The ambulance has an accident. I fly off the stretcher into my husband's arms, who is sitting there, and the gurney flies out of the ambulance like a comic strip. Four accidents in an hour. It was meant to be."

At the local hospital, doctors inserted a metal rod into Bella's neck to stabilize it. In this small hospital, however, no one knew much about treating spinal cord injuries. The staff didn't know how to turn Bella or even what pressure sores were. Bella heard staff say, "God will see." She later heard her mother repeat those words.

Bella has no memories of the first week in the hospital. When she awoke, she asked the nurse to "untie her," but, in truth, Bella couldn't move. She had an incomplete C4 injury, with partial movement in her right arm. She had sensation throughout her body but was paralyzed from the shoulders down. During the hospitalization she couldn't talk much because she had a tracheostomy tube and was on a ventilator.

Over the next few weeks, Bella's condition deteriorated. Against the wishes of her husband's family, her father arranged for Bella to be flown to a small clinic in another country that specialized in treating spinal cord injuries. Eight days later Bella was able to sit up, was taken off the ventilator, and breathed on her own. She found herself setting goals: "if I could just breathe" turned into "if I could just move my arm." In the beginning, says Bella, setting goals was essential motivation.

No one told Bella her injury was permanent, until her physical therapist said, "This is it. You'd better deal with it." Bella told the therapist she hated her and wanted a different physical therapist. She was assigned a "mellow" therapist who stopped treatment when it started to hurt. But Bella realized that pain during therapy was often paired with physical improvement, and she requested the return of the first physical therapist.

Bella found the rehabilitation program in the clinic invigorating. Everyone ate together and had occupational therapy, physical therapy, psychological counseling, and self-care classes. She remembers a saying from her stay there: "You have to live your life exactly as if you're ready to face the consequences."

While Bella was pursuing her rehabilitation in Europe, her parents were investigating various other treatment regimens and facilities. Bella returned to the United States after completing the program in Europe. She underwent testing at a famous rehabilitation institute to assess the extent of injury and whether she could benefit from additional medical or surgical intervention. Although her neck was "full of bone fragments," no further intervention was necessary.

In the meantime, Bella's mother, Lamar, found her a lovely one-level home in the same city where Lamar lived. Carpeting was ripped out, a few doors were moved to make the place more accessible, and the walls were painted in light colors.

A few months later, Bella's husband, who had accompanied her to the United States, returned to Europe. He and Bella have not communicated since. She says, "He left because he couldn't deal with the accident and didn't learn the *language." His family told him to forget the past, but Bella feels he blamed himself for the accident.*

Bella says image seemed to be all-important in Europe: "You played different roles in different groups." Some groups of friends accepted her disability, while others chose to ignore it. But when meeting with friends, she found it difficult to come up with her own image of being paralyzed and "confined to a wheelchair," no longer athletic and risk-taking as she'd been before the accident.

Back in the United States, Bella returned to university studies, earning her BA in public relations and languages at one university and earning a translation degree at another. She became a major force for increased accessibility on the latter campus. Bella is continuing her studies while freelancing, teaching people how to make museum collections accessible to disabled people, and creating databases and developing policy and manuals for museums. She also continues her advocacy.

Listening to her own body signals is important to Bella. Most people don't do this as much as they should, she says. She tries to figure out what is best for her comfort and physical well-being and does research into how to achieve what she needs. For example, she has devised a bedding system that reduces the number of position changes necessary at night. She uses a hospital bed with a flat platform and no springs, with a stiff orthopedic mattress. On top of this mattress is an air mattress and a geo-mat (a type of egg-crate mattress that allows air to flow horizontally, relieving pressure and giving support). She contends that with the air mattress under the geomat, her skin and bony areas have a change of pressure every four minutes. To transfer into or out of her bed, she uses a Trans-aid lifter, which requires only one hand and is small, transportable, and very sturdy.

Like Joan (see Chapter 4) and Nora (see Chapter 7), Bella encourages people with spinal cord injury to question the status quo and to figure out what works for their own situation.

When Bella's life was interrupted by spinal cord injury, she was a young woman on the cusp of adulthood. She had led an exciting life—crossing international boundaries, speaking several languages, and participating in a number of athletic and cultural events. Her story illustrates how one person coped, surviving both the adjustment to spinal cord injury and the loss of a relationship. Bella has both changed and remained the person she always was. She has reassembled, reordered, and substituted new pieces of the puzzle that make up a life, creating the life she now leads.

Some people's idea of really "doing" a jigsaw puzzle is to cover up the picture of the completed puzzle on the front of the box. This adds to the challenge of figuring out which notch fits into which groove, by matching colors, patterns, and shapes. The trial and error needed to arrange the pieces without knowing what the completed picture looks like can be frustrating, but the final feeling is one of triumph.

Much the same process has been going on as you "reemerge" after spinal cord injury. So many pieces to reconnect—and the final picture is an unknown. First there was the pre-disability you, then the trauma and its aftermath—hospitalization and (in most cases) rehabilitation—then your return home, perhaps to school or to work, or to a new home somewhere else. You resumed the daily rhythm of your life. You began to go out with friends again. Life, with its disability blip, continued.

This chapter is about finally having almost all the pieces of the puzzle connected and seeing what the picture looks like. You are beginning to feel like *yourself* again. It may have taken one, two, or even five years to arrive at this point. But at last you can say, "I'm back. I'm my old self." Or, "I'm my new self"—a surprising arrangement of your jigsaw puzzle.

As you begin to feel in control of yourself and your life again, you may be ready to chart where you are and what you'd like to do to make life more complete. Remembering the variety of experiences you have endured, survived, and mastered will give you the sense that "you can do it." Indeed, as your ability to deal with life and its adversities deepens, you may find a wellspring of strength and confidence for the years ahead. In short, you've discovered that life is a journey of "uncovery" and "discovery"—of the world and its possibilities, and of yourself, your talents, and your deepest resources.

ADJUSTING, ADAPTING, AND RECONCILING

As you put the puzzle pieces of your life together, you will adjust to your new situation, adapt to changing circumstances, and reconcile with reality. Adjustment is a balancing of all areas of life so as to bring about a more satisfactory situation. It includes the element of adaptation, the process of making modifications to deal with changing circumstances. Reconciliation is the recognition of the underlying consistency or congruity in your life, even when it has been disrupted by spinal cord injury.

However, before you can adjust, adapt, and reconcile to life with spinal cord injury, you may need to work through old, unresolved issues. Only then can you enjoy the present and better plan for the future. The resolution of issues and needs left festering from the past is a priority before moving on. It's like taking a car in for periodic tune-ups to correct what's gone wrong so that it will run smoothly in the future. Your looking-back-in-order-to-move-ahead assessment will include the following personal checkpoints:

1. Healing old wounds
2. Checking out coping patterns
3. Reframing your self-image
4. "Owning" your spinal cord injury
5. Integrating disability into your life
6. Relating to others

In each area, you need to look at the challenges ahead and the strengths you have to meet them.

Healing Old Wounds

The first step is to deal with old wounds that have not healed. Although disability brings a torrent of new issues, you have to face those old, unresolved matters from before the spinal cord injury so you can move on with adjustment to your new life. To make the most of your internal creativity and resiliency, old hurts need a chance to heal. Sometimes this means reopening the wound to allow the "inner tissues" to mend. The wound may include old "chips on the shoulder" that have resulted in your viewing life as a series of disappointments ("Everyone has it better than I do").

Forgiving, forgetting, or redefining will be the start of your healing process. This might require reformatting the way you view life and interact with others. Instead of interpreting other people's words and actions negatively, for example, you might want to listen to those words and see those actions as honest expressions of their feelings.

Lark (see Chapter 8) recalls her desire to repair relationships after her injury, to go back and ask for forgiveness. "I wanted to reach out, to make sure there was no negative energy." She reached out to her former husband, whom she had not spoken to for five years. Getting closure on the unfinished business of this and other relationships helped her "sleep well at night," says Lark, and gave her the energy to focus on developing a new social network.

In order to move on, you must unload your pre-disability trunk of old hurts and unresolved issues. Resolving these issues will allow you to refill and restock your mental and psychological reserves. Resolution will probably not be a quick fix. This is a gradually evolving process, full of insights, some dawning slowly and others occurring with the suddenness of flashbulbs popping. Don't hesitate to get the spiritual or psychological help you may need to do this work.

Jack dealt with intermittent bouts of anger after the automobile accident that caused his cervical spinal cord injury, anger that was interfering with his relationship with his wife. Jack had modeled himself after his father, a strict and emotionally unavailable parent. In Jack's eyes, his father had been perfect and powerful. In rehabilitation, when Jack found himself needing to ask for help, he felt demeaned and weak, imagining his father's disapproval. He fought against his weakness with bursts of anger.

After talking about his father in therapy, Jack learned other models of "fathering himself" and was able to unload the model he had grown up with. Having rid himself of this old baggage, he could invest all of his energy in dealing effectively with the demands of his current life. For example, before his injury Jack had been a foreman on an automobile assembly line, accustomed to making things happen. In the new, accessible apartment he and his wife had just moved into, he couldn't even open the front door himself—until he read about and purchased a remote control device. This experience led him to search for other technological innovations for his home. His mental power took over where his physical power left off. Freed of his old fear and anger, Jack had the energy to be creative, coming up with many other "light bulb" realizations.

Like Jack, you'll find that with each new insight, you're infused with the knowledge that change is possible, that you can find new ways to manage your life and environment.

Checking Out Coping Patterns

A recent article notes, "The way in which a person adjusts to spinal cord injury reflects his or her long-standing global perspective on life." The "global perspective on life" most often found in the people whose stories we've told in this book is optimism. Their disabilities were acknowledged, not denied, but the thrust was toward moving on with life. This optimistic adjustment often springs from a sense of who you are and what your competencies are. Your ego, or self, provides a powerful sense of continuity over time, as the essential elements of "you" do not change following the injury. What may change are patterns or ways of living and the ways in which you resolve problems—the adaptations to the new circumstances in your life. For example, perhaps you found jogging a great way of releasing stress. After spinal cord injury, you'll need to perceive stress in a new way, reframing and defusing it, or to find some new way to release it.

Adjustment is based in part on your past patterns of coping and adaptation. You'll have to reassess those patterns to see whether they fit your life as you begin once more to gain control and chart your course. Sometimes old patterns are helpful: your former drive and determination to become first cellist may help you work harder in your physical therapy. On the other hand, that same determination may go into overdrive, pushing you to attempt the impossible—with frustration, anger, or depression as a result. So your former styles of dealing with issues can be either helpful or hurtful as you reconcile the new factors that enter your life after injury.

We provide here some ideas to help you evaluate the patterns learned from your family and your own risk-taking behaviors to determine which can hinder and which can help you create the life you want.

Family Lessons

Pragmatic and philosophical attitudes that we've inherited from our families or carved out later in life help us shape the "stuff" of ourselves.

These core learnings and leanings are informative. Did your father say, "God helps those who help themselves"? Did you engrave it in your mind? Did Grandma say we were never given "a load too heavy for us to haul"? Musing on the importance of old sayings such as these, we find how important they are in our lives. They motivate us to recognize the deep reserves of mental and emotional strength with which we can meet difficult times. You might decide that these family lessons are "keepers." They become part of your self.

On the other hand, maybe Grandpa taught you to be stoic, "toughing it out" and never letting others know how you were feeling. From your experience with spinal cord injury, you know that sharing your feelings is helpful and necessary. After releasing pent-up feelings, you feel "lighter" and ready to tackle the next hurdle. You realize now that Grandpa's philosophy is not healthy for you, and you discard it.

Developing your own philosophy of life may mean examining your attitudes, belief systems, and general outlook. The optimism we've encountered in people with spinal cord injury seems to cut across ages— people injured during young adulthood, in middle age, or in their later years. And many people living with spinal cord injury have an intense appreciation of life's brevity, perhaps because they have faced near-death situations. This perspective has allowed them to set priorities, conserve energy for important issues, and reduce the impact of daily stress.

Another guiding principle is the belief in setting goals and striving to reach them. The process of working toward a goal, and the value of trying, may be more important than the final outcome. A related principle is the value of activity, involvement, or productivity. While not necessarily gainfully employed, many people who live successfully with spinal cord injury have something of a work ethic, a "get up and go" approach to life. An important part of this philosophy is the belief that doing something that benefits people or things outside oneself is essential to living.

Taking Risks

Some people with spinal cord injury take lots of risks, and risk-taking may have been an important part of their pre-disability behavior. And after injury, risk-taking can be important in allowing them to keep up their interests.

What is risk-taking? It's a bit like gambling. You weigh the odds that you can accomplish your goal against the odds that you will fail. For example, river rafters calculate the odds of safe passage through whitewater rapids against the odds that they will collide with hidden boulders and capsize. To "better" their odds, they prepare themselves and chart the passage carefully.

A willingness to take risks can be helpful in rehabilitation as you are challenged to test the limits of your physical abilities. If you're someone who likes to take risks, however, you may need to examine your pattern of seizing risky opportunities without adequately assessing the consequences. This is not to say that taking risks is to be discouraged—on the contrary, it is vital to living. The key is to weigh the potential benefit of the risky situation (achieving the goal, joy, excitement, growth) against the potential harm (physical damage, emotional pain, creating burdens for others).

> Sally was a seasoned sailboat operator, having sailed from the West Coast to Hawaii on several occasions. After a speeding car rammed her pickup truck at an intersection and left her with paraplegia, she dreamed of returning to the sea. But she was fearful about her abilities to do what was essential in helping to sail the boat. She talked with fellow nautical enthusiasts, and they worked with her to come up with safety precautions and tasks that she could perform. This, for Sally, was a reasonable way of doing what she loved to do, because the planning helped her control some of the risky variables.

Reframing Your Self-Image

At the same time that you're working on many other changes, you may be entering a new phase of dealing with external appearances and differences. Recall the time it took for you to get used to the change in your image after you started using assistive devices, such as braces or a wheelchair. Remember how Joan refused the power wheelchair for a couple of years because it looked stodgy and bulky (see Chapter 4)? As she re-entered life more fully, she realized that the power chair gave her greater freedom and autonomy to do the things she wanted to do. She began to adapt or modify her image of herself in the power chair. This is what reframing your self-image is all about.

As you gain more self-direction, you'll probably feel free to make the decisions that feel right to you, including decisions about how you present yourself to others. Have you learned the art of reframing your picture to highlight those aspects of yourself that you value most—a well-developed, muscular upper body, beautiful long hair, friendly eyes, nicely proportioned figure, big smile, or symmetrical features? Lee (whose story is in Chapter 10) is conscious of the cut of his suit jackets, preferring a shorter cut, which looks better when he's in his wheelchair. Lark (see Chapter 8) wears slacks because she feels she looks more attractive in them. She always dresses up, believing that "people treat you with more respect" if you are well dressed and that a good appearance creates positive attitudes and enhances relationships with others.

Remember: there are many "right" decisions. Listen to your inner voice to find out what you want. Some people proudly include their sports wheelchair or crutches or power chair in their photographs. Others do not. How you choose to see yourself is up to you. This is a part of the fine-tuning of your adjustment to spinal cord injury.

"Owning" Your Spinal Cord Injury

Each individual has a unique story about coming to terms, at last, with spinal cord injury. People talk about "coming to terms with," "accepting," "coping with," or "adjusting to" disability. It doesn't matter what words you use to describe "owning" your disability. What matters is that you did it, and that now you can redirect your energy toward other areas of life: relationships, family, creativity, or work.

You took the first steps in this direction during your rehabilitation, but the issue of adjustment usually comes up again from time to time, especially when passing from one life stage to another. In going through these passages (marital commitment or commitment to a single life; parenthood; choice of vocation; midlife changes; adapting to old age) new issues will arise. To deal with them successfully, you need to see yourself as a person worthy of receiving the investment required to forge ahead.

The extra physical effort associated with disability is required often, sometimes daily, as you live in a world constructed for people without disabilities. Physical needs have to be met before you can enjoy the fun things in life, such as having dinner with friends or attending a concert. As one recent article on adjustment stated, "You can't go out and look at the stars without taking care of the wheelchair or without attendant care."

People with a disability encounter many definitions that try to box them into a category: *crippled, disabled, person with a disability, physically challenged*. Do these terms define any of the people you have met in this book? Could you, for instance, say "Joan is disabled" and know what is essential about her? Wouldn't "Joan is a computer engineer, an artist, a philanthropist, a family member, a dancer, and, oh yes, she has a disability," be a better description?

Looking at yourself, you can assess the attributes or abilities you still have and acknowledge those you don't. And, as part of the creative discovery process, you may find ways to do those things you thought you'd never do again. Jerry, who was injured while mountain climbing, had a difficult time even thinking about no longer being a part of his pals' touch football team after he became paraplegic. He ached to be out on the field with them. One day he decided to talk with his friends about playing with the team in whatever way he could. His friends were excited about the prospect of Jerry's comeback and set about redesigning their game to include their old friend.

The qualities that defined you as a person without a disability—your sense of humor, purposefulness, friendliness, shyness, thoughtfulness, naivete, joyfulness, garrulousness, or ability to articulate—still define you as a person who happens to have a disability. Ownership of who you were before your spinal cord injury now extends to who you are as a person who happens to have a disability. It is the combination of all these aspects of yourself that leads to our next point.

Integrating Disability into Your Life

Where you were in life at the time of your injury (your age, relationship status, geographic location, education, job) has a crucial bearing on how you react, adapt, and reconcile to this new part of your life. People have different strengths and challenges. Bella's past included international travel and athletics. Would they be part of her future or influence her direction? Ray painted houses for a living and was the sole breadwinner for his family of five when, in his late fifties, he climbed the ladder to clean the gutters on his house and fell, injuring his spinal cord. How would he reconstruct his future?

How individuals build their lives depends on many variables. For a young person, the task is to define the direction for a lifetime. This will be aided or hindered by support or lack of support, such as family attitudes, education, economic means, and whether adequate rehabilitation facilities are available. An older person, on the other hand, has to deal with the disruption of an established lifestyle at a time when one usually expects life to be in a fairly stable pattern. The situation can be even more complicated for a person in a rocky relationship with few people who are able and willing to serve as a support network.

So, where you are at the time of injury helps you assess and understand yourself and the assets and deficits of your situation. It helps in explaining why your puzzle looks the way it does . . . and how you might change it.

Relating to Others

A large piece of the puzzle is social connections. Socializing, after all, is a primary activity for human beings. Will your disability be an impediment to communicating and socializing with others? Some people find that the injury has no impact at all, while others say that it does make a difference. If you find that it does, define the roadblocks that seem to separate you from others. Are they the steps into a friend's house or the lack of cut-outs in the pews at church so that you can fit your wheelchair next to your family? Or do you find a qualitative difference in how you and other people relate to each other? Are stereotypes or unrealistic expectations clouding or obstructing communication, on your side or other people's? Communicating with an old friend can be made difficult by both your friend's and your own image of disability.

Mike, who was paraplegic as the result of an automobile accident, owned a neighborhood bar. Before his disability, he was the jovial master of the bar and a good Samaritan in the community, sponsoring soccer teams and sending toys to children in the local hospital at Christmas. After the accident, Mike was depressed and withdrawn, seeing little hope that he would be able to return to his old way of life. He felt that no one would want to be with him.

After his acute hospitalization and three weeks in the rehabilitation center, Mike returned home to his wife and two teenage children. They became very concerned about his continuing depression and sought help for him. After several months of psychotherapy, Mike's depression lifted and he began to understand that he was still the same person. He might have to be creative in pursuing his pre-injury lifestyle, but he could arrange enough elements of it to be satisfying. At the same time he realized that he would have to "put himself out there," just being himself. If he saw himself as the same person he always was, others would see him that way, too.

While the core of your self remains unchanged, you may have an expanded awareness and appreciation of your life and of those around you. Having tended to old unresolved hurts, sorted through coping patterns, integrated spinal cord injury into your self-image, and worked on sorting through relationships with others, you may find that you can adjust, adapt, and reconcile to your new life. You may also have a new appreciation for life and its fragility.

THUS FAR WE'VE FOCUSED ON PUTTING TOGETHER THE PIECES of your life, solving the puzzle of who you are and who you can be. In the next section we explore the implementation of these personal "pieces" through the choice of lifestyle.

LIFESTYLES

As we've shown throughout this book, people with spinal cord injuries have many different styles of living, just as they did before injury. While individual diversity is often a consideration in planning rehabilitation goals, the development of overall lifestyle has not traditionally been a major focus of rehabilitation. Rehabilitation programs and society at large tend to view "successful" rehabilitation as a return to pre-injury functions and roles, perhaps with some modifications or assistance. Little emphasis is placed on assisting people who cannot return to pre-injury lifestyles in developing alternative pathways to meaningful and enjoyable living. For example, when Randy's insurance company discontinued coverage for vocational services because he was deemed "unemployable," no comparable services were available to help him develop volunteer activities or explore hobbies. (Randy's story is told in Chapter 10.)

Too often, the implicit message of society is that lack of gainful employment means failure, just as using a wheelchair means confinement. Fortunately, as social roles become more flexible, this is beginning to change. People with spinal cord injury have clearly been able to redefine life goals and lifestyles, sometimes even viewing the injury as an opportunity for positive change.

Non-Vocational Lifestyles

There are many reasons why people, with or without spinal cord injuries, decide not to make paid employment the major focus of their lives. Some people choose to stay home to care for children or other family members. Some pursue a life of volunteerism. Others involve themselves in hobbies, creative activities, political activism, or religious service. Many people—disabled or not—make several lifestyle shifts over a lifetime, depending on economic necessity, developmental stage, changing interests, or family needs. For example, most people now have some choice about when to retire. Some people work until they are no longer physically able, while others retire early in order to enjoy other interests or relationships. Some women and, increasingly, some men have a choice about how long to leave their jobs in order to care for young children and whether or not to devote themselves primarily to child-rearing or employment. There is no "right" decision about retirement age or child-care leave. Most people agree that individual preference is an important and legitimate factor in these and other lifestyle choices.

Lifestyle decisions and choices are just as important, and just as individual, after a spinal cord injury. You'll undoubtedly be faced with a changed set of circumstances and needs after your injury, and these changes may or may not result in a change of lifestyle. But if, by necessity or by choice, your focus of activity shifts away from work, keep in mind that able-bodied people often choose non-vocational lifestyles and that a wide variety of activities can shape a rich and productive life.

We discuss here several of these non-vocational activities. In order to highlight specific choices, we discuss them individually. But bear in mind that most people's lives are multidimensional and that it is a combination of activities that defines a lifestyle.

Hobbies

Steve (whom you met in Chapter 5) was a single man in his early thirties who lived with his parents and worked the nightshift at a factory. By day, Steve could be found at the local racetrack, avidly pursuing his hobby: watching horse races and placing bets. Steve did his job responsibly but was never emotionally involved in his work. It was simply a means to an end—a way to make a living. The real center of Steve's life was the track, and he spent as much time there as he could.

Steve was shot at work in a robbery attempt and became tetraplegic, with no mobility below the shoulders. During his hospital rehabilitation, Steve and his family were taught transfer techniques and bowel, bladder, and skin care. Steve was offered a variety of technologies that could have given him more personal control of his life, such as a power wheelchair and environmental control unit. And he was eligible for vocational services and could have returned to school, though employment prospects were limited.

But Steve declined these services, and on returning home he chose to use a manual wheelchair. By mutual agreement, his mother provided his personal care. Steve was content with this arrangement and felt that fancy gadgets were superfluous to his rehabilitation, because his family would take care of his needs.

The staff might have jumped to the conclusion that Steve was unmotivated. But Steve did want a van with a lift, which would enable his family to take him out—to the racetrack! Steve wanted to get back to his favorite pastime, and he made sure that he did so. He had no interest in returning to school and was not skilled in anything but manual work. He chose to build a lifestyle out of his hobby. Whenever possible, he spent his days at the track, where he enjoyed the excitement of the races and the companionship of other racing devotees.

Steve's family continued to provide care and transportation for him. His relationship with them was also an important aspect of his life, as they spent many hours together, had common interests, and were very close. Steve and his family never questioned whether his life was "productive." He enjoyed life, related lovingly to his family, and was at peace with himself.

Steve's story is just one example of how a particular interest or hobby can become even more important after spinal cord injury. The amount of free time you'll have if you don't return to work may let you immerse yourself more fully in leisure interests. Eugene, for example, was tattooed from neck to thigh, and before he became tetraplegic he regularly attended tattoo conventions. Following his injury, he decided to learn computer graphics in order to design tattoo art.

The Internet offers a wealth of recreational activities, such as a wide variety of games, discussion groups, music, videos, and news reports. Creative writing is possible for people with tetraplegia using voice-activated computers or other adaptive devices for writing or typing. Others participate in wheelchair sports (see Sports, below). Peter (introduced in Chapter 3) was an avid singer. After his injury, his immersion in singing as an avocation was central to his enjoyment of life. Involvement in recreational activities such as billiards (shooting pool), camping, games (for example, bridge and chess), flying, and gardening offers avenues for enjoyment and accomplishment. Noah, who was introduced in Chapter 8, loves computer chess, video games, and writing poetry. He notes that "success lies in finding something you enjoy. Then you have a lot of small-, medium-, and long-term goals. [Enjoyable activities] allow you to focus on what you can do." Having something you're "into" can be a great source of satisfaction, can bolster your self-esteem, and can provide the basis for "getting a life."

You can also use your mind and imagination to provide comfort, entertainment, and relaxation at times when you can't participate in the external world or choose to be alone. Pauline (whom you met in Chapter 8) uses classical music to "abstract" inside her own mind. She feels her intellectual bent makes her "the perfect person to have spinal cord injury, because I like living in my head." Though Pauline has a career and an active social life, expanding the "living space" in her mind has been important in making her life rich and meaningful.

Sports, Recreation, and Travel

Taking up old passions for sports (or becoming involved in a new sport), although requiring time and effort, is a great way to return a sense of balance to your life—with spinal cord injury being just one part of the package. Sports are a source of exercise, relaxation, pleasure, and achievement for many people, and numerous opportunities exist for participation in adapted sports after spinal cord injury. *Sports 'N Spokes* magazine, published by the Paralyzed Veterans of America, is a good source of information about sports for people with spinal cord injury. Many outdoor and indoor sports, such as hunting, fishing, scuba diving, skiing, tennis, basketball, volleyball, and cycling are possible after spinal cord injury, usually with adaptive equipment. Robert, who was introduced in Chapter 7, expresses his passion for life through sports. "I work hard, play hard. I don't sit around much; I try things." Robert has tried a variety of water sports, boating, all-terrain-vehicles, and sledding. Andrew, also introduced in Chapter 7, was a young tennis star before his spinal cord injury at age twelve. After his injury, he was introduced to wheelchair tennis and became an international competitor, earning a gold medal in the Junior Paralympics while still in his teens.

Several organizations specialize in accessible sports and recreation activities for the less serious athlete. For instance, if you like skiing or horses, the National Ability Center in Park City, Utah, provides an accessible lodge and cafeteria, and offers skiing, horseback riding, and yoga lessons. Families are welcome and some scholarships are available. (See the Resources section at the end of this book.)

For those who enjoy horses, but may not be able or want to ride them, driving a cart or carriage is another option, easily adaptable for people with disabilities. There are cart/carriage centers and competitions across the United States, run by the North American Riding for the Handicapped Association. (See the Resources section at the end of this book.) For those in wheelchairs, there are ramps allowing you to run your wheelchair up and into the cart or carriage. If you are looking at physical benefits, this activity helps with flexibility, balance, and muscle strength.

When you feel life is closing doors to you, what do you think about doing? Many people contemplate getting away, doing something unusual, visiting far-off family, or finding a place of tranquility. Although some doors may be closed to those with spinal cord injuries, options for travel are open.

There's a whole wide world out there to explore, people to meet, foods to savor, experiences to be had, and scenery to soak in. And there are cars and boats and trains and planes to get you to them (see Chapter 7).

Just because you use a wheelchair or crutches, a ventilator, or attendant care doesn't mean that you cannot travel. While technology has not opened up the entire world, it has created more opportunities to explore this earth than ever before in history.

Some people like the exotic, others tend toward nature, while others go for big-city life. Some find their travel most satisfying in day trips, long weekends, or a week in a cabin, while others will want two or three weeks of uninterrupted scaling-down time. The choice is yours. So uproot yourself from your own space and try out another.

Want a peaceful retreat? The West Virginia and Arkansas state park systems have accessible cabins and facilities; other state and private parks have similar accommodations. For a more remote, especially tranquil setting, the Mersey River Chalets in Nova Scotia offer the opportunity to "get into" nature with trails offering easy rolling for chairs into the woods and along the Mersey River. Wharfs allow access to swimming, kayaking, and canoeing with lifts available for transferring from chair to kayak, for instance. Totally accessible chalets have roll-in showers. This unique site was designed and built by a team that included several people with varying levels of spinal cord injury; one of the directors on site is a person with paraplegia (see the Resources section at the end of this book).

For some people, "getting there is half the fun," and the mode of transportation is an important factor in their decisions about travel and vacations. There are the cruise aficionados who have their tales of the Alaskan trip or the voyage through the Panama Canal. As discussed in Chapter 7, most cruise ships are accessible and provide a relaxing, less structured alternative to touring by land. In addition to getting you from place to place, cruise ships provide accessible entertainment, dining, fitness centers, swimming, lectures, and other activities. By contrast, train travel is far less luxurious, but devotees of train trips often enjoy meeting new people and share their tales of the various routes with the best scenery or "hottest" stops along the way. Some prefer to have more control over the route they take and the stops they make and they choose a vacation by car.

For those of you who want lots of hustle and bustle, action, noise, and movement, your choice of destination will probably be a big city. While travel to a city offers much in the way of entertainment, culture, education, and stimulation, it does require some advance work and preparation. For instance, you might choose the Big Apple—New York City! Or the Windy City—Chicago! If you use a wheelchair, know in advance that sidewalks are uneven, curb-cuts might have a big "drop off" from the sidewalk to street level, and because they are "old" cities, in American terms, steps can often be a challenge or a barrier. You may want to bring your own car or van, despite the cost of parking. Hailing a taxi cab from a wheelchair is not always successful. Be prepared to be picked up by some and passed by others who may not want to put your wheelchair into the trunk. If you plan to rely on taxi cabs, you probably need to make arrangements ahead of time, as you schedule the trip. Some cities have accessible taxi or private van services; most have wheelchair-accessible vans to take you from the airport to your hotel. These vibrant cities require additional energy from you or from your co-travelers to access all they offer. Make sure to request an accessible hotel room; most larger hotels can accommodate your needs with advance notice. The cost of lodging and meals is higher in big cities, but information from travel agents and travel books can help you plan a trip on a moderate budget.

Vacation doesn't necessarily mean travel, however. One person opted to take her vacation at home, exploring unknown parts of her own city. She explained that it was easier for her to have her home base from which to stretch out. And because she didn't "stress out" about planning and packing, she felt more relaxed, refreshed, and revitalized from her daytime outings. This type of vacation can be an opportunity to explore the cultural and entertainment centers of your own area, perhaps discovering new restaurants and clubs that are wheelchair accessible.

Creative Pursuits

In our work with people with spinal cord injury, we've repeatedly heard this advice from "old hands" to those just starting out: Find something to do. Be productive. Don't vegetate. Where there's a will, there's a way. Be creative!

Creative potentials and talents discovered after spinal cord injury can become the basis for a new lifestyle. Richard started painting watercolors in recreational therapy, initially as a distraction from pain and a way to relax. But painting soon became a consuming interest, which he continued long after returning home. People with high-level cervical cord injuries can learn to paint by mouth or to use computer programs to make drawings, paintings, graphic designs—or tattoos!

Many creative activities are open to you after spinal cord injury. Creative writing, playing an instrument, singing, gourmet cooking, sewing, and acting are some examples. Some of these may require adaptations. Computers, often touted as the panacea for vocational rehabilitation, are perhaps even more useful in the creative activities of people with severe limitations in mobility. You can find software programs to help you create artwork, musical compositions, sewing patterns, and numerous other things. Tape recorders, videotapes, and other technical aids can expand your opportunities to create.

One aspect of creativity is problem-solving and producing new tools or technologies to deal with obstacles in daily living. Necessity has been the mother of invention for many people with spinal cord injury: designing and creating their own tools, gadgets, wheelchair accessories, and so forth, or developing their own methods for transfers, pressure releases, baby care, and dressing. Developing your skill in creative problem-solving will help you generate ideas and solutions as your needs change.

The Association of Mouth and Foot Painting Artists provides a commercial outlet for artists who cannot use their hands. Many of the artists are people with tetraplegia who trained in art and learned mouth-painting after their injury. The association exhibits and sells the art produced by its members, and some members earn their living in this manner. *Kaleidoscope* is a magazine devoted to the interface of art, literature, and disability. It publishes articles and artwork by persons with disabilities and on themes relating to disability, as well as poetry written by and about people with disabilities.

Chuck Close is a famous artist who lives in New York City. He was well established in the art world before he developed incomplete tetraplegia at the age of forty-seven, caused by a collapsed spinal artery. He continues to paint with the aid of a simple hand brace made of metal and Velcro, which allows him to hold a paintbrush (he is otherwise unable to grip). He can use his teeth to put on the brace and place a paintbrush in it. A motorized easel allows him to turn his giant canvases so he can reach all parts of his paintings from his wheelchair. Close feels his portraiture has changed only in that it has "a celebratory aspect that wasn't there before, and that's because I feel so happy that I was able to get back to work after my illness."

Advocacy

As we've emphasized throughout this book, becoming an advocate and spokesperson for yourself and your needs is essential to successful living with a spinal cord injury. Some people find that advocating for themselves, especially when confronting legal rights or educational or employment problems, attracts the attention of others with similar problems, and this leads to advocating for a particular cause or group. Some individuals have made a career of advocacy for people with disabilities, and this is another lifestyle path you may choose.

> *Lee (see Chapter 10) has made advocacy both a personal and a professional commitment. The most overt discrimination he has confronted occurred as he was returning home from a professional trip on a national airline. After the plane had landed, he was told that he couldn't use the shuttle to the main terminal "without an attendant." He sued the Department of Transportation for not issuing the regulations implementing the Air Carrier Act. They were issued and implemented within thirty days.*

> *Noah (introduced in Chapter 8) was injured in a diving accident. Ten months after his injury he founded an organization to provide information about preventing beach injuries, ease the transition made by families of newly injured spinal cord patients, support and provide funding for spinal cord research and rehabilitation, and maintain a Web site of information and advice about spinal cord injury. Noah has also been involved in education about beach safety through public speaking, publishing and distributing brochures, and raising funds for programs to increase safety awareness. He has worked in political campaigns on behalf of candidates who support legislation that benefits people with disabilities, and has partnered with state agencies on increasing public insurance funding of medical equipment and attendant care. Noah's advocacy work has helped him channel his energy and talent toward helping others, retain a positive outlook on life, and meet new people, all of which have helped him to cope with his own injury.*

Vocational Lifestyles: Testing the Limits

Going back to your old job after a spinal cord injury is often possible, sometimes with physical modifications, always with emotional and social adjustments. Finding a new job or developing a new career are also possibilities. Each of these paths requires some "testing" as you try out new ways of doing old tasks, negotiate environmental barriers, and cope with the feelings and reactions of co-workers to the "new you."

Resuming a vocational lifestyle may be a relatively smooth process. If you have paraplegia and your line of work is not primarily physical, getting back on the job and resuming your identity as a worker may be easier. David, working in restaurant management, and Don, a stockbroker, resumed working life with minimal adaptations—as have many other people with paraplegia who are lawyers, doctors, office managers, and salespeople. They continue to gain self-esteem and a sense of purpose from their work. Aware that not everyone has the chance to return to work, David says, "I think I was one of the fortunate ones when I had my accident, because I did have the opportunity to go back to work." He believes that people with spinal cord injuries are often deprived of work because of the prejudices of some employers. In his volunteer peer counseling, David tries to encourage people to assert their rights to employment.

If you have a more severe disability (such as high-level tetraplegia), perhaps needing the assistance of a personal care attendant, or if your pre-injury job required full mobility, resuming a work-based lifestyle may be more challenging. It may take considerable effort and the courage to test the limits of your employer's attitudes, physical barriers in the workplace, and your own abilities.

Elliott (introduced in Chapter 6) was employed in construction before his injury. Although intelligent and able to return to college, he was unsure about what kind of job he could do with C5–C6 tetraplegia. Had he not been motivated by the need to support his new baby, Elliott might have floundered even longer in employment limbo. Fortunately, he was able to receive practical training in accounting and financial planning, which was then a fast-growing field. He got a job immediately after finishing his training and was soon employed full-time.

But Elliott's return to work life required some important adjustments and was not always easy. There were days, for example, when he had to skip work because of bowel problems or other medical issues. He ultimately developed a way to work from home via a computer modem on days when he couldn't get to his workplace, and his boss was willing to adjust Elliott's hours as long as he got the work done.

Elliott started his new job while still using a manual wheelchair. He could drive to work, park in the garage under the building, and take the elevator to his office. But going out to lunch was impossible, because in the downtown area "there were no curb-cuts, nothing. I could barely get off the block without some-one's help." In order to use a motorized wheelchair, Elliott had to save up enough money to buy a van with a lift. But he now considers the power chair a must for a tetraplegic who wants to work: "The real world out there is not set up like a hospital." The power chair has given him the freedom to go anywhere he wants without having to take along a co-worker. And without expending so much physical energy on pushing, he has more to give to his job.

Elliott had to "push" more than his wheelchair to re-create a good work situation. He had to push himself to complete retraining, save money, and adapt to new technologies, and he had to push his boss and co-workers to accept his limitations while valuing his capabilities. But twenty years later, Elliott enjoys his career and continues to develop his skills. "I used to make things with my hands, and now I make them with computers," he says.

David, who has paraplegia, had to make similar adjustments. He says, "A lot of people I worked with felt uncomfortable seeing me in a wheelchair." He had to tell his story and explain his injury to many co-workers. "But once I got that over with, everyone got comfortable—and I got comfortable with it." Now David's co-workers respect his competence and enjoy his company on the job.

LIFE IN A NURSING HOME

A very small minority of people with spinal cord injuries (about 5 percent) are discharged from acute hospital or rehabilitation to nursing homes (not including subacute rehabilitation units), and probably fewer live permanently in nursing homes. Individuals with high-level tetraplegia who need full-time attendant care, fully accessible housing, and perhaps ventilator monitoring, and who cannot get these in their community, may have to live in a nursing home. And people who are capable of some self-care but lack accessible, affordable housing and have no one available to assist them may also need to live in a nursing home. If you are unable to work, and do not have assets to pay for care, Medicaid may pay for a nursing home. Sometimes individuals are temporarily unable to take care of themselves at home because of medical complications such as skin ulcers or a kidney infection. A short-term stay in a nursing home can be a solution. After the complication is taken care of, they resume life on their own.

Life in a nursing home has many institutional routines and rules. Times for meals and times for personal care may be largely out of your control. But your ability to advocate for yourself can substantially improve your quality of life while in a nursing home. For example, you may have to negotiate with the nursing staff about when you want to get up, where you would like to be seated at different times of the day, and what activities are "allowed" when you have visitors. If you are able and want to perform certain aspects of your own care, communicate this clearly to the nursing staff. Let the staff know that you are an independent, thinking adult with a physical, not a mental, disability and that you expect to be treated accordingly. If you believe your rights have been violated, request a conference with the nursing home administrator. Make sure you read the residents' rights pamphlet. And, if possible, enlist a family member or friend to act as your co-advocate. You can also call a lawyer, if necessary, to get advice or assistance.

Your level of social support on the "outside" will be an important factor in determining the quality of your life in a nursing home. Unlike a hospital, a long-term-care nursing home is considered your place of residence, and you may come and go from the facility as you like, for visits with family or community outings. If you have little support from family and friends, you can request social services from the nursing home. These services may include volunteer companions, assistance with developing friendships with other residents, or contacting organizations that enrich your life through access to computers, trips outside the nursing home, correspondence courses, and so forth.

Pauline was single, in her late twenties, and an executive in a large corporation when she sustained her C4 injury. She didn't think her parents would be able to provide the extensive care she needed, nor did she want to leave her job and move back to her hometown in another part of the country. Although she was able to afford a personal care attendant, Pauline chose to live in a nursing home, where she could receive "built-in" medical and attendant care. Her nursing home room became the base from which she traveled to her full-time job and attended frequent dinners and concerts with her boyfriend.

Pauline has lived in the nursing home for many years and finds it a satisfactory arrangement. The ready access to care gives her peace of mind and frees her mental and physical energy for work and social and leisure activities.

A nursing home is often thought of as a last resort, a place to live if you have no financial resources or home care options. But Pauline's unusual experience shows that a nursing home can also be a base from which to conduct a busy and varied life.

SO THE PUZZLE IS COMING TOGETHER. The notches are fitting into the grooves as you find, like Joan, that a power wheelchair gives you a greater range of activity and more flexibility, or decide, like Steve, that the manual chair better suits your lifestyle. As some doors close, new ones open, as when Nora developed a career devoted to disability issues following her own experience with spinal cord injury. You will discover your own way to incorporate the puzzle pieces that spinal cord injury has added to your life.

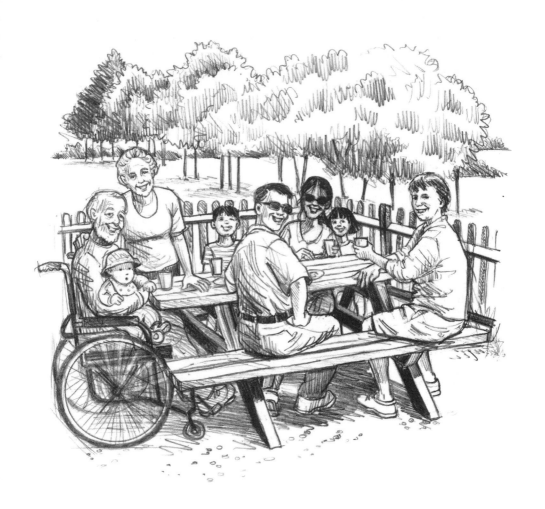

Concluding Thoughts

The path to finding yourself can be long and rocky, but it can lead to a place where life feels secure, relatively stable, and full of possibilities. The future is uncharted territory. You'll encounter beautiful vistas, long, hard climbs, welcome rest stops, and unanticipated bumps in the road. With or without spinal cord injury, there is no magic formula for successful living.

In this final chapter we summarize some ways for making your life easier and more enjoyable: building on your unique strengths, adapting to new stresses and demands, and sharing your wisdom with others. We include some thoughts on living with a disability as you get older.

We begin with stories about two men, with very different backgrounds before injury and very different life experiences afterward, who worked to overcome obstacles to adjustment and to live successfully.

Lee was returning to college after spending the Christmas holidays with his family. He had piled his MG convertible with his clothes and books and packed in the shotgun shells he planned to use for duck hunting. After he'd been on the road for many hours, snow began to fall—unusual for this border state. Driving at fifty-five to sixty miles an hour, Lee suddenly hit a patch of black ice. The car cartwheeled repeatedly down a steep embankment, then blew up and broke in half.

A passing motorist approached the smoldering car, saw the young man trapped inside, and, assuming he was dead, left the scene. The next person to stop was a young soldier, a paramedic, just returned from a second tour of duty in Vietnam. He could feel Lee's pulse, and he dragged him from the smoking car, shielding him with his own body. The shotgun shells, detonated by the fire, began to explode. The explosions triggered flashbacks for the soldier, but he managed to drag Lee from the car and, with the help of another motorist, carry him up to the road. Here they waited for an ambulance to arrive.

Lee was taken to the local hospital, where his uncle, already notified about the accident, was waiting. His parents were called and arrived after a day of driving. They learned that Lee had sustained a T7 spinal cord injury.

The local hospital was a "holding place" for Lee. With the record snowstorms that year, he had to wait to be flown to a hospital nearer his home. Finally, a short break in the weather allowed the transfer. At the hospital in his home-town, surgeons implanted Harrington rods (metal rods attached to the verte-brae) to stabilize Lee's spinal bones and protect his spinal cord. He was in the hospital for almost six months, then transferred to a rehabilitation hospital. Here, Lee says, he rehabbed himself in one month.

Just before Lee's accident, his parents had put their home up for sale and were planning to build a two-story colonial house. After the accident, on learn-ing that Lee would be using a wheelchair, they opted for a ranch house. Con-struction began while Lee was still in the hospital.

Lee had a relatively easy adjustment to spinal cord injury. "I never had a hard time dealing with it because . . . just look at the alternatives, which are not so good. I knew things wouldn't change, so I moved on." But he needed time to "acclimate" to the disability, and with the support of family and friends, he took off a semester from college. He bought a van with hand controls and took a driver's training course.

After this break, still living with his family, he transferred to the local univer-sity. Because he felt he needed to be realistic about his physical limitations, he switched his major from wildlife management to psychology. He excelled in all his subjects and graduated with honors.

It was during his undergraduate days that he first encountered insensitivity to people with disabilities. He had signed up for a geology course that was taught on the second floor of a building on the old campus of the university. Before approaching the professor to ask that the class be moved, Lee talked to a friend who had a spinal cord injury and was active in the disability rights movement, and he learned about Section 504, a federal law that mandates equal access to education for students with disabilities. The professor refused to move the class. "No, this is my classroom," he said. He offered to ask some stu-dents to haul Lee's wheelchair up and down the two flights of stairs to the classroom. Lee declined, saying that this method was both unequal access and dangerous for everyone involved! The professor was forced to move the class, but he was quick to pick on Lee in class when he had a particularly difficult question to ask. Lee says this was his first foray into self-advocacy.

Lee was planning to become a rehabilitation counselor, but when a couple of friends started to study for the law school entrance exam, he became intrigued with the idea of becoming a lawyer. He was accepted into the law school at his university.

During Lee's third year of law school, and after a two-year courtship, he married Tricia (see Chapter 5). They met while snow skiing. Lee used "sitskis," which are adapted for skiing in a seated position, and Tricia was his "tetherer," the person holding the safety lines.

Lee says it was wheelchair basketball, which he began playing in law school, that helped him deal more effectively with his disability. He saw how other men managed their disabilities and learned from them. They taught him tricks, such as where to get supplies, how to deal with "male things" such as condoms coming off, and where to get leg bags (urine collection bags). He says, "You can't talk about those things with doctors or family members."

Through his basketball contacts, Lee found his first job after law school, working for a national advocacy organization. "I was thrilled. It was my first job, $21,000 a year!" Lee and his wife were active socially and in sports and they traveled frequently. But since becoming parents, they've stayed home more.

Lee's younger son had severe medical problems since infancy. Lee kept the boy's medical reports in a three-ring binder and created charts to track his lab results. In this way, when going to a new doctor he could present all the data, which would have been impossible to remember. From his own experience as a patient, Lee has learned to make sure he is part of the decision-making. He knows how to be an advocate and is not intimidated by doctors.

Lee has had some medical complications related to his spinal cord injury. The most troublesome is a chronic urinary tract infection that has become resistant to antibiotics. Lee has worked closely with a trusted urologist and has learned not to self-medicate with "leftover" antibiotics. When possible, rather than getting a prescription over the telephone, he takes a urine sample to the doctor's office for analysis—and he encourages other people to do the same. Specific bacteria respond to specific types of antibiotics.

Another medical problem for Lee is pressure sores. He now sits on a one-half-inch-thick plywood cutout with a cushioned covering, placed on the wheelchair seat. This avoids uneven distribution of his body weight when the wheelchair seat sags in the middle. He also sits with his knees lower than his hips so that more pressure is on the backs of his legs than on his buttocks. Since adopting these methods he's had only one pressure sore.

Although an expert in technology, Lee continues to limit its use in his life as best illustrated by his progressive use of less technology over the years in his vehicles. For instance, when the cable lift in his first van kept breaking down, he tried a hydraulic lift. He found this to be slow and also prone to breakdowns. The van itself presented a problem because people frequently parked too close to the accessible door, blocking his exit or entrance. He then purchased his "dream come true," a pickup truck! This was fun to drive but it had limited space for his children. He is now driving a sports utility vehicle that has doors opening from the center on each side of the vehicle so that he can easily pull his wheelchair into the back seat space without having a center post or door in the way. Though technological aids are helpful, Lee finds it liberating not to have the worry about their use and upkeep.

Finding an affordable and accessible house for a family with a wheelchair user and four young children was a challenge. Although Lee and Tricia wanted a single-level home, a two-story home with an elevator was more affordable. The elevator is not ideal, and Lee has had to "bump" his way up or down steps or sleep on the couch on the main level when the power has gone out. But it was worth the savings.

Maintaining the house is a joint venture. Both Lee and Tricia work on repairs. Lee delegates to his father bigger projects that are beyond Lee's physical capability. Tricia is a stay-at-home mother, and Lee pitches in after work. "I changed diapers, got the kids ready for bed, helped with homework." Until their younger son's successful operation, Lee would prepare the multiple medicines the boy had to take each night and sleep with him so that he could monitor the special medical equipment the boy had to use.

When the children were young and out in the community with Lee, the triplets sat on his lap or stood on his footrest as they crossed streets. The older son held onto the armrest. The children learned never to run from their father while in the street. Lee has helped with the coaching of his children's sports teams. On weekends, the family likes to explore accessible nature trails in the wilderness.

Lee tends to be an optimist. "I try to be fair to everybody and expect the same in return. I try to bring the kids up to be honest and to explore and try different things. I want them to question things and always understand why, not just accept things." Lee says that spinal cord injury changed his life. "I learned life is too short and not worth getting upset over. Not worth bad blood. It changes your outlook. Things are put into perspective after a life-changing experience. If I had not had the injury I would never have met my wife. Its a good life. I wouldn't change it."

Randy was in his late thirties and just pulling his life together when disaster struck: a factory accident broke his neck, resulting in incomplete tetraplegia. This felt like the final crash of his roller coaster life.

Randy had been raised in a big city in the Midwest and exposed to street crime and drugs at an early age. His father, an alcoholic, abandoned the family when Randy was a child. Largely through his mother's support and strong values, Randy did well in school, despite having to work part-time to help support his family. He received a scholarship to attend an Ivy League college, but when his mother became ill in his freshman year, he had to leave school and work full-time to help provide for his mother and siblings. He eventually got a steady job working for a major transportation company. Randy married and had a daughter. His mother recovered, and she and most of his siblings moved to the extended family "compound" in a southern state.

Randy was friendly, outgoing, and bright. He moonlighted as a minister/counselor, and he studied accounting and helped friends with their taxes. But he was plagued by unresolved anger at his father and deep fears of abandonment, which made it difficult for him to assert himself or express anger constructively in a relationship. He tended to hold in his feelings or express them passively, by withdrawing. He often turned to alcohol to ease his tensions and anger.

When his daughter was about twelve, Randy's marriage fell apart. His wife took their daughter and moved out of state. Randy was devastated and began drinking heavily, isolating himself from friends and family. He lost his job and sank into despair. Eventually he hit rock bottom—homeless, drunk, and with no resources, Randy ended up in a men's shelter run by the city.

From this low point, Randy had nowhere to go but up. In the shelter, he "dried out" and was offered job training in a city program. His friendly manner, intelligence, and physical strength made Randy an attractive prospect, and after training he got a job operating machinery in an auto manufacturing plant. It

was low-paying but steady work, and he did well at it. He rented a small apart-
ment and began to make some friends in his neighborhood. His life seemed to
be coming together again. And then it was blown apart by the accident.

Randy's early recovery and rehabilitation went well. Because his accident
was work related, all expenses connected with his injury were covered by his
worker's compensation insurance, including medications, psychotherapy, and
transportation to medical appointments. He had a small paycheck each month,
and a nurse case manager was assigned to coordinate his care. Returning home
as a wheelchair user with limited hand function, Randy qualified for a home
health aide, who came three times a week to help him with laundry, cooking,
and other chores. He had outpatient physical therapy and vocational counsel-
ing. Everyone who worked with Randy was impressed by his warm and engag-
ing personality, his ability to bounce back from disaster, and his intelligence.

But despite the services at his disposal and the encouragement of his rehab
nurse, Randy felt alone. His wife and child were long gone, his family was out of
state, his old friendships were over. He was filled with rage about his accident
but unable to express his anger in a constructive way.

Randy's recovery was another series of ups and downs. He seemed to make
progress physically and emotionally, only to regress. He had begun a friendship
with a neighborhood woman shortly before his injury, and she moved in with
him after his return home. She provided companionship and practical assis-
tance, but she was often verbally abusive and took advantage of Randy finan-
cially. Randy was afraid to lose her, seeing himself as dependent and needy, but
when she left he began to recover his self-esteem and to do more for himself
physically. Randy did well in computer programming training, but he couldn't
find a job in this area because his hand function was too impaired. Another
setback for Randy was a fall in which he broke a hip. Though his recovery from
surgery was remarkably quick, this episode delayed his pursuit of his social and
vocational goals.

Randy struggled with alcohol abuse throughout the two years after his in-
jury. He drank when he was angry or sad, then felt ashamed and tried to keep
his drinking a secret. He succeeded in hiding his drinking, though his therapists
were puzzled by the waxing and waning of his progress in walking and other
physical tasks. He struggled with depression and couldn't seem to start any
social relationships or to pursue financial benefits that would make life easier.
Ultimately, Randy's drinking increased and became noticeable. A confronta-
tion by his therapists and psychologist led to a treatment contract in which

Randy agreed to stop drinking and attend Alcoholics Anonymous. This was a turning point in his life.

Over the next year, Randy gradually took charge of his life. He finally took steps to get the economic benefits he'd been eligible for all along—food stamps, subsidized rent, and a pension from the transportation company, supplemented by Social Security Disability. Qualifying for Social Security Disability entitled him to Medicare insurance, which meant that all his medical problems could finally be covered, not only those that had resulted directly from his injury.

Randy took hold psychologically as well. He volunteered to participate in a medical study at his local rehabilitation hospital, which included relaxation and mental imagery techniques. He practiced diligently and learned better control of his anxiety as well as his physical discomfort. He worked in individual psychotherapy on managing his anger, asserting himself, and resolving emotional issues stemming from his relationship with his father and his ex-wife. He increased his contact with his family and got in touch with his daughter after many years of not communicating with her.

Randy's physical progress continued. He could walk with a walker and sometimes a cane. He used the wheelchair at home, because it was safer for him in the kitchen and bathroom. He learned to make decisions for himself about what equipment to use, finally rebelling against the idea that any use of the wheelchair was a sign of "failure." Randy knew he had reached an important landmark, physically and emotionally, when he took a train trip out of state to visit his mother and family. He went alone, using only his walker, and had a successful trip. He began to think more about leaving the city and returning to his family, whose love and support were so uplifting for him.

Randy had continued to work with a vocational counselor after he'd realized that a job in computer programming wouldn't be possible. He looked at many other possibilities, but the jobs were generally low paying and not easily adapted to his unique abilities and disabilities. He considered returning to college but felt that, at age forty-five, he wouldn't be able to give academics his all. Randy went through the difficult process of giving up on competitive employment, deciding instead to become a volunteer, perhaps also doing some freelance computer work at home.

At last, Randy was finding his own way, choosing his own path to recovery. He became a volunteer for a children's recreation program, reading books to small children and helping others with homework. He offered his math and accounting skills to friends and neighbors who needed help with budgets, paying bills, or figuring out tax payments, and he tutored a friend who was preparing for the high school equivalency diploma exam.

Randy was able to disentangle himself from several social relationships in which friends were taking advantage of him by "borrowing" money or imposing on his time or privacy. He began to date a woman who had been his aide but was now working elsewhere. Randy was able to have an enjoyable sex life, taking Viagra to sustain erections. He met other people through his girlfriend and soon had a small social circle. With his pension money, he could go out to movies and restaurants on occasion and could buy things that made his life easier and more enjoyable.

Four years after his injury, Randy finally feels he's out of the woods. He has a life that is radically different from what he'd imagined or hoped for in his youth. But he has a life that works, a life that is full, and a future that holds potential for usefulness, creativity, and love.

No matter how difficult your life, you can do things to improve it. You can use your intellect, talents, and emotions to increase your enjoyment of life and build a sense of purpose and meaning. Taking an active role in directing, planning, conducting, and managing your life will increase your success in living with spinal cord injury. The quality of your life will depend in large part on your ability to maintain an active, dynamic posture and to stay in the arena, not get "sidelined" by your family, your caregiver, your medical providers, or your friends. Stay focused on getting your voice heard and being responsible for your own life.

BUILDING ON YOUR STRENGTHS

Each person reading this book is at a particular point in life's journey. You may be young, middle-aged, or old. You may be newly injured or you may have lived with your injury for many years. You may be at peace with yourself or you may be still struggling with difficult adjustments and unsettling emotions. We hope that the ideas and stories in this book have shown that adjustment to spinal cord injury is possible and that, whatever your stage of life, you can reach the point in the road where recovery ends and real life begins again.

The future holds many challenges, of course, some anticipated and some unknowable. As you get older you'll face new tasks, changes in health, and declines in strength. Medical problems related to your spinal cord injury may require you to adjust to additional losses or adapt to new technological aids. You'll have highs and lows in your personal and social life, achievements and disappointments in your work life, losses and additions in your family.

What strengths can you build on to meet these and other challenges? How can your life be gratifying and full of joy in the years ahead? Everyone has unique character strengths, talents, ideas, and dreams, and these can be your building blocks. We've already discussed the importance of maintaining old interests and finding new ones, using your ingenuity and creativity, and developing a positive, optimistic approach to life (see Chapter 9), as well as the important role of spirituality, in its many forms (see Chapter 3). Here we discuss some other tools that people have found helpful: humor and the creation and pursuit of dreams.

Humor

Humor is an invaluable tool in dealing with adversity and in celebrating life's joys. Humor releases tension, eases pain, soothes sorrow, and enhances communication and bonding between people. It helps people feel they have some control during seemingly uncontrollable or overwhelming events. People who can see the funny side of life often cope better with stressful or even catastrophic situations, and they may be able to elicit more support from others. Not only is laughter "the best medicine," it can give you the strength to endure life's many stresses and disappointments.

Reading joke books, watching funny movies, visiting a comedy club, reading the "funnies" and cartoons, or listening to comedians on audiotape are some ways of stimulating humor. You might try writing an account of a humorous experience, sharing jokes with friends, or even performing as a comedian or comic actor. Several people with disabilities have been highly successful as comedy entertainers, such as Gene Mitchner, a wheelchair user once referred to as a "sit-down comic." One Hollywood agency caters specifically to comics and entertainers with disabilities. Being able to find humor in the ups and downs of everyday life and to laugh at yourself is a real gift. Terry Galloway, a deaf performance artist, tries to communicate "Joy! Absolute joy! That jolt of love for life in its infinite complications." Humor helps us accept those complications with a laugh.

Pursuing Your Dreams

Dreams or passions evolve out of our interests, creativity, relationships, and values. They can be specific and personal, like Franklin's dream to learn scuba diving and parachuting after he became paraplegic. Or they may be general and altruistic, like Nora's passion for disability advocacy after her spinal cord injury. Sometimes dreams evolve from personal passions to entire movements. Ed Roberts's dream of going to college eventually led not only to his admission as the first tetraplegic at his school, but to a campus-wide, then community-wide, movement for independent living. Sometimes dreams that are purely personal, such as accomplishing difficult athletic feats, can change the attitudes or behavior of others simply by setting inspirational examples.

More "ordinary" dreams—to find a steady, loving relationship, get married, have children, go to graduate school, help other people, play an instrument, run for local office, and so on—are just as important. Not everyone dreams of extraordinary accomplishments, but most people who live happy lives are able to look beyond their present circumstances, imagine where they would like to be in the future, and find the means to get there.

ADAPTING TO NEW STRESSES AND DEMANDS

Your initial rehabilitation prepared you to meet your immediate physical and social needs. As life continues, you'll need to "rehabilitate" yourself many times, to readjust, readapt, renew your energies, and reset your priorities. Adjustment is a *process*, not an end point.

Resetting Your Timetable

In the workaday world we need to adhere to schedules, to be on time, and to organize our day to be as productive as possible. In our hectic society, even stay-at-home parents, retirees, and volunteers seem pressured to follow rigid schedules and cram more and more events into their lives.

But after a spinal cord injury, you may need more "in-between" time—to get from place to place in your wheelchair, to catheterize yourself every four hours, or to navigate the cafeteria line. You have to adjust your timetable to accommodate these parts of your routine.

You may also need to spend more time just getting prepared for the day. Joan, an artist with tetraplegia, spends two hours with her attendant each morning, getting dressed and ready for work. Don, a successful businessman with paraplegia, gets up at 5:00 each morning to spend two hours on his bowel care before leaving for the office.

Making the time for ordinary self-care can be one of the most difficult adjustments after a spinal cord injury. You must learn to pace yourself, to respond to your body's need for extra time and attention. Slowing down may feel frustrating at first, as you see others rushing around and remember when you, too, could be a master of efficiency. These increased demands may seem to rob you of time you'd rather spend on more exciting activities.

> Lark, who has tetraplegia, is acutely aware of this. "You realize how precious time is after spinal cord injury. Everything just takes longer." She has calculated that it takes her eighteen times longer to go to the bathroom and one hundred and twenty times longer to get out of a taxicab! She's solved the problem, in part, by getting additional help to speed up tasks that are necessary to living but not interesting or fun. Allowing others to give her more help actually adds to her independence and the amount of time she has for other activities.

> Pauline, who uses a ventilator and requires full-time attendant care, chose to live in a nursing home so that she'd get the most efficient care and have enough time for her career. She believes in conserving time and energy for the business of living. "Never try to do anything for yourself that someone else can more easily do for you," she says. "You don't need to struggle."

Even with the best possible assistance, physical care needs and changes in mobility will slow you down. Yet with more "down time" between work, social, and domestic activities, each part of your life can become more intense and distinct. You may have more time to observe the world around you, to attend to the emotional nuances of others, and to savor the esthetic high points of daily life—to smell the roses.

While doing your best to conserve time for the activities you value, you can also improve the quality of the time spent in self-care and other necessary chores. You can improve your relationship with your attendant. You can enhance the environment in which your care takes place. And you can do "multitasking," such as listening to the news or a book on tape while you're being dressed or bathed, or conducting business on a speakerphone while you are cooking or putting on braces.

Apart from the many technological devices for saving energy, many people find they can use ordinary, inexpensive items to make everyday tasks easier and can make simple changes in daily routines to save energy.

> *David discovered that dressing is a lot simpler if he lays out all his clothes and catheter supplies on his wheelchair, next to his bed, before going to sleep. In the morning, he can catheterize, fully dress in bed, transfer to the wheelchair, wash his face, and be ready for the day in record time. Elliott has a hard time getting his socks on and off. Rather than wasting valuable energy each day, he chooses to sleep in his socks, changing them every three days with his wife's help. He also discovered that he can elicit a spasm in his trunk that allows him to get his pants on and off easily in the wheelchair.*

Recharging Yourself

Living with a spinal cord injury requires more energy, at work and at home. Dealing with the additional demands in self-care, mobility, transportation, and social stress is sometimes draining. You have to find ways to recharge, mentally and physically, and to relax, take time for yourself, and rest.

Where do you find pleasure, solace, and respite? How do you relax and unwind? Take stock of what has helped you in the past. You may be able to find activities parallel to those you used before your injury, or you may develop new ways to recharge. Nora finds sewing, reading, and family visits to be relaxing. Elliott likes to get into the woods and has found parks and trails he can navigate with his electric wheelchair. Randy periodically takes a "mental health day"; he turns off the phone, watches movies, eats his favorite snacks, and takes a nap. The next day, he's ready to face the world again.

Adjusting Your Goals with Age

The aging process brings changes in health, strength, flexibility, and mental stamina that can compound the challenges of coping with spinal cord injury. Aging can also bring the wisdom and perspective to help you adapt gracefully to these changes. Perhaps you'll greet these changes more easily than your able-bodied peers because of your greater experience in adjusting to changes and losses in function.

Adjusting your goals and accepting additional technological or human assistance are two important aspects of dealing with aging. Many able-bodied people initially resist changing their ways when confronted with changed abilities and may avoid facing reality until necessity forces them to adjust. You may find similar resistance in yourself. If you have incomplete paraplegia and are used to walking everywhere with crutches, you may find that, as you get older, you need a wheelchair to navigate the mall or museum. If you've used a manual chair for years, you may find that arthritis in your shoulders or hands makes a power chair essential. You used to toss your wheelchair in the back of the car; now you may need a lift or chair topper to get the chair in and out. These changes may feel defeating at first, but if you can stay focused on the goal of making the most of your function and independence, you may find the savings in pain and energy expenditure to be well worth the adjustments.

Other changes may be needed because of social changes with aging, such as relocation, retirement, or the loss of your spouse or friends. If you are suddenly living alone in late middle age or old age, you may need to move to a fully accessible apartment, or hire an aide, or reorganize your kitchen, or use a motorized wheelchair. Openness to these and other changes will help you maintain your independence.

As you age, you'll find that more people of your generation are also using wheelchairs as they acquire disease-related disabilities. Your disability may then seem more socially "normal" or acceptable, and you may experience less stigma associated with wheelchair use. Peter, who became independent after a spinal cord injury at the age of sixty-seven, has had to confront the challenges of aging. Now in his late seventies, he senses that other people's expectations of him are lower and that a retreat from life's demands and responsibilities would be socially acceptable. But Peter tries to stay well so he can continue to live productively. "The things that bother me now are those that threaten my independence," he says. He doesn't worry about dying, but he wants to be an active participant in life as long as possible. He tries to avoid situations where he needs physical assistance from others, preferring accessible venues where he can be in charge of himself. "That's my little hang-up," he says. "Many people my age who are in wheelchairs are frail; it's because they're ill." He doesn't identify with this group of seniors and is more comfortable with his able-bodied friends or the somewhat younger group he worked with on a disability advisory committee.

Medical problems that arise with aging can interact with or complicate the problems associated with spinal cord injury. Pay special attention to medical care and preventive health measures as you get older. Regular medical checkups are necessary, just as they are for able-bodied people. Don't assume that every symptom is connected with your spinal cord injury, but do coordinate your medical care with an internist and physiatrist in order to get the best possible treatment. Keep careful records of your medications, changes in diet, and new symptoms. Interactions between the normal and pathological changes associated with aging and the problems associated with chronic spinal cord injury are not well understood. Providing your doctor with detailed information will help in the diagnosis and treatment of problems that may be associated with menopause, osteoporosis, diabetes, or high blood pressure.

Finally, you may need to adjust your day-to-day goals as you age because of greater limitations in strength or endurance. You may have to give yourself more time, plan a less intensive schedule, or switch from more physical to more sedentary hobbies. Continue to reset priorities and redefine what is important to you.

Changing Perspectives

In Chapter 3 we discussed the process of life review as a method for making emotional sense of your injury. This process is useful at intervals throughout life, and especially in later years. Perspectives on major life events evolve with time. For many people whose stories we've told in this book, their spinal cord injury at first seemed completely devastating. But months or years later, they saw it as the turning point to a better life or an opportunity for becoming a better person.

Franklin was only twenty-one years old when he became paraplegic follow-ing a shooting. Almost immediately, he experienced his injury as a wake-up call to get his life in order. After only a month in the rehabilitation hospital, he al-ready felt his life had changed for the better. "I'm going back to school now, try to get my GED. I've got a lot of opportunities to do other things now." Franklin's injury encouraged him to be responsible for himself and to use his intelligence constructively. He was so enthusiastic and adventurous in his approach to wheelchair mobility training that his physical therapist said she should put a sign on his chest that read "No Fear"! Franklin's success in rehabilitation gave him the confidence that he could learn fast, be responsible for his body, and set his own goals, inspiring him to get out of his rut and move into a better life for himself and his family.

Noah, only a few years from his injury, interprets it as "bad luck" but also feels that the injury "put me onto another plane," one where he had an oppor-tunity to make a difference. He has done this through volunteering, public speaking, fundraising, and political advocacy.

Elliott, looking back over the twenty years since his injury, says, "I'm a better person because of it. I had to grow up. Because of being in a chair, I had to look at things differently. I'm more accepting. Now, when I look at someone, I tend not to make judgments on the physical. I want to know you. Physical doesn't mean anything. I grew up in a very biased family. Because of my disability, I had to deal with other people, especially in the hospital. Color, religion . . . not something I think about anymore. But coming from my background, I probably would've been something of a racist. I'm definitely different!"

Art has also lived his entire adult life with incomplete tetraplegia. Living with a spinal cord injury enhanced his personality, says Art. "I use eye contact, my personal qualities, to let people know I'm interested in them." He sees spinal cord injury as a "magnifier" that can enlarge positive personality traits, making the good person even better.

Nora emphasizes the opportunity that spinal cord injury gave her for a career in advocacy work. Had she not been injured, says Nora, she would have had more children and lived most of her adult life as a homemaker. Though this was indeed her original plan, she now feels that her career was a change for the better, adding a welcome new dimension to her life and an outlet for her enormous energies.

Of course, feelings of loss, anger, or frustration about your spinal cord injury may resurface periodically. But in the wake of this life-altering event, you may feel stronger and cope better if you can reassess your life in terms of the positive changes. In discussing their overall adjustment to living with a spinal cord injury, many people point out that everyone has bad days and, if you feel depressed at times, that's part of being human.

The perspective that life after spinal cord injury is just as good as or better than before comes from the active processes of *reassessing* the past in the light of accumulated experience and *moving forward* into the future by welcoming each day and focusing on those aspects of life that are positive and enjoyable.

SHARING YOUR WISDOM

As you develop emotionally, grow older, and evolve, your life with spinal cord injury may give you a unique perspective. You may discover special knowledge about practical techniques for living optimally with physical limitations, special insights about emotional adjustment and coping skills, a personal philosophy of living, a method for enhancing communication and social effectiveness, or a particular path to increased spiritual awareness. Finding a way to share your personal wisdom with others can be an important part of self-validation and personal fulfillment.

One way to share your ideas is by writing about them. Articles about the experience of living with a disability and coping are generally welcomed by others who are going through similar difficulties, and they are often enlightening and inspiring for able-bodied people as well. Even if you are not a professional writer, try writing a letter to the editor, a brief human-interest article for your local newspaper, or a short opinion piece for a magazine. You can also share your ideas on the Internet, where you'll find Web sites for chatting about spinal cord injury, obtaining research information, and exchanging practical tips (see the Resources section at the end of this book).

Don discovered one such site while looking for information on sexuality and spinal cord injury. He ended up "meeting" a young woman with a new spinal cord injury and was able to give her some helpful information and ideas. Temporarily forgetting his own quest for information, Don found that sharing his insights about spinal cord injury made him feel better about himself, and the insights were clearly useful to and appreciated by his Internet friend.

Another outlet for sharing is through peer counseling. Some rehabilitation hospitals have formal programs that train people living with a spinal cord injury to counsel newly injured patients. These programs can be enormously helpful, providing a positive role model, hopefulness, and practical guidance for the new patient. David jumped at the chance of becoming a peer counselor. He realized that not everyone would be as outgoing or comfortable as he was about talking to professionals. And he empathized with people who were injured earlier in life than he was. "I think younger guys really take it hard. They give the therapists a hard time. They're more angry. They think, 'I'm only twenty years old, my life is over.'" David felt his own injury was somewhat easier to bear because, at forty-one, he'd already done things, traveled, and had more experience of life. He was eager to share his perspective that life can be fulfilling after a spinal cord injury.

Participating in community advisory boards is a way to get your ideas across to people who make policies that affect the lives of people with spinal cord injury and, as we've seen, some people make careers of advocacy work for people with spinal cord injury. Not everyone can run for office or work for a government agency devoted to disability policy, of course. But you can participate in advocacy work by supporting national or local disability organizations, writing letters to legislators, or working to expand opportunities for people with spinal cord injury within your own professional organization, house of worship, or community center.

Direct involvement in education is another outlet for sharing your knowledge. Joan, for example, participates in conferences where she describes and demonstrates the functional electrical stimulator that has enhanced her hand and arm mobility. Elliott gave presentations at his daughter's elementary school, teaching children not to be afraid of people with disabilities. Vanessa returned to her high school to talk about the dangers of piloting a boat while drinking and to educate students about prevention of spinal cord injury.

Even if you do nothing deliberate or structured to share your wisdom, just striving to live fully and successfully with spinal cord injury can make you a role model, an inspiration, a challenge for other people. If "living well is the best revenge," it may also be the best teacher. Elliott observes that sometimes you can do more good by "just being out there," going about your business in the world like anyone else. When able-bodied people interact with teachers, doctors, musicians, and salespersons with spinal cord injuries and see models, reporters, actors, and politicians with spinal cord injuries, their attitudes begin to change. They begin to see that people with spinal cord injuries are, above all, *people*. When newly disabled individuals see their peers in these roles, they may feel more encouraged, hopeful, and motivated to participate fully in life.

REMEMBER THE OLD SAYING, "everything changes and everything stays the same"? Life is a constant process of adaptation, a paradox of perpetual change and continuity. In some ways, your life after a spinal cord injury is completely different from before, yet you are the same person. At times, your injury may seem to define you. At other times, your identity transcends the injury completely.

After nine years with a spinal cord injury, Peter says that whenever he passes a mirror and sees himself in the wheelchair, he's shocked. "Is that me? I don't think about myself as being in a wheelchair even when I'm in it, except when I see it." Elliott, tetraplegic for twenty years, says that, on the whole, he rarely thinks of himself as disabled. Forty years after becoming paraplegic, Hannah says, "I go about the day knowing that I'm a person. I have a personality aside from my wheelchair." David, only two years after injury, says, "I'm a human being. I feel great about myself," and Noah, also recently injured, notes that "it changed my life; I've learned to adapt and roll with the punches." Robert, more than two decades after the injury that caused his paraplegia says, "Early on I made the decision to move forward, not back. I've accomplished a lot . . . Great job, kids, exercise. I've had twenty-three years in a chair; it's been a great life."

Your humanness, your personality, your spirit, your self are central to surviving, coping, and living with your injury. The challenges of managing, integrating, and transcending the consequences of spinal cord injury are shared by everyone who has had such an injury. And everyone can meet these challenges with proper rehabilitation, medical care, and psychological, social, and economic supports. But to live a successful and satisfying life, these external supports must be integrated with the unique strengths, interests, and characteristics that define you as an individual.

You are the same person you were before your spinal cord injury, yet you'll develop and change throughout your life. Be yourself. Let yourself grow to meet the ever-changing challenges of life, as a person with a spinal cord injury and as a human being.

Resources

Listed here are resources of interest to people with spinal cord injury and their families. Resources of general interest (books and pamphlets, periodicals, organizations) are listed first, followed by various types of resources grouped by topic area.

GENERAL

Books about Spinal Cord Injury

Hammond, M. C., R. I. Umlauf, B. Matterson, and S. Perduta-Fulginiti, eds. *Yes You Can! A Guide to Self-care for Persons with Spinal Cord Injury.* Washington, DC: Paralyzed Veterans of America, 1989.

> Available from PVA Distribution Center, P.O. Box 753, Waldorf, MD 20604-0753.

An Introduction to Spinal Cord Injury: Understanding the Changes. 3rd ed. Washington, DC: Paralyzed Veterans of America, 1997.

> Available from PVA Distribution Center, P.O. Box 753, Waldorf, MD 20604-0753.

Karp, Gary. *Life on Wheels: For the Active Wheelchair User.* Sebastopol, CA: O'Reilly & Associates, Inc., 1999.

Maddox, Sam. *Paralysis Resource Guide.* Springfield, NJ: Christopher and Dana Reeve Paralysis Resource Center, 2003.

> Available free online, www.paralysis.org.

Resource Connection. Washington, DC: Paralyzed Veterans of America. Updated periodically.

> Available from PVA Distribution Center, P.O. Box 753, Waldorf, MD 20604-0753.

Secondary Conditions, Prevention and Treatment. Lawrence, KS: The Research and Training Center on Independent Living, 1993–1998.

> Series of pamphlets. Topics include Spinal Cord Injury and Depression; Spinal Cord

Injury and Aging; Deconditioning and Weight Gain; Bowel Function; Joint Problems; Chronic Fatigue; Chronic Pain Management; Urinary Tract Infections; Pressure Sores; Contractures; Spasticity. Available from The Research and Training Center on Independent Living, 4089 Dole Life Span Institute, Lawrence, KS 66045-2930.

Memoirs and Personal Stories of Living with Spinal Cord Injury

Cole, Jonathan. *Still Lives: Narratives of Spinal Cord Injury.* Cambridge, MA: MIT Press, 2004.

Hockenberry, John. *Moving Violations: War Zones, Wheelchairs, and Declarations of Independence.* New York: Hyperion Press, 1995.

Holicky, Richard. *Roll Models: People Who Live Successfully Following Spinal Cord Injury and How They Do It.* Victoria, BC: Trafford Publishing, 2004.
Available through the Paralyzed Veterans of America (see listing under Organizations).

Karp, Gary, and Stanley D. Klein, eds. *From There to Here.* Horsham, PA: No Limits Communications, Inc., 2004.

Kumin, Maxine. *Inside the Halo and Beyond: The Anatomy of a Recovery.* New York: W. W. Norton & Company, 2000.

Reeve, Christopher. *Still Me.* New York: Random House, 1998.

Williams, Margie. *Journey to Well: Learning to Live after Spinal Cord Injury.* Newcastle, CA: Altarfire, 1997.

Periodicals about Spinal Cord Injury and Disability

Ability. Published bimonthly. C. R. Cooper Publishing, 1682 Langley Avenue, Irvine, CA 92714.
Covers a wide range of medical, social, and lifestyle topics of interest to people with various disabilities.

Action. United Spinal Association, 75-20 Astoria Boulevard, Jackson Heights, NY 11370. Telephone: 800-404-2898. Web site: www.unitedspinal.org.
Available in audio format, by request.

Active Living: The Adapted Lifestyle Resources Guide. Published biannually. Disability Today Publishing Group Inc., 2276 Rosedene Road, St. Ann's, ON LOR 1Y0 Canada. Telephone: 905-957-6016.

Disability Rag. Published six times a year. Avocado Press, Inc., Box 145, Louisville, KY 40201.

En-able Magazine. Published six times a year. En-able Magazine, Inc., 3657 Cortez Road West, Suite 120, Brandenton, FL 34210.

Horizons, News by and for People with Disabilities. Published monthly. P.O. Box 985, Gambrills, MD 21054.

Mainstream: Magazine of the Able-disabled. Published ten times a year. Box 370598, San Diego, CA 92137.

New Mobility: Disability Culture and Lifestyles. Miramar Communications Inc., 23815 Stuart Ranch Road, P.O. Box 8987, Malibu, CA 90265. Web site: www .newmobility.com.

Orbit. Published monthly. United Spinal Association, 75-20 Astoria Boulevard, Jackson Heights, NY 11370-1177. Telephone: 718-803-3782.
    Available in audio format, by request.

Paraplegia News. Paralyzed Veterans of America, 2111 East Highland Street, Suite 180, Phoenix, AZ 85016-4702. Web site: www.pvamagazines.com/pnnews.

SCI Life Newspaper. National Spinal Cord Injury Association, 6701 Democracy Boulevard, Suite 300-9, Bethesda, MD. Telephone: 800-962-9629.

We Magazine. Park West Station, P.O. Box 20553, New York, NY 10125-0214. Telephone: 800-WE-MAG-26.
    New lifestyle magazine for people with disabilities.

Working! Published quarterly. Goodwill Industries International Inc., 9200 Rockville Pike, Bethesda, MD 20814.

Organizations

American Paralysis Association, 500 Morris Avenue, Springfield, NJ 07081. Telephone: 800-225-0292. Web site: www.apacure.com.

Christopher and Dana Reeve Paralysis Resource Center, 636 Morris Turnpike, Suite 3A, Short Hills, NJ 07078. Telephone: 800-225-0292. Web site: www .paralysis.org.

National Paraplegia Foundation, 4617 Houghton, Fort Worth, TX 76107-6175. Telephone: 817-737-6661. Web site: www.basicomputer.com.

National Spinal Cord Injury Association, 6701 Democracy Boulevard, Suite 300-9, Bethesda, MD. Telephone: 800-962-9629. Web site: www.spinalcord.org.

Paralyzed Veterans of America, 801 Eighteenth Street NW, Washington, DC 20006. Telephone: 800-795-4327 TTD. Web site: www.pva.org.

Spinal Cord Injury Information Network, UAB Model SCI System, Office of Research Services, 619 19th Street, Birmingham, AL 35249-7330. Telephone: 205-934-3283. Web site: www.spinalcord.uab.edu.

Spinal Cord Injury Network International, 3911 Princeton Drive, Santa Rosa, CA 95405. Telephone: 800-548-CORD (548-2673). Web site: www.spinal@sonic.net.

United Spinal Association, 75-20 Astoria Boulevard, Jackson Heights, NY 11370. Telephone: 708-803-3782. Web site: www.unitedspinal.org.

ACCESSIBLE DESIGN

Amherst Homes, Inc., 7378 Charter Cup Lane, Westchester, OH 45069. Telephone: 513-891-3303.

The Center for Universal Design, North Carolina State University, Box 8613, Raleigh, NC 27695-8613. Telephone: 800-647-6777. Web site: www.design.ncsu.edu.

Concrete Change, 600 Dancing Fox Road, Decatur, GA 30032. Telephone: 404-378-7455. Web site: www.concretechange.home.mindspring.com/.

Internet sites for information on accessible housing and accessible design:
www.universaldesignonline.com/index.html
www.wiredonwheels.org/about.asphttp/
www.ableproject.org/ableproject/
www.disabilityinfo.gov

Lifease, Inc., 2451 Fifteenth Street, NW, New Brighton, MN 55112. Telephone: 612-636-6869. Web site: www.lifease.com.

Standards for Accessible and Usable Buildings and Facilities, 2003. Available from International Code Council/American National Standards Institute, 500 New Jersey Avenue NW, 6th floor, Washington, DC 20001-2070.
   Contact the ICC Store, 800-786-4452 or order from the Web site: www.iccsafe.org.

ARTS AND LEISURE

Computer-Disability News. National Easter Seals Society, 5120 South Hyde Park, Chicago, IL 60615. Telephone: 312-667-7400.
   Newsletter functions as a computer resource for people with disabilities.

Kaleidoscope: International Magazine of Literature, Fine Arts and Disability. Published semiannually. United Disability Services, 701 South Main Street, Akron, OH 44311.
   This magazine explores the experience of disability through literature and the fine arts.

Mouth and Foot Painting Artists, 2070 Peachtree Court, Suite 101, Atlanta, GA 30341. Telephone: 770-986-7764. Web site: www.mfpusa.com.

National Institute of Art and Disabilities, 551 23rd Street, Richmond, CA 94804. Telephone: 415-620-0290.

> A comprehensive visual arts center for people with disabilities, featuring a creative art studio, exhibition, teaching, consultation, publications.

Open Circle Theatre, 500 King Farm Blvd., #102, Rockville, MD 20850. Telephone: 240-683-8934. Web site: www.opencircletheater.com.

> A theater company that includes the talents of actors with disabilities.

That Uppity Theatre Company, 4466 West Pine Blvd., Suite 13C, St. Louis, MO 63108. Telephone: 314-995-4600. Web site: www.uppityco.com.

> A theater company for actors with and without disabilities.

VSA Arts, 818 Connecticut Avenue NW, Suite 600, Washington, DC 20006. Telephone: 800-933-8721. Web site: www.vsarts.org.

> This nonprofit organization provides opportunities for people with disabilities to learn through, participate in, and enjoy visual and performing arts.

ECONOMIC, LEGAL, POLITICAL, AND SOCIAL PERSPECTIVES

ADA Home Page. Web site: www.ada.gov.

> Information and technical assistance on the Americans with Disabilities Act (ADA) with links to related agencies.

ADA Information Line. U.S. Department of Justice. Telephone: 800-514-0301 (voice) or 800-514-0383 (TYY).

> For information on the ADA.

Charlton, James I. *Nothing about Us without Us.* Berkeley: University of California Press, 1998.

Detlets, Dale R., Robert J. Myers, and J. Treanor. *Mercer Guide to Social Security and Medicare.* Louisville, KY: William M. Mercer, Inc., 2002.

Disability Rights Education and Defense Fund (DREDF), 2212 Sixth Street, Berkeley, CA 94710. Telephone: 415-644-2555.

> Provides information on disability rights laws and policy. Publishes a free newsletter, *Disability Rights News.*

Fair Housing: How to Make the Law Work for You. Washington, DC: Paralyzed Veterans of America, 1997.

Johnson, Mary, and Editors of the *Disability Rag. People with Disabilities Explain It All for You: Your Guide to Public Accommodations Requirements of the Americans with Disabilities Act.* Louisville, KY: Avocado Press, 1992.

On the Move: A Financial Guide for People with Spinal Cord Injury.
 Available from the Paralyzed Veterans of America or the National Spinal Cord Injury
 Association (see listing under Organizations).

Shapiro, Joseph. *No Pity: People with Disabilities: Forging a New Civil Rights Movement.* New York: Times Books, 1993.

U.S. Department of Housing and Urban Development, Office of Fair Housing and Equal Opportunity, 451 Seventh Street SW, Washington, DC 20410. Telephone: 202-708-1112. Web site: www.hud.gov.
 Provides information on housing rights and resources for people with disabilities and for
 those who encounter discrimination in housing.

What You Should Know About Health Insurance: Guidelines for Persons Living with SCI.
 Available from the National Spinal Cord Injury Association (see listing under Organizations).

EQUIPMENT AND TECHNOLOGY

Abledata, 8455 Colesville Road, Suite 935, Silver Spring, MD 20910. Telephone: 800-227-0216. Web site: www.abledata.com.
 Maintains a database with over fifteen thousand listings of adaptive devices for all disabilities.

Axelson, Peter, Jean Minkel, and Denise Chesney. *A Guide to Wheelchair Selection: How to Use the ANSI/RESNA Wheelchair Standards to Buy a Wheelchair.* Washington, DC: Paralyzed Veterans of America, 1996.

Easy Street, Inc., 8 Equality Park West, Newport, RI 02840.
 Offers a free catalog of products to make daily living easier, such as items for household
 activities, mobility, writing, recreation, and incontinence.

The First Whole Rehab Catalog: A Comprehensive Guide to Products and Services for the Physically Disadvantaged. Crozet, VA: Betterway Publications, 1990.
 Available from Betterway Publications, Box 219, Crozet, VA 22932.

Kettelkamp, Larry. *High Tech for the Handicapped: New Ways to Hear, See, Talk, and Walk.* Hillside, NJ: Enslow, 1991.

Sammons Preston and Enrichments, P.O. Box 5071, Bolingbrook, IL 60440-5071. Telephone: 800-323-5547. Fax: 800-547-4333.
 A mail-order catalog for accessibility aids.

Teeter, Jeanne O., Caroles Kantor, and Denise L. Brown. *FES: Functional Electrical Stimulation Resource Guide.* Cleveland: FES Information Center, 1995.
 Available from FES Information Center, 11000 Cedar Avenue, Cleveland, OH 44106.

FAMILY RESOURCES: PARENTS, CHILDREN, AND TEENS

Accidents Stink! (video).
> A film to educate caregivers about bowel function and methods for providing assistance with bowel movements. By Steven Stiens, M.D., Tammy Piddle, R.N., and Brenda Veland. Available from Concepts in Confidence, 800-822-4050.

Family Caregiver Alliance, 180 Montgomery Street, Suite 1100, San Francisco, CA 94104. Telephone: 800-445-8106. Web site: www.caregiver.org.

Holicky, Richard. *Taking Care of Yourself While Providing Care: A Guide for Those Who Assist and Care for Their Spouses, Children, Parents and Other Loved Ones Who Have Spinal Cord Injuries.* Englewood, CO: Craig Hospital, 2000.

Internet sites for families and children:
www.kidsonwheels.us
www.nichcy.org
www.yellowpagesforkids.com

Krementz, Jill. *How It Feels to Live with a Physical Disability.* New York: Simon & Schuster, 1992.

Kriegsman, Kay H., Elinor L. Zaslow, and Jennifer D'zmura-Rechsteiner. *Taking Charge: Teenagers Talk about Life and Physical Disabilities.* Rockville, MD: Woodbine House, 1992.

National Family Care Givers Association, 10605 Concord Street, Suite 501, Kensington, MD 20895-2504. Telephone: 800-896-3650. Web site: www.nfcacares.org.

Through the Looking Glass: National Resource Center for Parents with Disabilities, 2198 Sixth Street, #100, Berkeley, CA 94710-2204. Web site: www.lookingglass.org.

RESEARCH AND EDUCATION

Center for Research on Women with Disabilities (CROWD), One Baylor Plaza, Houston, TX 77030. Telephone: 713-798-5782 or 800-44-CROWD (800-443-7693) (toll-free). Fax: 713-798-4688. Web site: www.bcm.edu/crowd.

Christopher and Dana Reeve Foundation, 636 Morris Turnpike, Suite 3A, Short Hills, NJ 07078. Telephone: 800-225-0292. Web site: www.christopherreeve.org.

The George Washington University HEATH Resource Center, 2011 I Street NW, Suite 200/Rooms 208 and 215, Washington, DC 20036. Telephone: 202-973-0904 or 800-544-3284 (toll-free). Web site: www.heath.gwu.edu.
> Clearinghouse on postsecondary education for individuals with disabilities. A variety of publications is available.

The International Center for Spinal Cord Injury, Kennedy Krieger Institute, 707 N. Broadway, Baltimore, MD 21205. Telephone: 888-923-9222. Web site: www .spinalcordrecovery.org.

Lanza, R., and N. Rosenthal. "The Stem Cell Challenge." *Scientific American*, vol. 290, 2004.

Miami Project to Cure Paralysis, University of Miami School of Medicine, 1600 NW Tenth Avenue, R-48, Miami, FL 33136. Telephone: 800-782-6387. Web site: www.miamiproject.miami.edu.

National Center for the Dissemination of Disability Research. Web site: www.ncddr .org.
> Information developed for the public from National Institute of Disability and Rehabilitation Research (NIDRR) research. Topics include assistive technology, employment, women with disabilities. Includes listings of Model Spinal Cord Injury Systems; disability statistics; links to other NIDRR sites.

National Rehabilitation Information Center. Web site: www.naric.com/naric.
> Research results, audiovisuals, and publications about disability research. Publications available include guide to the ADA and directory of national information resources.

SEXUALITY, PREGNANCY, AND FERTILITY

American Society of Reproductive Medicine, 1209 Montgomery Highway, Birmingham, AL 35216-2809. Telephone: 205-978-5000. Web site: www.asrm.org.

Baer, John. *Is Fred Dead?: A Manual on Sexuality for Men with Spinal Cord Injuries*. Pittsburgh: Dorance Publishing Company, 2004.

Bregman, Susan. *Sexuality and the Spinal Cord Injured Woman*. Minneapolis: Sister Kenney Institute, 1975.

Ducharme, Stanley H., and Kathleen M. Gill. *Sexuality after Spinal Cord Injury: Answers to Your Questions*. Baltimore: Paul Brookes, 1997.
> This book also has a listing of independent living centers in the United States and Canada (Appendix C).

A Guide and Resource Directory to Male Fertility Following SCI/D: A Miami Project Resource. Web site: www.themiamiproject.org.

Guter, B., and J. R. Killacky. *Queer Crips: Disabled Gay Men and Their Stories*. New York: Harrington Park Press, 2004.

Rogers, Judith. *The Disabled Woman's Guide to Pregnancy and Birth*. 2nd ed. London: Demos Publishing, 2006.

Sexuality Reborn (video, 48 minutes). Produced by Kessler Institute for Rehabilitation, 1199 Pleasant Valley Way, West Orange, NJ 07052. Telephone: 800-248-3321, ext. 6977.

> This video explores the relationships and sexuality of four couples in which at least one partner has a disability. They demonstrate and share their experience on self-esteem, sexual functioning, and intercourse.

SPORTS AND FITNESS

For camping and wilderness experiences, see Travel (below).

Murderball (film, available on DVD and video). Co-directed by Henry Alex Rubin and Dana Adam Shapiro. Produced by Jeffrey Mandell and Dana Alex Shapiro.

> This is a documentary about wheelchair rugby and the journey of the American "quad" rugby team to the Olympics. For more information on this sport, including locating a team, contact the United States Quad Rugby Association at www.quadrugby.com.

National Ability Center, Parks City, UT. Telephone: 435-694-3991. Web site: www .nac1985.org.

> Specializes in accessible recreation, sports, and leisure activities.

National Association of Handicapped Outdoor Sportsmen, Inc., R.R. 6, Box 25, Centralia, IL 62801.

National Center on Physical Activity and Disability. Telephone: 800-900-8086. Web site: www.ncpad.org.

> Hosted by the University of Illinois, this group provides resources on outdoor activities for people with disabilities, including canoeing and horseback riding.

National Foundation of Wheelchair Tennis, 940 Calle Amanecer, Suite B, San Clemente, CA 92672.

National Wheelchair Basketball Association, 110 Seaton Building, University of Kentucky, Lexington, KY 40506. Web site: www.nwba.org.

North American Riding for the Handicapped Association, Inc. (NARHA) (horse riding), P.O. Box 33150, Denver, CO 80238. Telephone: 800-369-RIDE (7433). Web site: www.narha.org.

Shake-a-Leg, Inc., 76 Dorrance Street, Suite 300, Providence, RI 02903. Telephone: 401-421-1111. Web site: www.shakealeg.org.

> Offers therapy and recreation services to people with disabilities, with an emphasis on independent living and leisure/fitness; an Adaptive Sailing program; and a summer camp program for children with disabilities ages seven to fourteen.

Sports 'N Spokes magazine. Paralyzed Veterans of America, 2111 East Highland Street, Suite 180, Phoenix, AZ 85016-4702. Telephone: 602-224-0500.

The Steadward Centre, University of Alberta, Edmonton, Alberta, Canada. Web site: www.steadwardcentre.org.

Fitness, lifestyle, and activity programs for people with disabilities.

United States Driving for the Disabled. Therapeutic carriage driving (horse carriage) for people with disabilities. Web site: www.usdfd.org.

SUPPORT AND ADVOCACY

Determined 2 Heal, 8112 River Falls Drive, Potomac, MD 20854. Telephone: 703-795-5711. Web site: www.determined2heal.org.

Provides information on spinal cord injury prevention, support, and research.

National Association of Governors' Committees on People with Disabilities. Telephone: 916-654-1764. Web site: www.nagcpd.com.

Promotes equal access to employment, programs, and services for people with disabilities. Provides monthly updates of information and resources on the following: grants, scholarships, internships, and other funding opportunities; publications, media resources, and releases; conferences, events, meetings, and courses; Web sites on disability topics and issues, including accessible living, advocacy, laws, education, employment, funding, government, Internet disability job board, policy-related information, sports and recreation, statistics, transportation, travel, veterans, women, and youth; and resolving issues.

United Spinal Association's Peer-Mentoring Program. Telephone: 800-404-2898.

Connects newly injured persons with people experienced in living with spinal cord injury, to provide role modeling and support. Contact Jerome Kleckley, LMSW, director of social services, United Spinal Association.

TRANSPORTATION

The Air Carrier Access Act: Make it Work for You. Washington, DC.

Available from Paralyzed Veterans of America (see listing under Organizations).

New Horizons: Information for the Air Traveler with a Disability. Washington, DC: U.S. Department of Transportation, 2004.

Available from U.S. Department of Transportation, Aviation Consumer Protection Division, C-75, 400 Seventh Street SW, Washington, DC 20590. Web site: www.faa.gov. The Web site has the full text of the document. The URL for the document is http://airconsumer.ost.dot.gov/publications/Horizons_Printable.doc.

TRAVEL AND WILDERNESS TRIPS

Access-Able Travel Source, P.O. Box 1796, Wheat Ridge, CO 80034. Web site: www.access-able.com.

Accessible Europe. Telephone: 011-39-011-30-1888. Web site: www.accessible europe.com.
> Travel agencies in Italy specializing in accessible tourism.

Accessible Journeys. Telephone: 1-800-846-4537. Web site: www.disabilitytravel .com.
> Organizes wheelchair travel, including cruises, for groups and individuals.

Emerging Horizons, P.O. Box 278, Ripon, CA 95366. Web site: www.emerging horizons.com.

International Association for Medical Assistance to Travellers. Telephone: 716-754-4883. Web site: www.iamat.org.
> This organization provides access to English-speaking medical care providers for English-speakers traveling in foreign countries.

Mersey River Chalets, Nova Scotia, Canada. Web site: www.merseyriverchallets .ns.ca.
> Accessible accommodations and nature activities.

Roth, W, and M. Tompane. *Easy Access to National Parks.* San Francisco: Sierra Club, 1998.
> A guide to accessible places in national parklands. Available from Sierra Club Books, 100 Bush Street, San Francisco, CA 94101.

Society for Accessible Travel and Hospitality, 347 Fifth Avenue, Suite 610, New York, NY 10016. Web site: www.sath.org.

Travelin' Talk Network, 130 Hillcrest Plaza, Suite 102, P.O. Box 3534, Clarksville, TN 37043. Telephone: 615-552-6670. Web site: www.travelintalk.net.
> A network of over a thousand people who offer help and services to travelers with disabilities. Its Membership Benefits Program includes discounts at various motels.

Wilderness Inquiry, Inc., 1313 Fifth Street, P.O. Box 84, Minneapolis, MN 55414. Telephone: 800-728-0719. Web site: wwwwildernessinquiryorg.
> Wilderness (land and water) excursions for people with and without disabilities.

Wilderness on Wheels Foundation, 7125 W Jefferson Ave., No. 155, Lakewood, CO 80235.
> Accessible camping, hiking, and fishing.

Notes

p. 47 For further information on depression rates and suicide risk in people with spinal cord injury, see the pamphlet "Depression: What You Should Know," available from the Paralyzed Veterans of America.

p. 66 For further discussion of the role of case managers, see the "Case Management" issue of *Topics in Spinal Cord Injury Rehabilitation*, Spring 1999.

p. 81 The concept of attribution of responsibility is from J. Scott Richards et al., "Attributions of Responsibility for Onset of Spinal Cord Injury and Psychosocial Outcomes in the First Year Post-Injury," *Rehabilitation Psychology*, Summer 1997. Further references to the concept of attribution of responsibility can be found in this article.

p. 82 The relevance of internal versus external locus of control to adjustment to disability has been described in numerous sources. For further discussion of the application of this concept to spinal cord injury and a review of relevant literature, see Roberta Trieschmann, *Spinal Cord Injuries: Psychological, Social, and Vocational Adjustment* (New York: Pergamon Press, 1980).

p. 83 John Hockenberry's description of his rehabilitation is from his autobiography, *Moving Violations: War Zones, Wheelchairs, and Declarations of Independence* (New York: Hyperion Press, 1995), 78.

p. 83 The problem-solving model in rehabilitation is described in an article by Steven A. Stiens et al., "Spinal Cord Injury Rehabilitation, 4. Individual Experience, Personal Adaptation, and Social Perspectives," *Archives of Physical Medicine and Rehabilitation*, March 1997.

p. 83 Ralf Hotchkiss is quoted in an article by Michael Ryan, "I've Been Liberated by a Wheelchair," *Parade Magazine*, August 3, 1997.

p. 89 Hockenberry's description of the Palestinian youth with spinal cord injury is from *Moving Violations*, 244.

p. 90 Hugh Gregory Gallagher's comment on disability is from his article "This Thing Has a Happy Ending . . . Right?" *New Mobility*, March–April 1995.

p. 90 Vash's comment on disability and spirituality is from *Personality and*

Adversity: Psychospiritual Aspects of Rehabilitation (New York: Springer, 1994), 47.

p. 90 Vash's comment on the longing for spiritual growth is from *Personality and Adversity,* 115.

p. 108 The iBOT Mobility System is available from Independence Technology. This motorized wheelchair allows people to stand up and climb stairs. For more information, contact 866-813-0761 or www.ibotnow.com.

p. 110 An ACE (antegrade colonic enema) stoma is a surgically created opening (stoma) from the outside of the abdomen into the bowel. This enables a person with limited hand function to give himself or herself an enema through the stoma and evacuate the bowel while sitting on the toilet. This method will not work for every patient; you should consult your physician if interested in learning more about this procedure.

p. 151 Objections raised by family members to marriage between an able-bodied woman and a man with spinal cord injury are discussed in an article by Maureen Milligan and Alfred Neufeldt, "Postinjury Marriage to Men with Spinal Cord Injury: Women's Perspectives on Making a Commitment," *Sexuality and Disability,* Summer 1998.

p. 159 The information on women's wish for their disabled husbands to share responsibility is from Milligan and Neufeldt, "Postinjury Marriage."

p. 166 Christopher Reeve describes his experience with spinal cord injury in *Still Me* (New York: Random House, 1998). The quotation here is from page 275.

p. 172 Conceptual distinctions between sexuality, sex drive, and sex acts are further described in Trieschmann, *Spinal Cord Injuries,* 129–139.

p. 177 Dating recommendations for teens are from teenagers interviewed by Kay H. Kriegsman et al., reported in *Taking Charge: Teenagers Talk About Life and Physical Disabilities* (Rockville, MD: Woodbine House, 1992).

p. 181 The story of the man who fell out of his wheelchair while on a date is from Alan Troop, "Falling On Love," *New Mobility,* February 1997.

p. 181 The story of the difficult transfer is from Donald Dinsmore, "This Is Crazy," *Accent on Living,* Winter 1997.

p. 181 Recommendations for dating skills are from Susan Bregman, *Sexuality and the Spinal Cord Injured Woman* (Minneapolis: Sister Kenney Institute, 1975).

p. 183 Ed Gallagher's account of his sexual experiences after spinal cord injury is excerpted from *Queer Crips: Disabled Gay Men and their Stories* (Binghamton, NY: Harrington Park Press, 2004), 112–116.

p. 184 John R. Killacky's description of the change in his relationship with his husband after spinal cord injury is excerpted from *Queer Crips,* 57–59.

p. 193 Women's recommendations for a variety of sexual positions are from Bregman, *Sexuality and the Spinal Cord Injured Woman,* 9.

p. 206 Guidelines for access are given in ANSI (American National Standards Institute), *Standards for Accessible and Usable Buildings and Facilities,* 2003. Available from International Code Council (ICC). See the Resources section in this book for the address.

p. 206 Recommendations for accessibility are from "Universal Design of the Future," *En-able Magazine,* January–February 1998.

p. 206 Ron Mace's comment is from "Universal Design of the Future."

p. 208 *Fair Housing: How to Make the Law Work for You* (Washington, DC: Paralyzed Veterans of America, 1997). Available from the Paralyzed Veterans of America. See the Resources section in this book for the address.

p. 209 The story of Naomi Shoemaker and Jason Fleckenstein appeared in two articles by Ernest F. Imhoff, " 'Average' Family Deals with Two Grievous Wrecks," *Baltimore Sun,* December 18, 1997; and "An 'Overwhelming' Kindness," *Baltimore Sun,* January 9, 1998.

p. 211 The story of Kelsie Collins and her real estate agent are from James Cavanaugh, "Moving Past Hurdles," *Baltimore Sun,* August 14, 1997.

p. 213 Hockenberry's description of problems with taxis is related in *Moving Violations,* 302.

p. 214 *New Horizons: Information for the Air Traveler with a Disability* is available from the U.S. Department of Transportation; *The Air Carrier Access Act: Make It Work for You* is available from the Paralyzed Veterans of America. See the Resources section in this book for the addresses.

p. 220 Jerome Lee's story appeared in his autobiographical article, "A Good Investment," *Newsweek,* June 23, 1997.

p. 221 The story of Keith Thompson appeared in *Working!* Spring 1998.

p. 229 The "essential functions" stipulation for nondiscrimination in employment under the ADA is quoted from *The Americans with Disabilities Act: Your Employment Rights as an Individual with a Disability,* booklet number EEOC-BK-18 (Washington, DC: U.S. Equal Employment Opportunity Commission, 1991).

p. 229 Information on the ADA is from *Voices of Freedom: America Speaks Out on the ADA: A Report to the President and Congress* (National Council on Disability, July 26, 1995), 233–335; and *The Americans with Disabilities Act: Your Personal Guide to the Law,* 3rd ed. (Washington, DC: Paralyzed Veterans of America, 2002). (There is now a 4th edition available on-line only, at www.pva.org.)

p. 249 More information regarding spinal cord regeneration, stem cells, and activity-based restoration therapy can be found in the following articles: J. W. McDonald and the Christopher Reeve Paralysis Foundation, "Spinal Cord Injuries: New Hope for Treating Paralysis," *Scientific American,* vol. 281, 1999; and V. Belegu, M. Oudega, D. S. Gary, and J. W. McDonald, "Restoring Function after Spinal Cord Injury: Promoting Spontaneous Regeneration with Stem Cells and Activity-based Therapies," *Neurosurgical Clinics of North America,* vol. 18, 2007.

p. 260 Several ABRT programs are currently available at rehabilitation centers in the United States, including the following: The International Center for Spinal

Cord Injury at the Kennedy Krieger Institute in Baltimore, MD; The Shepherd Center, Atlanta, GA; Craig Hospital, Denver, CO; Shriners Hospital, Philadelphia, PA (specializing in children); and Courage Center, Minneapolis, MN.

p. 289 The comment on global perspective and adjustment to spinal cord injury is from "Life Stories of People with Spinal Cord Injury," *Rehabilitation Counseling Bulletin,* September 1997.

p. 293 The statement on the necessity for adjustment is from Boni B. Boswell et al., "Quality of Life as Defined by Adults with Spinal Cord Injuries," *Journal of Rehabilitation,* January–March 1998.

p. 302 Chuck Close was profiled and quoted in an article by Deborah Solomon, "The Persistence of the Portraitist," *New York Times Magazine,* February 1, 1998.

p. 317 Gene Mitchner's comic career is described in an article by Lisa M. Kramer, "Have You Heard the One About . . . ?" *Kaleidoscope,* Winter–Spring 1998.

p. 317 Terry Galloway is quoted in an article by Nathan S. Hipps, "Portrait of an Artist," *Kaleidoscope,* Winter–Spring 1998.

p. 318 The story of Ed Roberts and the development of the independent living movement is described in Joseph P. Shapiro, *No Pity: People with Disabilities Forging a New Civil Rights Movement* (New York: Times Books, 1993).

Index